Promoting Child and Adolescent Mental Health

Carl I. Fertman, PhD, MCHES

Associate Professor
School of Education
University of Pittsburgh
Pittsburgh, Pennsylvania

Myrna M. Delgado, MEd

Chief, retired
Division of Student and Safe School Services
Pennsylvania Department of Education
Harrisburg, Pennsylvania

Susan L. Tarasevich, EdD

Clinical Educator
Center for Addiction Medicine
Western Psychiatric Institute and Clinic
University of Pittsburgh Medical Center
Pittsburgh, Pennsylvania

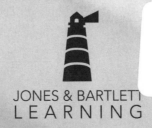

JONES & BARTLETT
LEARNING

D1088038

World Headquarters
Jones & Bartlett Learning
5 Wall Street
Burlington, MA 01803
978-443-5000
info@jblearning.com
www.jblearning.com

Jones & Bartlett Learning books and products are available through most bookstores and online booksellers. To contact Jones & Bartlett Learning directly, call 800-832-0034, fax 978-443-8000, or visit our website, www.jblearning.com.

Substantial discounts on bulk quantities of Jones & Bartlett Learning publications are available to corporations, professional associations, and other qualified organizations. For details and specific discount information, contact the special sales department at Jones & Bartlett Learning via the above contact information or send an email to specialsales@jblearning.com.

Production Credits

Publisher: William Brottmiller
Executive Editor: Cathy L. Esperti
Editorial Assistant: Agnes Burt
Editorial Assistant: Kayla Dos Santos
Associate Director of Production: Julie Champagne Bolduc
Production Assistant: Stephanie Rineman
Senior Marketing Manager: Andrea DeFronzo
VP, Manufacturing and Inventory Control: Therese Connell

Composition: Lapiz, Inc.
Cover Design: Theresa Day
Rights & Photo Research Assistant: Joseph Veiga
Cover and Title Page Images: (yellow image) © yxiwert/ShutterStock, Inc.; (purple image) © Creatas/Thinkstock
Printing and Binding: Edwards Brothers Malloy
Cover Printing: Edwards Brothers Malloy

Library of Congress Cataloging-in-Publication Data

Fertman, Carl I., 1950- author.
  Promoting child and adolescent mental health / by Carl I. Fertman, Myrna M. Delgado, and Susan L. Tarasevich.
    p. ; cm.
  Includes bibliographical references and index.
  ISBN 978-1-4496-5899-1 — ISBN 1-4496-5899-7
  I. Delgado, Myrna M., author. II. Tarasevich, Susan L., author. III. Title.
  [DNLM: 1. Community Mental Health Services—organization & administration—United States.
2. Adolescent—United States. 3. Adolescent Psychology—methods—United States. 4. Child—United States. 5. Child Psychology—methods—United States. 6. Health Promotion—methods—United States. 7. School Health Services—United States. WM 30.6]

362.19689—dc23

6048

2012048917

Printed in the United States of America
17 16 15 14 13   10 9 8 7 6 5 4 3 2 1

Dedication

For my parents, Frances and Lester Fertman, with gratitude and love.
—Carl I. Fertman

For Felicita Alvarez Rivera, Doris Cristina Cortijo, Edith S. Shilling, Celia S. Lipovsky, and Helen A. McLain who taught me about giving, loving, working, and caring for others.
—Myrna M. Delgado

To Theo Allyn Finnie for her unconditional love, support, encouragement, and unwavering faith in me.
—Susan L. Tarasevich

Brief Contents

Contents

Preface

Opportunities to promote mental health of children and adolescents are abundant. Promoting youth mental health helps young people lead socially and economically productive lives. The goal of *Promoting Child and Adolescent Mental Health* is to provide a comprehensive introduction to mental health promotion programs by combining theory and practice. Each of the 12 chapters in this text corresponds to a key step identified through research and practice to promote the mental health of youth. Throughout *Promoting Child and Adolescent Mental Health*, text and resources are drawn from the real-world experiences of professionals working in schools and feature course materials currently used in schools and human service agencies.

Each chapter of this textbook is designed to engage students in thought, discussion, and action, and direct the student to achieve a specific mental health outcome or an improvement in the overall mental health status of youth. Using clear, relatable language and evidence-based methods, we emphasize the development of individual responsibility through active involvement with diverse communities, by focusing on the practical application of programs for youth mental health promotion. Where possible, we use examples about real programs, communities, and organizations that relate to common elements of life, as well as practical questions and a conversational tone to engage the reader in a personal way. Throughout the text we provide students with useful tools as they seek additional information to expand their knowledge about the variety of mental health-related organizations for promoting adolescent mental health programs, including: action-based tips for promoting child and adolescent mental health, extensive information on networking with educational and human services professionals to develop a larger framework of support for children and adolescents, and information on referrals, teams, partnerships, and collaborations.

Special pedagogical features included in each chapter explore ideas, test recommended approaches, and develop knowledge and competencies that will inform students' youth mental health promotion efforts. These features include the following:

- ❖ **Learning Objectives** at the beginning of each chapter highlight the central concepts covered in the chapter as well as how they apply in real-world settings.

- ❖ **Scenarios** at the beginning of each chapter are real-world vignettes that inspire critical thinking and promote further discussions and thought on the practical aspects of working in schools and communities to promote youth mental health.

- ❖ **For Practice and Discussion Questions** at the end of each chapter provide activities for both the classroom and community and are designed to engage students in discussion and application of the knowledge and competencies described in that chapter. They can be assigned as individual or group activities to promote teamwork, leadership, and professional growth. Activities include developing a professional resume or portfolio, as well as visiting a local neighborhood or community organization for a strong real-world experience.

- ❖ Bolded **Key Terms** appear throughout the text and are defined in a comprehensive glossary. A Key Terms list is found at the end of each chapter for additional review.

To the Instructor

The accompanying Instructor's Resources are a valuable resource to help instructors spend more time teaching and less time planning:

- ❖ PowerPoint lecture outlines,
- ❖ Test Bank, and
- ❖ Instructor's Manual.

A Special Note from the Authors to the Student

The need to promote the mental health of children and adolescents is all around us. Staff in schools, colleges, day care centers, government offices, centers of worship, health clinics, community centers, youth organizations, and local health departments are all thinking about how to improve the lives and productivity of children and adolescents where they live, learn, worship, and play. If you are working or planning to work in education, public health, counseling, social work, community health, psychology, medicine, or nursing, you are probably going to be involved with promoting the mental health of youth at some time. In the process, you will use your clinical and professional expertise as well as academic training to develop and implement a plan to improve the mental health of children and adolescents as well as reduce the risk of youth having mental health problems. You will most likely be part of a team that is organizing a mental health promotion program. At first, the concept of a program to improve or promote the mental health of youth may sound a little intimidating. Ultimately, it becomes clear that although the idea of a mental health promotion program is appealing and seems worthwhile, turning the idea into reality demands work and expertise. In other words, it is easy to say that something should be done or needs to be done. It is very different to know how to design and implement a program to actually achieve a specific mental health outcome or an improvement in the overall mental health status of youth. It is a complex process.

Promoting Child and Adolescent Mental Health examines how to address the mental health problems and concerns of youth. We hope that the guidance and resources in this book leave you feeling empowered to make a difference in the lives of young people. We wish you success as you apply your knowledge, tools, and skills in your schools and communities. We hope that this book helps guide and inspire a healthier world for all children and adolescents.

Acknowledgments

Promoting Child and Adolescent Mental Health has been a team effort. We thank the multitude of students preparing for careers in education, public health, counseling, social work, community health, psychology, medicine, and nursing whose input identified the need for and shaped the content of this book. We recognize the staff of the Maximizing Adolescent Potentials Program in the University of Pittsburgh School of Education for their support and effort on behalf of the text. Additionally, we are grateful to the Prevention Education staff of the Addiction Medicine Service line of Western Psychiatric Institute and Clinic, University of Pittsburgh Medical Center for their encouragement and good example. We thank the staffs of the Allegheny County Department of Human Services, as well as schools and community agencies in Pittsburgh and the surrounding communities for their support and insights. Additionally appreciated are members of the Pennsylvania Association of Student Assistance Professionals and Pennsylvania Commonwealth Approved Student Assistance Program Trainers who support our work and advocate every day for mental health promoting schools and communities. We recognize the Pennsylvania Network for Student Assistance Services, a collaborative venture between the Pennsylvania Departments of Public Welfare, Education, and Drug and Alcohol Programs to promote child and adolescent mental health. We thank for their input and support the school and community professionals with whom we have had contact over the years, working to promote the mental health of children and adolescents across Pennsylvania, as well as throughout New Jersey, New York, Rhode Island, Vermont, Illinois, Tennessee, Florida, Texas, California, and Washington. Acknowledged and thanked is Erin Hasinger for her editing and preparation of the figures, tables, and manuscript.

We are grateful to Cathy Esperti, executive editor, and editorial assistants Agnes Burt and Kayla Dos Santos. Senior marketing managers Andrea DeFronzo and Jennifer Stiles were great sources of support and guidance. Stephanie Rineman, production assistant, was meticulous in her care of the manuscript.

We thank the variety of colleagues whose encouragement and honest critique helped us reach our goal.

- Howard Adelman, University of California
- Laura Campbell, SUNY Cortland
- Kendra P. DeLoach, University of South Carolina
- Steven Evans, University of Ohio
- Melissa George, University of South Carolina
- Annette Giovanazzi, Baldwin-Whitehall School District.
- Patricia L. McDiarmid, Springfield College
- Michael McGaughey, Sr., Titusville Area School District
- Elizabeth Mellin, Pennsylvania State University
- Connell O'Brien, Pennsylvania Community Providers Association
- David Osher, American Institutes for Research
- Betty Rothbart, New York City Schools
- Sean Slade, ASCD
- Linda Taylor, University of California
- Mark D. Weist, University of South Carolina

Finally, appreciated and acknowledged are the hundreds of children, adolescents, and their families who shared their stories, time, thoughts, and feelings with us, all of which made this book a reality. Every day young people learn, live, worship, and play in their schools, communities, and families to achieve personal goals with enthusiasm, energy, and excellence.

Thank you.

Carl I. Fertman, *Pittsburgh, Pennsylvania*
Myrna M. Delgado, *Harrisburg, Pennsylvania*
Susan L. Tarasevich, *Pittsburgh, Pennsylvania*

About the Authors

Carl I. Fertman, PhD, MCHES is an associate professor and executive director of the Maximizing Adolescent Potentials (MAPS) Program in the School of Education at the University of Pittsburgh. His expertise is working with schools and communities to prevent tobacco, drug, and alcohol problems among youth, and to promote the mental health of children, adolescents, and families. He has worked for more than 30 years in designing, implementing, and evaluating health programs and services for children, adolescents, and adults both locally (human service agencies and health departments) and statewide (Pennsylvania Departments of Education and Health, and Rhode Island, Vermont, North Carolina, and California Departments of Education). His research interests are in designing and evaluating evidence-based health programs and services in schools, workplaces, community organizations, and healthcare organizations.

Myrna M. Delgado, MEd, is a consultant, retired from the Pennsylvania Department of Education as chief of the Division of Student and Safe School Services and chair of the Interagency Committee of the Network for Student Assistance Services. During her tenure she provided leadership for alternative education, juvenile correction education, Safe and Drug Free Schools and Communities, Safe Schools Initiative, Center for Safe Schools, and Bullying Prevention, among others. Ms. Delgado's career includes teaching in secondary school, adult evening school, and college and serving as an interpreter/translator. She has been a small-business owner and has worked in social service settings. She enjoys volunteering in her professional and social community and has twice received formal recognition as a visionary by the Pennsylvania Association of Student Assistance Professionals for her work on behalf of student assistance programs.

Susan L. Tarasevich, EdD, is a clinical educator with Addiction Medicine Services at the Western Psychiatric Institute and Clinic, University of Pittsburgh Medical Center. She worked in schools as a teacher and administrator before coming to her current work as a preventionist. For more than 20 years she has been engaged in design, implementation, and evaluation of school-based substance abuse prevention programs and services for youth at all levels. She provides training and technical assistance to local and regional education and human service agencies. Statewide, she has consulted with Pennsylvania Departments of Education, Health, and Welfare. She served with the Northeast Regional Expert Team, Center for Substance Abuse Prevention providing technical evaluation assistance. Her areas of expertise include the interactive training and teaching of undergraduate, graduate, and professional educators and clinicians related to the many facets of effective substance abuse prevention.

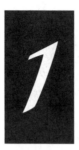

Foundations

In this chapter, we will:

✦ Summarize child and adolescent mental health concerns and problems

✦ Explain five approaches to address the mental health concerns and problems of youth

✦ Discuss the benefits of the approaches

Scenario

Even the best students get depressed, use drugs, don't come to school, or lose interest in learning. For some children and adolescents, schools are the safest places. No fights, no drugs, no alcohol. Close to the end of my second year of teaching, a favorite student of mine was almost killed in a drive-by shooting at a popular nearby park. All of my students were touched by that event. The climate of the school changed. Teachers like me didn't know what to do to help the students, let alone teach them English. I used to think I could help students myself. I can't; I just don't have the skills. I need the support personnel, I need colleagues in the community, and professionals working in different systems who are connected to organizations bigger than me—people who know how to navigate the systems. The good news is that through this experience, I've found we have a lot of resources and support for children and their families. I realized that it is not all about the school, but effective prevention programs and social-emotional skills can help. Yes, there can be a shooting at the school, but there can also be a shooting at the mall or the movie theatre. Yes, there can be drugs at the school, but drugs are everywhere. And yes, we can do a lot in the school to help students develop physically and mentally but we cannot think schools can do it all. I know our community will help us through it. Effective prevention of problems and promotion of kids' mental health cannot wait until there is a gunman in a school parking lot. Our schools must not become fortresses. These issues require attention and work at the school and community levels and beyond.

Source: Vince Linger, a third-year teacher in a large urban New York school district

Mental Health Concerns and Problems of Children and Adolescents

Children and adolescents struggle if they are depressed; concerned about a family member or friend; abusing tobacco, alcohol, marijuana, prescription medicines, or other drugs; struggling with the loss of a loved one; victims of abuse and violence and bullying; anxious about their futures; questioning their sexual or gender identity; or trying to address any one of a host of mental health concerns and problems. Conversations with school superintendents, board members, principals, teachers, counselors, psychologists, social workers, and nurses about young people's social and emotional health show how actively these professionals and community members work to help youth confront difficult issues. Equally important, and of great concern, is developing competent young people who are socially and emotionally healthy and can build positive relationships and resolve conflicts peacefully.

The 1999 Surgeon General's Report on Mental Health defined **mental health** as "successful performance of mental function, resulting in productive activities, fulfilling relationships with other people, and the ability to change and to cope with adversity. Mental illness refers to diagnosable mental disorders that are characterized by alterations in thinking, mood, or behavior (or a combination thereof) associated with distress and/or impaired functioning." A 2004 report by the World Health Organization (WHO) includes a similar distinction between mental health and mental illness. With children, this includes a wide range of mental, emotional, and behavior problems that, in lay terms, may not be considered mental or psychiatric disorders.

Common disorders include mood disorders such as depression; anxiety disorders; behavioral problems such as oppositional defiant disorder and conduct disorder; eating disorders such as anorexia nervosa and bulimia; addictive disorders; and other disorders commonly seen in childhood and adolescence such as autism, learning disorders, and attention-deficit/hyperactivity disorder (AD/HD). Research suggests that co-occurrence of disorders is not uncommon in adolescence. According to the Surgeon General's report (1999), "children with pervasive developmental disorders often suffer from AD/HD. Children with a conduct disorder are often depressed, and the various anxiety disorders may co-occur with mood disorders. Learning disorders are common in all these conditions, as are alcohol and other substance use disorders."

According to the Surgeon's General's report and WHO, mental health encompasses positive aspects of well-being and healthy functioning as well as negative aspects of mental disorder and dysfunction. Ideally, a comprehensive overview of child and adolescent mental health status would reflect both positive and negative aspects. A comprehensive overview would also recognize that family, community, and social contexts influence mental health status. For example, exposure to violence can have adverse consequences for mental health status.

The National Research Council/Institute of Medicine published a comprehensive review of the state of child and adolescent mental health in the United States in 2009 (O'Connell, Boat, & Warner, 2009). It found that almost one in five young people have one or more mental, emotional, or behavioral (MEB) disorders at any given time. Among adults, half of all MEB disorders were first diagnosed by age 14 and three-fourths by age 24. This provides a window of opportunity to prevent, reduce frequency, and reduce intensity of these issues through earlier intervention (O'Connell, Boat, & Warner, 2009).

Proponents who argue for mental health programs and services in schools and communities focus on the gap between child and adolescent mental health concerns and problems, and children's utilization of these services. Most children with mental health challenges do not get the help they need. The most recent prevalence study, published in 2011 by Merikangas et al., reveals that:

❖ One in three adolescents (ages 13 to 18) with mental disorders receives services for their diagnosis.

❖ Almost half of adolescents with severely impairing mental disorders never receive treatment.

❖ Service rates are highest for adolescents with AD/HD (59.8%) and behavior disorders (45.4%).

❖ Fewer than one in five adolescents with anxiety, eating, or substance use disorders receives treatment for those disorders.

❖ Hispanic and black adolescents are less likely than their white counterparts to receive services for mood and anxiety disorders.

The National Research Council and Institute of Medicine estimate the total economic costs of mental, emotional, and behavioral disorders among youth in the United States at approximately $247 billion (2009). This study also documents that more than 6 in 10 U.S. youths have been exposed to violence within the past year, including witnessing a violent act, assault with a weapon, sexual victimization, child maltreatment, and dating violence. Nearly 1 in 10 was injured.

Schools, communities, and families can address this chasm between young people and the mental healthcare system by making connections critical to linking children, adolescents, and families with the resources they need, as well as developing new resources to meet unfilled needs.

Mental Health, Also Known as Behavioral Health

The term **behavioral health** is often used in place of saying mental health. In fact, *behavioral health* is used interchangeably with *mental health* because both terms refer to the promotion of practices that deal with the prevention, diagnosis, intervention, and treatment of mental illness. The term *behavioral health* recognizes that mental health now includes addictive disorders (such as substance abuse, addiction and gambling) as well as behaviors related to neurological conditions from AD/HD to autism, fetal alcohol spectrum disorders, and traumatic brain injury. In this text, we will use the term *mental health* to encompass the range of positive aspects of well-being and healthy functioning, the negative aspects of mental disorder and dysfunction, as well as the increasing number of identified neurological conditions. In this text, *behavioral health* and *mental health* are synonymous.

Addressing Mental Health Concerns and Problems of Youth

Five approaches provide the foundation to address mental health concerns and problems of children and adolescents. They help us know what might be available within any particular school, district, and community. Given the changing nature of young people's mental health concerns and problems, all of the approaches are dynamic, fueling how we identify new and recurring needs, and creating, implementing, and evaluating new programs and services. Together the approaches form a social ecological model that spans children and adolescents, families, school and community, health systems, and the larger environment, including local, state, and federal governmental programs, services, and public policy.

Institute of Medicine Intervention Classifications Focused on Preventing Problems

The Institute of Medicine (IOM) classification for mental health promotion and problem prevention interventions helps us think about how to enhance individuals' ability to achieve developmentally appropriate tasks (competence) and a positive sense of self-esteem, mastery, well-being, and social inclusion, and strengthen their ability to cope with adversity. Interventions can occur in schools, homes, community centers, or other community-based settings that promote emotional and social competence through activities emphasizing self-control and problem solving. The **Institute of Medicine (IOM) intervention classification** organizes the necessary action (interventions) into three categories based on the health needs of three different populations of individuals. **Table 1-1** shows the classifications. Universal interventions are for general population groups without reference to those at particular risk. Selective interventions are for individuals who are at greater-than-average risk for mental health problems. Indicated interventions are for individuals who may already display signs of mental health problems.

TABLE 1-1	IOM Mental Health Promotion and Preventive Intervention Classifications		
Universal preventive interventions:	**Selective preventive interventions:**	**Indicated preventive interventions:**
Focus on the general public or a whole population that has not been identified on the basis of individual risk. The intervention is desirable for everyone in that group. Universal interventions have advantages when their costs per individual are low, the intervention is effective and acceptable to the population, and there is a low risk from the intervention.	Focus on individuals or a population subgroup whose risk of developing mental disorders is significantly higher than average. The risk may be imminent or it may be a lifetime risk. Risk groups may be identified on the basis of biological, psychological, or social risk factors that are known to be associated with the onset of a mental, emotional, or behavioral disorder. Selective interventions are most appropriate if their cost is moderate and if the risk of negative effects is minimal or nonexistent.	Focus on high-risk individuals who are identified as having minimal but detectable signs of symptoms foreshadowing a mental, emotional, or behavioral disorder, or biological markers indicating predisposition for such a disorder, but who do not meet diagnostic levels at the current time. Indicated interventions might be reasonable even if intervention costs are high and even if the intervention entails some risk.
Example: School-based programs offered to all children to teach social and emotional skills or to avoid substance abuse. Programs offered to all parents of sixth graders to provide them with skills to communicate to their children about resisting substance use. The Olweus Bully Prevention Program is offered to promote a bully-free culture in schools. PATHS, the Positive Alternative Thinking Strategies program, promotes self-control, social competence, and positive peer relations.	*Example:* Programs offered to children exposed to risk factors, such as parental divorce, parental mental illness, death of a close relative, or abuse, to reduce risk for adverse mental, emotional, and behavioral outcomes. CARE, or Care, Assess, Respond, Empower, exists to help decrease suicidal behaviors, decrease related risk factors, and increase personal and social assets in adolescents.	*Example:* Interventions for children with early problems of aggression or elevated symptoms of depression or anxiety. Parenting Through Change is a theory-based intervention program that works to promote healthy child adjustment and prevent children's internalizing and externalizing conduct behaviors and problems. Parents are coached in effective parenting techniques such as skill encouragement, limit-setting, problem-solving, positive involvement, and monitoring.

Source: Republished with permission of National Academies Press, from Institute of Medicine. Mrazek, P.J., & Haggerty, R.J. (Eds.). (1994). *Reducing risks for mental disorders: Frontiers for preventive intervention research.* Washington, DC: National Academy Press, Committee on Prevention of Mental Disorders, Division of Biobehavioral Sciences and Mental Disorders. Copyright © 1994; permission conveyed through Copyright Clearance Center, Inc.

Coordinated School Health Programs

Schools are a natural setting to address the mental health needs of children and adolescents. Health promotion programs proposed in the 1980s to address many of the health-related problems of children and young people were designed to take advantage of the pivotal position of schools in reaching children and families by combining—in an integrated, systemic manner—health education, health promotion, and disease prevention; access to health-related services at the school site; and advocacy to change local and national policy.

Coordinated school health programs (**Figure 1-1**) include eight components (Centers for Disease Control and Prevention, 2008). These eight components are disciplines and services that most schools would have but that have not necessarily been organized to work together. A school health program coordinating council is formed with members from the school staff, teachers, nurses, guidance counselors, and administration as well as community members to oversee the day-to-day operations of the program. Frequently at the district level there is a staff position (e.g., director, coordinated school health program) with responsibility for the program's operation. The eight components are as follows:

1. *Health education:* Classroom instruction that addresses the physical, mental, emotional, and social dimensions of health; promotes knowledge, attitudes, and skills; is tailored to each age or developmental level; and is

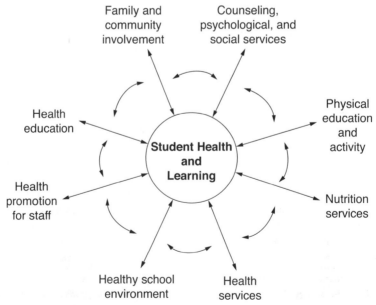

FIGURE 1-1   Coordinated school health components.
Source: Centers for Disease Control and Prevention. (2008). Components of coordinated school health. Retrieved from http://www.cdc.gov/healthyyouth/cshp/components.htm

designed to motivate and assist students in maintaining and improving their health and to reduce their risk behaviors.

2. *Physical education and activity:* Planned, sequential instruction that promotes lifelong physical activity. Designed to develop basic movement skills, sports skills, and physical fitness as well as to enhance mental, social, and emotional abilities.

3. *Health services:* Designed to promote the health of students, identify and prevent health problems and injuries, and ensure appropriate preventive services, emergency care, referral, or management of acute or chronic health conditions.

4. *Nutrition services:* Integration of nutritious, affordable, ethnically and culturally diverse, and appealing meals and nutrition education in an environment that promotes healthy eating habits for all children. Diet review and counseling for disordered eating and diet-related concerns.

5. *Counseling, psychological, and social services:* Designed to prevent and address problems, facilitate positive learning and healthy behavior, and enhance healthy development by providing services that focus on cognitive, emotional, behavioral, and social needs of students.

6. *Healthy school environment:* Designed to provide both a safe physical plant and a healthy and supportive environment that fosters learning, including the physical, emotional, and social climate of the school.

7. *Health promotion for staff:* Assessment, education, and fitness activities for school faculty and staff. Designed to maintain and improve the health and well-being of school staff members, who serve as role models for students.

8. *Family and community involvement:* Partnerships among schools, families, community groups, and individuals. Designed to maximize resources and expertise in addressing the healthy development of children, youth, and their family members.

The work of Ramona Valles, who directs her school district's coordinated school health program, illustrates how the approach works to address students' mental health needs and concerns. She has worked with each component to put in place a range of curricula, programs, and services. **Table 1-2** shows Ramona's efforts for each of the components. To be successful, she has had to build her network of contacts across the school and larger community. For example, she works with Latino centers (as well as other culturally relevant centers) that reach out to families to inform and educate them about available mental health services. A range of universal, selective, and indicated preventive programs is offered at the schools. She works with the county law enforcement agency to increase school safety, which has helped decrease violence in school and the community. Teachers have been trained to identify and refer students for whom the teachers have a mental health concern.

TABLE 1-2   Using a Coordinated Approach to Address Mental Health Issues in Schools

◆ Stigma is addressed and reduced. ◆ School policies address mental health issues. ◆ Students feel supported/respected. ◆ Create a safe and drug-free school building. ◆ Create safe and drug-free school-sponsored activities, sports events, and school buses. ◆ Maintain ongoing school climate assessments.	◆ Offer adaptive physical education. ◆ Emphasize lifelong recreational activities, such as yoga, walking, dancing, swimming, biking, and golf. ◆ Offer health programs for student athletes (e.g., pain management, performance enhancements). ◆ Provide concussion awareness and management.	◆ School curriculum mental and emotional health content area aligned with National Health Education Standards. ◆ Provide mental health promotion service learning activities. ◆ Educate student body on mental health to help increase understanding and decrease stigma. ◆ Provide interventions to reduce bullying.
HEALTHY ENVIRONMENT	**PHYSICAL EDUCATION AND PHYSICAL ACTIVITY**	**HEALTH EDUCATION**
◆ Provide free breakfast and lunch. ◆ Provide healthy school lunch choices following USDA standards. ◆ Lunchroom and schedule are conducive to relaxed eating. ◆ Limit sugary snacks and drinks. ◆ Offer ethnic and vegetarian/vegan choices. ◆ Provide diet management and screening.	**Promoting Child and Adolescent Mental Health**	◆ Make referrals for a continuum of care beyond the school. ◆ Offer school-based health clinics that help with STD/HIV, pregnancy, asthma, immunizations, and physical exams. ◆ Provide medication management. ◆ School nurses are engaged in primary prevention programs.
NUTRITION SERVICES		**HEALTH SERVICES**
◆ Actively involve families in the coordination of services.	◆ Assess student needs and available mental health programs and services.	◆ Provide smoking cessation programs and support.

◆ Recognize families as advocates. ◆ Welcome families in the school. ◆ Schedule meetings at times that are convenient for families. ◆ Offer mental health fairs. ◆ Create a resource center for parents. ◆ Link parents and caregivers for networking and support.	↔	◆ Make referrals for a continuum of care beyond the school. ◆ Offer student support services such as support and development groups for anger management and conflict resolution. ◆ Student support teams operate K–12.	↔	◆ Provide stress management skill workshops. ◆ Provide employee assistance programs (EAPs). ◆ Staff model conflict resolution and mediation skills. ◆ Provide supervisory training. ◆ Include recreational staff activities such as volleyball, basketball, and softball.
YOUTH, PARENT, FAMILY, AND COMMUNITY INVOLVEMENT		**SCHOOL COUNSELING, PSYCHOLOGY, AND SOCIAL SERVICES**		**STAFF HEALTH PROMOTION AND WELLNESS**

USDA = U.S. Department of Agriculture; STD/HIV = sexually transmitted disease/human immunodeficiency virus

Source: Adapted from Maine Coordinated School Health Program Departments of Education and Health and Human Services.

System of Care

A **system of care** is an adaptive network and interfacing of different systems, organizations, and groups that provides children and youth with serious emotional disturbance and their families with access to services and supports (Hodges, Ferreira, Israel, & Mazza, 2006). The system of care is an important approach to address the mental health needs of children and adolescents. It moves beyond the school to the community. Schools are one part of a system of care, but it is much broader and larger than any one system or organization.

The system of care values and principles initially articulated by Stroul and Friedman (1986) for the federal Child and Adolescent Service System Program (CASSP) were developed with the population of children with serious disorders in mind. The core values of the system of care philosophy specify that services should be community-based, child-centered and family-focused, and culturally and linguistically competent. Services need to be comprehensive, individualized, provided in the most appropriate setting, coordinated at the system and service delivery level, include family and youth as partners, and emphasize early intervention. **Box 1-1** illustrates a case example for a system of care for a 13-year-old child.

Box 1-1
Illustration of a System of Care Approach

Monte is a 13-year-old boy in the child welfare system. His mother has a history of substance abuse and child neglect. Due to a shoplifting charge, Monte has recently become involved with the juvenile justice system as well.

Thanks to the system of care approach in his community, local agencies and organizations partnered with the family in a coordinated way to keep Monte in his home and help his family access services that address their strengths and needs:

◆ By arranging to meet Monte and his mother in their home at a time that does not conflict with the family's schedule, agency representatives are able to work in partnership with the family to ensure the goals of their individualized service plan can be met.

◆ By working with the school system, the care coordinator is able to arrange alternative busing for Monte during a recent stay with family members while his mother participated in a residential treatment program, allowing him to continue at his current school. He was matched with a school mentor for school service learning projects occurring in the community.

◆ By working as a liaison with the juvenile justice and dependency court judges, a family advocate ensures Monte's family is able to adhere to multiple agency requirements and expectations. He participated in an anger management program at school, thereby avoiding having to travel to the agency.

◆ With the support of flexible funding, Monte is able to attend music lessons, which he identified as an interest, while his mother participates in weekly mandatory substance abuse counseling, reducing the need for child care.

The system of care concept holds that *all* life domains and needs need to be considered rather than addressing mental health treatment needs in isolation; therefore, systems of care are organized around nine overlapping dimensions:

1. Operational services
2. Mental health services
3. Social services
4. Recreational services
5. Child and family services

6. Educational services

7. Vocational services

8. Substance abuse services

9. Health services

The system of care requires communication and coordination among and across organizations and systems. The systems differ in what they offer and how they operate.

Public Health Approach

The **public health approach** to addressing the mental health concerns and problems of youth is organized into the three categories of **primary prevention**, **secondary prevention**, and **tertiary prevention** (**Table 1-3**). It is a proactive approach that covers all youth. The public health focus on population encourages us to think big. When we are implementing primary, secondary, and tertiary prevention interventions (Table 1-3), the public health approach works across systems to forge connections that promote child and adolescent mental health in varied types of sites (e.g., schools, communities, workplaces, and hospitals). Recognized in the approach is the diversity of program sites, real world challenges, how different professions understand the underlying determinants of mental health problems and concerns, and the larger understanding of how demographics and social transitions affect mental health and disease.

Four public health approach key concepts are defined in **Table 1-4**. Three process concepts, although less consistently identified as definitive, repeatedly emerge in discussions about a public health approach and naturally ensue when the first four concepts are implemented.

TABLE 1-3 Public Health Approach: Key Concepts		
Intervention category, population, and purpose		
Category	**Priority Population**	**Purpose**
Primary prevention	Whole population	Prevent new and future incidents of concerns and problems
Secondary prevention	Subpopulation with elevated risk and/or with concern and problem, but often undetected and with mild manifestations	Identify concerns and problems early, reduce symptoms, treat problem, and/or limit negative consequences; reduce frequency
Tertiary prevention	Subpopulation with concern and problem, experiencing severe negative consequences; diagnosable mental illness	Address, treat, and resolve concern and problem; slow progression of negative consequences, minimize complications, and reduce intensity

The public health conceptual framework places a special emphasis on intervening by building on and expanding prior models of intervening in the area of mental health. By incorporating the public health concepts of a population-level focus and a balanced emphasis on optimizing mental health and addressing mental

TABLE 1-4 Concepts of a Public Health Approach	
Concept	Definition
Four Defining Concepts	
Focuses on populations	Public health thinks about, intervenes with, and measures the health of the entire population and uses public policy as a central tool for intervention.
Emphasizes promotion and prevention	In public health, the focus includes preventing problems before they occur by addressing the sources of those problems, as well as identifying and promoting conditions that support optimal health.
Addresses determinants of health	Interventions guided by a public health approach focus on addressing determinants of health. Determinants are malleable factors that are part of the social, economic, physical, or geographical environment; can be influenced by policies and programs; and contribute to the good and poor health of a population.
Engages in a process based on three action steps	A public health approach requires implementation of a series of action steps. In the most widely recognized public health model, those action steps are assessment, policy development, and assurance, although some models place more emphasis on intervention. In this process, data are gathered to drive decisions about creating or adapting policies that support the health of the population, and efforts are made to make sure those policies are effective and enforced.
Three Process Concepts	
Intervention often means changing policies and broad environmental factors	Focusing at a population level requires addressing determinants that affect whole populations. Sometimes determinants can be addressed one child at a time through individual- or family-level interventions, but it is often more effective to make changes at broader levels by changing policies at the school, community, state, or national level, or by changing environments to which large numbers of children have exposure.
Uses a multi-system, multi-sector approach	There is no single entity that has sole responsibility for impacting children's mental health. Children are constantly impacted by many formal and informal systems and sectors, so changing environments in a meaningful way to positively impact children necessitates the involvement of all of those systems and sectors.

Implementation strategies are adapted to fit local needs and strengths	The three process/action steps support the integration of local needs and strengths. Public health recognizes that population-level change is not achieved by a one-size-fits-all approach because populations are made up of communities with divergent needs, resources, values, and the like. Activities like what to measure and how to intervene are examples for which local adaptation is not only appropriate, but fostered.

Source: Miles, J., Espiritu, R.C., Horen, N., Sebian, J., & Waetzig, E. (2010). *A public health approach to children's mental health: A conceptual framework—Expanded executive summary.* Washington, DC: Georgetown University Center for Child and Human Development, National Technical Assistance Center for Children's Mental Health. Reprinted by permission.

health problems, an intervening model emerges that organizes interventions into four categories. Two of the categories, promoting and re/claiming, optimize and measure *positive mental health*; two others, preventing and treating, reduce and measure *mental health problems*. **Table 1-5** shows the distinctions for the four intervention categories based on the action, timing of the intervention, and ultimate goal of the intervention for the population of focus. The intervening model also reflects the cyclical nature of the process. The first three categories reflect primary, secondary, and tertiary prevention. The fourth category (re/claiming) can be thought of as a mix of primary and tertiary prevention focused on positive mental health (primary prevention), while taking into consideration an identified mental health problem (tertiary prevention). It also reflects a recent blending and collaboration among education, health, and medical professions to promote and improve people's quality of life (Fertman, Allensworth, & Auld, 2010).

The public health approach recognizes that addressing the mental health needs and concerns of children is a process. At times it is full of struggles, frustration, conflicts, competing interests, and often no clear solutions. The process is dynamic, occurring over time (a number of years). It does not happen all at once and will not proceed smoothly. At the same time, it provides a framework and direction for how best to address the mental health concerns and problems of youth. An example of how the approach provides such a framework is illustrated by a recent communication from Dr. Marc Norman, superintendent of a south Florida school district. Writing to the school staff as well as the many staff members within agencies, programs, and services working with the school district, he summarized five keys of the public health approach to addressing the district students' mental health concerns and problems. He wrote:

❖ Taking a population focus requires us to emphasize the mental health of *all* children. Data needs to be gathered at population levels to drive decisions about interventions and to ensure the interventions are implemented and sustained effectively for entire populations.

❖ We want to create environments that promote and support optimal mental health and on developing skills that enhance resilience.

TABLE 1-5 Public Health Approach Intervention Model			
	Action	**Timing**	**Population Goal**
Promote …is to intervene…	To *optimize* positive mental health by addressing determinants* of positive mental health	*Before* a specific mental health problem has been identified in the individual, group, or population of focus	With the ultimate goal of improving the positive mental health of the population
Prevent …is to intervene…	To *reduce* mental health problems by addressing determinants of mental health problems	*Before* a specific mental health problem has been identified in the individual, group, or population of focus	With the ultimate goal of reducing the number of future mental health problems in the population
Treat …is to intervene…	To *diminish* or end the effects of an identified mental health problem	*After* a specific mental health problem has been identified in the individual, group, or population of focus	With the ultimate goal of approaching as close to a problem-free state as possible in the population of focus
Re/Claim …is to intervene…	To *optimize* positive mental health while taking into consideration an identified mental health problem	*After* a specific mental health problem has been identified in the individual, group, or population of focus	With the ultimate goal of improving the positive mental health of the population of focus

*Determinants of health are factors from biological, physical/geographical, social, and economic realms that positively or negatively influence the health of a population.

Source: Miles, J., Espiritu, R.C., Horen, N., Sebian, J., & Waetzig, E. (2010). *A public health approach to children's mental health: A conceptual framework—Expanded executive summary.* Washington, DC: Georgetown University Center for Child and Human Development, National Technical Assistance Center for Children's Mental Health. Reprinted by permission.

❖ We want to balance our focus on children's mental health problems with a focus on children's "positive" mental health—increasing our measurement of positive mental health and striving to optimize positive mental health for every child.

❖ We need to work collaboratively across a broad range of systems and sectors, from the child mental health care system to the public health system to all the other settings and structures that impact children's well-being.

❖ We want to think big and look across the county, state, and nation at programs and services while adapting our implementation to our local district and community—taking local needs and strengths into consideration as we implement our programs and services.

Individual Mental Health Concerns and Problems Intervention Process Approach

The **individual mental health concerns and problems intervention process approach** is concerned with addressing the mental health and problems of individual children and adolescents, one at a time, within the larger population of youth at a site (e.g., school, community program, camp). By definition, it is intense and time consuming to focus on attending to a single child or adolescent and his or her family and caregivers. It is a process with standard operating procedures, forms, and assigned staff members who are responsible for working with staff, community members, families, and students that identify and link children and adolescents to mental health programs and services. It represents a continuum of activities to link students to necessary programs and services. The Center for Mental Health in Schools at UCLA (n.d.) includes initial problem identification, clarifying need, consultation with child and family, management of care, and ongoing monitoring as key elements of the activity continuum. Student assistance programs (Fertman, 2004; Fertman et al., 2001) modeled after workplace employee assistance programs use four phases of activity to link students and their families to the behavioral healthcare system in the school and community—referral, planning and recommendations, intervention and implementation, and follow-up and support. **Figure 1-2** illustrates the continuum of activities with accompanying actions. The activities across the continuum may overlap, build on each other, and at times require stepping back to a previous action to gather additional information, ask a question, or address a new concern or problem.

First is an initial school-based mental health system connection with the child. Anyone (e.g., teacher, parent, administrator, bus driver, student) who identifies that a child or adolescent may be suffering with a mental health concern and problem can use an easily accessible form (everyone is informed regarding the availability of forms, where to turn them in, and what will happen after they do so) that is routed to a designated school employee to initiate the process. The form also serves as a reminder to staff to implement an immediate crisis response if the child or adolescent is believed to be in active crisis (e.g., suicidal, intoxicated). Initial information can be collected, and parent and caregiver contact is made both to get consent and to engage the parent and caregiver in the process.

Second is planning and recommendations, which include additional information collection; clarification of needs; consultation with youth, family, and caregivers; goal setting; and plan development, including recommendations. A mental health screening may be one of the options exercised during this step as a means to gather more information. As part of the screening, the information can be used to trigger immediate action (e.g., substance abuse evaluation) hospitalization or feedback to the family to use to formulate the goals and plan.

Third is the plan implementation and interventions. Implementation of the plan and interventions are difficult and not without challenges and struggles. It may not be a linear process, but rather nonlinear with twists and turns and at times unclear and unpredictable outcomes. It is best viewed from two points of view: staff, and child and family. The staff point of view is broad, with knowledge and

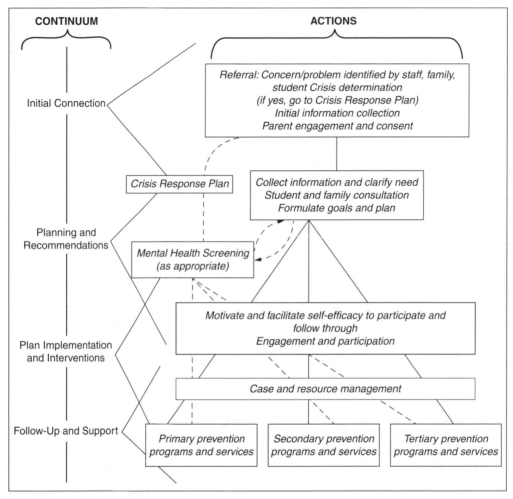

FIGURE 1-2 Individual mental health concerns and problems intervention process approach continuum and accompanying actions.
Source: Adapted from Center for Mental Health in Schools at UCLA. (n.d.). Guidebook: Common psychosocial problems of school-aged youth: Developmental variations, problems, disorders and perspectives for prevention and treatment. UCLA Department of Psychology School Mental Health Project. Retrieved from http://www.smhp.psych.ucla.edu

information on the range and diversity of available services and programs as well as the established procedures to participate. Staff members facilitate the engagement of the student and family in the process and continue to motivate them to follow through on recommended services. The child and family point of view focuses on the engagement and participation of the child or adolescent critical to achieve the agreed-upon goals. Frequently, the child and family point of view of the programs and services is narrow and concerned only with those aspects relevant to their particular situation.

Fourth is follow-up and support. The focus of this stage is case and resource management, the systematic procedure of continual feedback and monitoring of participation in planned activities and progress toward stated goals. Case management is how to attend to the children, adolescents, and their families who are participating in secondary and tertiary prevention programs. It lets them know, as individuals, they are important and deserve attention as they address their concerns and problems. Resource management is about looking at the system, identifying the gaps and places where the process breaks down, and fixing it. Resource management is about making sure that the system wraps around the child and family and meets their needs instead of requiring them to fit into an existing box. It is also about identifying new needs and providers and avoiding duplication of services by different entities.

The individual mental health concerns and problems intervention process approach reflects the reality that the mental health concerns and problems facing many students and their families are too numerous and too large for them to successfully confront and ameliorate without support. In addition, navigating the behavioral healthcare system, with its fragmentation, diverse funding streams, and eligibility requirements, adds layers of complexity that are often a barrier in themselves. Hoagwood (2004) describes the approach as a 180-degree turn from clinic- and office-based practices toward high quality, consumer-driven, empirically based services in the practical setting (i.e., school) in which the service is ultimately to be delivered.

Benefits of the Various Approaches

Although many programs and services fit in more than one of the approaches, overall, the approaches provide guidance about the full array of mental health interventions that are needed to serve all children and adolescents. They can serve as an organizational tool to help you develop a comprehensive, coordinated approach to addressing children and adolescents' mental health.

The approaches derived from behavioral and social science, education, and public health help teachers, counselors, principals, nurses, agency staff, program directors, and parents to address young people's mental health concerns and problems in several ways. First, the approaches help in developing program objectives. For example, schools use the IOM classifications to decide on the population of children and adolescents they want to serve. Community mental health agencies and government programs (e.g., child welfare, health, mental health, drug and alcohol) using the public health matrix of promote, prevent, treat, and re/claim can do likewise to decide on the population of children and adolescents to serve. This information is then used to determine the objectives for the mental health programs and services that will be planned, implemented, and evaluated.

Second, the approaches help to identify the specific programs and services to use to address the mental health concerns and problems. For example, using a system of care approach, the juvenile justice system, child welfare programs, community recreation, and afterschool services might be utilized with a population of youth who have previous and current legal system involvement. Third,

TABLE I-6   Benefits of Approaches to Address Children and Adolescents' Mental Health Concerns and Problems
I. Help to discern program outcomes
2. Specify programs and services for addressing concerns and problems
3. Identify the timing for interventions
4. Help in choosing the right mix of strategies
5. Enhance communication between professionals
6. Promote critical thinking and creative problem solving
7. Improve replication of programs
8. Improve program efficiency and effectiveness

the approaches help to decide the timing of the intervention. For example, interventions that prevent use of tobacco should be implemented at the upper elementary level (grades 4 and 5) because that is when the behavior is beginning. Fourth, the approaches help in choosing the right mix of strategies and methods. In the previous tobacco example, community recreation and afterschool programs provide the young people with additional support in their communities and within their families while augmenting school-based interventions.

Fifth, the approaches aid communication between professionals. The approaches provide frameworks that remain constant with each new initiative, so we can talk with colleagues and peers who are using the approaches with different groups of children and adolescents to compare and contrast implementation and outcomes. Sixth, using the approaches encourages us to think critically about the real world challenges that we face. Conflict and struggles are expected. The approaches help us to be creative in how we solve problems and face challenges.

Seventh, the use of approaches helps in replication of the programs because the same frameworks can be used from one intervention and population to another. Finally, approaches help in designing programs that are more effective (have greater impact) and more efficient (take less time). These benefits are summarized in **Table 1-6**.

Summary

Mental health concerns and problems among children and adolescents encompass a range of positive aspects of well-being and healthy functioning, negative aspects of mental disorder and dysfunction, and an increasing number of identified neurological conditions. The term *behavioral health* is often used in place of *mental health*. In fact, *behavioral health* is used interchangeably with *mental health* because both terms refer to the promotion of practices that deal with the prevention, diagnosis, intervention, and treatment for mental illness and the promotion of emotional well-being.

Five approaches provide the foundation to address mental health concerns and problems of children and adolescents. They help us know what might be available within any particular school, district, and community. Together the approaches form a social ecological model that spans children and adolescents, families, school and community, health systems, and the larger environment including local, state, and federal governmental programs, services, and public policy. The approaches are the Institute of Medicine intervention classifications focused on preventing problems, coordinated school health programs, the system of care, the public health approach, and the individual mental health concerns and problems intervention process approach. Although many programs and services fit in more than one of the approaches, overall, the approaches provide guidance about the full array of mental health interventions that are needed to serve all children and adolescents.

For Practice and Discussion

1. The five approaches discussed in this chapter help us to address the mental health concerns and needs of young people. In your own words, explain how the five approaches fit together. How do they complement each other? Are there places where they potentially conflict with and contradict each other?

2. Working in a small group, identify and reflect on primary, secondary, and tertiary mental health prevention programs that operated in your local school community as you progressed from elementary to high school. Share your experiences and reflections on participating or watching your friends participate in the programs.

3. In order for children and adolescents to receive adequate mental health care, 10 considerations need to be addressed. In your local school community programs and services, which of the considerations are most in need of attention?

   a. *Availability:* Are the programs and service available and at a time when needed? For example, do services exist after 6 p.m. for families in crisis? Do program hours coincide with parents' work hours, making it difficult to schedule appointments for fear of work reprisals?

   b. *Accessibility:* Are transportation services available? For example, would it be difficult for a single parent with four children to make three bus transfers to get one child to a counseling session?

   c. *Affordability:* Are programs and services available, and can a family with few financial resources afford them?

   d. *Appropriateness:* Are services available for all grade levels (K–12)?

   e. *Adaptability:* Can parents of a child receiving services also receive counseling at the agency, or must they go to a different agency?

f. *Acceptability:* Are services offered in a language preferred by the family?

g. *Awareness:* Are families, school staff, and community members aware that needed services exist in the community?

h. *Attitudes:* How do programs and services validate the importance of a child's home-based traditional beliefs and norms?

i. *Approachability:* Do young people and families feel welcomed at agencies? Do providers and receptionists greet children and teenagers in the manner in which they prefer? This includes greeting them with their preferred names.

j. *Additional services:* Are child- and adult-care services available if a parent must bring children or an aging parent to the appointment with them?

4. The individual mental health concerns and problems intervention process approach is different from the other four approaches in that it is concerned with addressing the mental health and problems of individual children and adolescents, one at a time, within the larger population of youth at a site (e.g., school community program, camp). By definition, it is intense and time consuming to focus on attending to a single child or adolescent and his or her family and caregivers. Compare and contrast how working with children and adolescents one on one is the same as and different from working with children and adolescents in small groups and classroom settings.

Key Terms

Behavioral health   4

Coordinated school health   6

Indicated preventive interventions   5

Individual mental health concerns and problems intervention process approach   15

Institute of Medicine (IOM) intervention classification   4

Mental health   2

Primary prevention   11

Public health approach   11

Secondary prevention   11

Selective preventive interventions   5

System of care   9

Tertiary prevention   11

Universal preventive interventions   5

References

Center for Mental Health in Schools at UCLA. (n.d.). Guidebook: Common psychosocial problems of school-aged youth: Developmental variations, problems, disorders, and perspectives for prevention and treatment. UCLA Department of Psychology School Mental Health Project. Retrieved from http://www.smhp.psych.ucla.edu

Centers for Disease Control and Prevention. (2008). Components of coordinated school health. Retrieved from http://www.cdc.gov/healthyyouth/cshp/components.htm

Fertman, C. (2004). Student assistance program practitioners talk about how to link students to behavioral health care. *Report on Emotional and Behavioral Disorders in Youth*, 4(4): 87–92.

Fertman, C., Allensworth, D., & Auld, E. (2010). What are health promotion programs? In C. Fertman & D. Allensworth (Eds.), *Health Promotion Programs: From Theory to Practice* (pp. 3–28). San Francisco, CA: Jossey-Bass.

Fertman, C., Fichter, C., Schlesinger, J., Tarasevich, S., Wald, H., & Zhang, X. (2001). Evaluating the effectiveness of student assistance programs in Pennsylvania. *Journal of Drug Education*, 31(4): 353–366.

Hoagwood, K. (2004). Evidence-based practice in child and adolescent mental health: Its meaning, application, and limitations. *Report on Emotional and Behavioral Disorders in Youth*, 4(1): 7–8, 24–26.

Hodges, S., Ferreira, K., Israel, N., & Mazza, J. (2006). *Strategies of System of Care Implementation: Making Change in Complex Systems: A Framework for Analysis of Case Studies of System Implementation: Holistic Approaches to Studying Community Based Systems of Care* (Research and Training Center Study 2). Tampa, FL: University of South Florida, Louis de la Part Florida Mental Health Institute, Department of Child and Family Studies.

Merikangas, K.R., He, J.P., Burstein, M., Swendsen, J., Avenevoli, S., Case, B., . . . Olfson, M. (2011). Service utilization for lifetime mental disorders in US adolescents: Results of the National Comorbidity Survey—Adolescent Supplement (NCS-A). *Journal of the American Academy of Child and Adolescent Psychiatry*, 50(1), 917–925.

Miles, J., Espiritu, R.C., Horen, N., Sebian, J., & Waetzig, E. (2010). *A public health approach to children's mental health: A conceptual framework—Expanded executive summary.* Washington, DC: Georgetown University Center for Child and Human Development, National Technical Assistance Center for Children's Mental Health.

National Research Council and Institute of Medicine. (2009). Preventing Mental, Emotional, and Behavioral Disorders Among Young People: Progress and Possibilities. Committee on the Prevention of Mental Disorders and Substance Abuse Among Children, Youth, and Young Adults: Research Advances and Promising Interventions. Mary Ellen O'Connell, Thomas Boat, and Kenneth E. Warner, Editors. Board on Children, Youth, and Families, Division of Behavioral and Social Sciences and Education. Washington, DC: The National Academies Press.

Stroul, B., & Friedman, R. (1986). *A System of Care for Children and Youth with Severe Emotional Disturbances* (rev. ed.). Washington, DC: Georgetown University Child Development Center, National Technical Assistance Center for Children's Mental Health.

U.S. Surgeon General. (1999). *Mental Health: A Report of the Surgeon General.* Retrieved from http://www.surgeongeneral.gov/library/mentalhealth/chapter3/sec8.html

World Health Organization. (2004). *Prevention of Mental Disorders: Effective Interventions and Policy Options. Summary Report.* Retrieved from http://www.who.int/mental_health/evidence/en/prevention_of_mental_disorders_sr.pdf

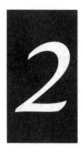

CREATING A MENTAL HEALTH PROMOTING SCHOOL COMMUNITY

In this chapter, we will:

✦ Discuss being a champion and advocate for students' mental health

✦ Describe a school community culture and climate to promote mental health

✦ Share what is important to youth in a mental health promoting school community

✦ Present a model for a mental health promoting school community

Scenario

After a couple of years of teaching, I found it useful to reflect on the difference between being a "good person" and being a "good teacher." It is important to be nurturing and supportive of young people, but it's also important to challenge them to work hard and to help them assume responsibility for making their lives successful. If you're able to take time to reflect on situations and not internalize or personalize everything, it will help smooth out the emotional ups and downs, which can get pretty intense. Having a shared vision of what we are working toward helps a lot. I want to encourage the young people with whom I work as well as my colleagues to think critically and to learn to take action to create a more caring school community.

Source: Ana Flores, a student support team member at a middle school in the Miami–Dade school system

Being a Champion and Advocate for Students' Mental Health

You will be a champion and advocate for child and adolescent mental health. What does that mean? It means you are going to provide leadership and passion. As a **champion**, you will know the setting, the mental health concerns, and the problems faced by children, adolescents, and their families. As programs and services are planned, implemented, and evaluated, you will provide insight into how the many organizations, groups, and individuals (also called *stakeholders*) involved with addressing young people's mental health interact and work together. You will be supportive and help address potential challenges to implementing programs and services. You will know the history of the concerns and problems and what has worked before in solving them, as well as what has not worked. (Frequently, a champion is also called a **key informant** because he or she knows important or key information about an organization.) Champions are the people who have initiated the effort to start the program, identify the health issue, or try to solve the problem.

As an **advocate**, you will fight for resources, time, funding, and space for the program's operations. By building trusting and honest relationships, you will form the foundation for the work of planning, implementing, and evaluating effective mental health programs and services. You know the system, all of the people who have a stake in getting the programs up and running, sustaining and expanding existing programs and services, and creating and adding new ones. You fight for policies that are supportive within the organization and beyond. Talking at school board meetings, community meetings, and serving on boards of organizations are all part of being an advocate. Being involved with public policy is a critical part of advocacy. You will have opportunities to learn and use skills to change public legislation at the local and state (maybe even national) levels to protect and promote the mental health of children and adolescents.

The work is endless. It is not your role or responsibility to finish the work, but rather to help it continue with its many twists and turns, ups and downs. The work is not stagnant; it constantly changes and requires us all to change, too. It is what will make you a good professional. However, you cannot do it alone. It requires too much time and energy. Staff get tired, frustrated, change jobs, and leave. Political and economic changes occur in the community. Staff get burned out. It is only natural.

In the long run, the mental health of young people and their families will most likely result from the work of active school and community teams, partnerships, and collaborations. Although in some cases a single teacher, principal, or counselor has a significant impact on the way students' problems and concerns are addressed, rarely does one person have enough knowledge, time, expertise, or energy to do everything required to prevent students from having mental health concerns and problems. This chapter sets the stage for you to move beyond instruction, counseling, and mentoring to create and build school teams, partnerships, and collaborations that ultimately make the difference in children and adolescents addressing their mental health concerns and problems and becoming competent young people.

Working together with other professionals across organizations and systems has a distinct advantage over solo efforts, namely the mutual support that develops among people. It is all too easy for one person's commitment and enthusiasm to flag over time, particularly because mental health concerns and problems are not likely to be considered the school's and community's number-one priority. The synergy that results when people work together on a team, partnership, and collaboration helps to sustain enthusiasm and support for the effort, even through difficult times.

Teams, partnerships, and collaborations enhance the skills of individuals and promote effective and creative work as a whole. Perhaps most important, over time, the teams, partnerships, and collaborations learn what works, and improve their performance to promote, develop, and support competent and capable young people as they develop and grow.

Mental Health Promoting School Community Culture and Climate

Throughout the text, we refer often to the school community culture and climate. But what do we mean by these terms? What is a school community? What is the difference between school community culture and school community climate? And why are they important to you as you work to address the mental health concerns and problems of young people?

The **school community** is the product of students, school staff, community professionals, parents, caregivers, families, residents, community organizations, public health agencies, government, hospitals, and businesses in a local community working to benefit young people. Schools are part of and reflective of their communities. Schools seek out community resources and experts to work with them to develop programs for the students. A healthcare organization, for example, might team up with its local school to provide a program to students and families. Individual schools team up with families, the district, and community members and organizations, and school districts create partnerships within the local community to develop programs and services. Working in a school or community agency, you are part of a school community. Living in a community, you are part of a school community.

School culture refers to a school's persona, which is made up of the attitudes of those within the school, as well as how people relate to each other and how they treat and feel about one another. School culture reflects the norms of the school, what happens within the school, and what the people within the school community care about and pay attention to. **Table 2-1** shows the Association of California School Administrators **school culture survey** that principals in that state complete to help them better understand their school's culture. School culture also describes the school's guiding beliefs and how it promotes learning and mental health. Knowing the culture of the school tells us what is important to the school community. You probably cannot find a school in which the students' mental health is not a value held by everyone. However, it is one of many values

TABLE 2-1 Association of California School Administrators School Culture Survey

Directions: Rate each norm/value on the following scale: 1 = Almost always characteristic of our school; 2 = Generally characteristic of our school; 3 = Seldom characteristic of our school; 4 = Not characteristic. For each norm/value, please provide a recent illustrative example of how that norm is demonstrated through individual or organizational behavior.

Norm/Value	Rating	Recent Illustrative Examples
Moral Purpose: The school community is driven by a commitment to make a positive difference in the lives of students and their community.		
Professional Learning Community: Commitment to examining practice with a focus on improving student achievement.		
Experimentation: Ongoing professional development with an interest in trying new practices and evaluating the results.		
High Expectations: A pervasive push for high standards-based performance for students and all staff, using multiple data sources to inform assessments and personnel processes.		
Public Service: Staff understands that their role is to serve the community. Staff respects and honors community values, culture, and contributions.		
Trust and Confidence: A pervasive feeling that people will do what's right between and across groups. No "us vs. them."		
Support for Personal and Professional Growth: Individual coaching and mentoring are pervasive.		
Tangible Support: Financial and material assistance aligned to the goals determined within a cycle of continuous improvement. People have what they need to do their work.		
Reaching Out to the Knowledge Base: Use of research, reading of professional journals, attending workshops.		

Appreciation and Recognition: Acknowledgment of quality student and faculty work and effort.		
Caring, Celebration, Humor: A sense of community with shared purpose and joy. Personal balance and health are values.		
Appreciation of Leadership: Specifically, leadership provided by teachers, principals, and other professional staff.		
Clarity of Goals and Outcomes: There is a coherent vision and action plan tied to measurable goals that members of the community could articulate and relate to their own work.		
Protection of What's Important: School goals, priorities, and core cultural values.		
Involvement of Stakeholders in Decision Making: Those who will be affected by decisions are involved in making them; diverse points of view are included and honored.		
Traditions: Rituals and events that celebrate and support core school and community values.		
Honest, Open Communication: Teaching and learning is public practice with multiple opportunities for peer and administrative observation and feedback. Coaching and feedback are valued among all practitioners.		
Willingness to Confront the "Brutal Facts": A pervasive culture in which multiple data sources are used to expose student achievement gaps as well as gaps in instructional expertise, within the context of fostering "critical friendships."		
Source: From Association of California School Administrators. (2010), School Culture Survey. Retreived from http://www.acsa.org		

that compete for people's time and energy to uphold and champion. We need to know and respect the other values and norms within the school community. We need to show and demonstrate how diverse, distinct norms and values are complementary and synergistic, championing and reflecting a broad, diverse range of values.

School climate describes the quality of everyday life at the school and the way people feel inside the school, and how these factors affect learning and mental health. It is what students, parents, teachers, and other school staff experience within the school and how teachers engage students and parents in education and promoting mental health. It refers to the sense teachers, staff, and students have of feeling included and appreciated. School climate also refers to the physical and emotional safety of a school campus and how the environment around the school affects the school itself.

How students, parents, community members, and school staff perceive a school's climate can be measured using surveys that ask participants about their experiences in the school. **School climate surveys** can be given to students, school staff and administration, parents, and community members. The surveys are similar, although questions are tailored for the particular audience. For example, school personnel are asked to indicate how much they agree with the statement, "Teachers encourage students to think independently," whereas parents are given the statement, "My child's teachers encourage him/her to try out new ideas (think independently)." Differences between surveys for elementary students and middle and high school students are found in word choice. Whereas elementary school students are asked about the statement, "Students in this school respect differences in other students (for example, if they are a boy or girl, where they come from, what they believe)," middle and high school students are asked about the statement, "Students in this school respect each other's differences (for example, gender, race, culture, etc.)." Surveys for school personnel include questions on school leadership and professional relationships that are not included on the other surveys.

These tools are used to learn about personal experiences in the school with issues such as bullying, race, and interpersonal relationships. Surveys can be used to find out what a school's strengths and needs are, and can be used both for needs assessment and to evaluate changes over time. One example of a student survey is from the Australia MindMatters program (**Table 2-2**), which asks students about a number of areas in order to get a sense of the students' school building climate.

Information gathered from school climate surveys can be used to help school leaders make decisions that help improve the school climate for students, staff, parents and guardians, and community members. If safety, for example, is noted as a problem area for students or staff, schools should note areas of particular concern and review their policies, ensuring that the student code of conduct, school crisis plans, and school bullying policies address the concerns noted in the surveys. Schools may also consider simple changes that can be implemented immediately, such as adding security to or closing off a stairwell, training staff at metal detectors to greet students warmly in the morning, creating a cell phone locker system, or the like.

Surveys such as the Gay, Lesbian and Straight Education Network (GLSEN)'s National School Climate Survey can be helpful for addressing the particular concerns of a priority population. The National School Climate Survey asks lesbian,

TABLE 2-2 MindMatters Student Survey—Short Version					
Dear Student, We are interested in finding out what you think about mental health and well-being, that is, your feelings, thoughts, relationships, and behavior. We greatly appreciate your time and effort in completing this survey.					
	Strongly Agree	**Agree**	**Disagree**	**Strongly Disagree**	**Do Not Know**
1. I like coming to school.					
2. I feel safe at my school.					
3. I have someone to talk to at school if I need help or advice.					
4. I think the school rules are fair.					
5. Our school deals fairly and quickly with bullying and harassment problems.					
6. I get information about mental health and well-being issues.					
7. I learn about different health issues, including mental health and well-being.					
8. I feel like I belong.					
9. I get to do work that I enjoy and find interesting.					
10. I have friends at school.					
11. I know who to go to for help with mental health and well-being issues if I need it.					
12. I am comfortable speaking with and getting help from the school counselors.					
13. There are teachers and other staff who understand my issues.					
14. Teachers show that the mental health and well-being of students is important.					

Source: Reprinted by permission of Principals Australia Institute MindMatters. (2012). Student Survey—Short Version. Retreived from http://www.mindmatters.edu. MindMatters is funded by the Commonwealth Department of Health and Ageing, Australia, 2011.

gay, bisexual, and transgender (LGBT) students about their experiences in school regarding biased and homophobic remarks, feeling unsafe at school because of personal characteristics, missing school for safety reasons, and the experience of harassment and assault at school (GLSEN, 2009). Results from this kind of survey can help school administrators develop policies that address LGBT students specifically, including adopting bullying policies covering harassment and assault due to sexual orientation.

Entering a school building, school district, and school community, you want to be aware of the culture and climate. There are a number of approaches for addressing students' mental health concerns and problems that can help us to understand the programs and services that we need to have in place to service children and adolescents and their families. The benefit of knowing the culture and climate is that it provides a framework and larger environment for our work. **Table 2-3** provides a list of values for mental health promoting school communities. Imagine working in a school community with this level of commitment to addressing the mental health concerns and problems of young people. Being aware of a school community culture and climate, even before we start talking about the specifics of our work, gives us a sense of how the school community operates and how the people involved might perceive us. We have a guide to how hard we can challenge staff to create programs and services; engage young people, families, and caregivers; and advocate for policies and procedures to promote and protect mental health.

TABLE 2-3   Mental Health Promoting School Community Culture and Climate

1. A school community that promotes mental health and well-being
   - ❖ School community staff understand the importance of mental health and well-being, its impact on learning, and the significant contributions the school community makes to improving student mental health.
   - ❖ School community staff have an understanding of their school community.
2. Respectful relationships, belonging, and inclusion
   - ❖ School community staff expect and model respectful and responsive relationships within the school community.
   - ❖ Belonging and inclusion for all school community members is specifically addressed in school strategic planning, policies, and practices.
   - ❖ The school community environment and communication reflect the diversity of the school community.
   - ❖ Leadership and staff create opportunities for students, staff, families, and the wider school community to be involved in a range of activities and contribute to school community planning.

3. Collaborative working relationships with parents and caregivers
    ❖ School community planning, policies, and practices support collaborative working relationships with parents and caregivers.
    ❖ School community staff implement strategies to proactively develop collaborative working relationships with parents and caregivers to promote children's mental health, well-being, and learning.
4. Support for parenting
    ❖ School community staff have knowledge and skills to communicate effectively with parents about their children in areas related to child development, learning and mental health, and well-being.
    ❖ School community staff communicate effectively with parents and caregivers about child development, learning, and mental health and well-being.
    ❖ Policies and practices support staff to identify and, where appropriate, facilitate access for parents to resources and services that support parenting.
5. Parent and caregiver support networks
    ❖ The school community provides opportunities for parents and caregivers to connect with each other and develop support networks, and actively seeks to minimize barriers to participation.
    ❖ The school community identifies and promotes community groups that may act as a source of support for parents and caregivers.
6. Understanding mental health difficulties and improving help-seeking
    ❖ School community staff have an understanding of childhood mental health difficulties including common signs and symptoms, their impact on children and families, and factors that put children at risk.
    ❖ School community staff understand that getting help and support early is important for students and families experiencing difficulties.
    ❖ The school community provides an inclusive and accepting environment for community members who may be experiencing difficulties with their mental health.
7. Responding to students experiencing mental health difficulties
    ❖ School community staff have a shared understanding of their role, and its boundaries, in addressing the needs of students experiencing mental health difficulties.
    ❖ The school community has protocols and processes for recognizing and responding to students experiencing mental health difficulties, including helping students to remain engaged in their education.
    ❖ Staff have knowledge and skills for recognizing and supporting students experiencing mental health difficulties, including how to access and connect to support.
    ❖ The school community has effective working relationships and clear pathways with services, and supports families to access these services.

Source: Adapted from KidsMatter Australian Primary Schools Mental Health Initiative. (2012). KidsMatter primary framework. Retrieved from http://www.kidsmatter.edu.au/primary/kidsmatter -overview/framework/. Used by permission of the Australian Government.

Creating the Mental Health Promoting School Community

A **mental health promoting school community** offers a range of programs and services, in both the school and the community, from primary prevention to tertiary prevention (**Figure 2-1**). These programs and service offerings combine and merge the Institute of Medicine prevention categories of universal, selective, and indicated with public health's primary, secondary and tertiary prevention classifications. The culture and climate of the school community supports, maintains, and nourishes the programs and services. The programs and services reflect the merger of public health and medicine to promote the quality of life for all individuals and populations, regardless of their health status (Fertman & Allensworth, 2010).

A mental health promoting school community has programs and services that span both school and community with primary, secondary, and tertiary prevention. Surrounding and supporting the school and community are partnerships and collaborations (**Figure 2-2**). You need to navigate and work across systems (each of which has its own unique role, norms, rules, and challenges) to create opportunities and resources for young people to get the consistent relationships, supports, and structures they need to address their concerns and problems. You need to work to make mental health promotion part of the school community values and norms. You need to create the infrastructure to address the mental health problems and concerns of children and adolescents.

Your work to create and support a school community culture and climate that promotes mental health is not easy. You do not just wake up one day to find that your school community with all of its schools and community organizations have the programs, services, staff, money, and support they need to address the mental health needs of their children and adolescents. Likewise, you cannot expect on day one of your job in a school, community organization, public health agency, or hospital to find such a culture or climate. You are going to be part of the teams, partnerships, and collaborations that create and support the mental health culture and climate. You and your colleagues will face struggles and challenges. **Figure 2-3** illustrates the dynamics and ever-changing environment that you will face. It is complex, and when considered from an ecological perspective, even more complicated and challenging.

What Is Important to Youth in a Mental Health Promoting School Community?

Including the voice of young people (**youth voice**) is central to our work to promote the mental health of children and adolescents. We want to know how adults in the school community make all youth feel supported. We also want to know young people's perceptions of how adults respond to youth with mental health concerns and problems. This information helps us to tailor and fit programs and

Intervention Continuum	Examples of Focus and Types of Intervention
	(Programs and services to build a mental health school community culture and climate)

Primary Prevention[1]

Universal Programs and Services[2]

1. Public health protection, promotion, and maintenance to foster opportunities, positive development, and wellness

   - Economic enhancement of those living in poverty (e.g., work/welfare programs)
   - Safety (e.g., instruction, regulations, lead abatement programs)
   - Physical and mental health (e.g., healthy start initiatives, dental care, immunizations, bullying prevention, substance abuse prevention, violence prevention, health/mental health education, sex education and family planning, recreation, social services to access basic living resources)

2. Preschool-age support and assistance to enhance mental health and psychosocial development

   - Enhance systems through student support teams, partnerships, and collaborations
   - Education and social support for parents of preschoolers
   - Quality day care
   - Quality early education
   - Appropriate screening and amelioration of physical and mental health and psychosocial problems

3. Early-schooling

   - Orientations, welcoming, and transition support into school and community life for students and their families (especially immigrants)
   - Support and guidance to ameliorate school adjustment problems
   - Personalized instruction in the primary grades
   - Additional support to address specific learning problems
   - Parent involvement in problem solving

Secondary Prevention[1]

Selected and Indicated Programs and Services[2]

   - Comprehensive and accessible psychosocial and physical and mental health programs (e.g., a focus on community and home violence prevention, conflict resolution, and other problems identified through school-community needs assessment)

4. Improvement and augmentation of ongoing regular support

   - Enhance systems through student support teams, partnerships, and collaborations
   - Preparation and support for school and life transitions
   - Teaching "basics" of support and remediation to regular teachers (e.g., use of available resource personnel and peer and volunteer support)
   - Parent involvement in problem solving
   - Resource support for parents-in-need (e.g., assistance in finding work, legal aid, ESL, and citizenship classes)
   - Coordinated school health program with accessible psychosocial and physical and mental health interventions
   - Priority population focus (e.g., GLBT, immigrants, individuals with a disability)
   - Special education and rehabilitation
   - Emergency and crisis prevention and response mechanisms

5. Short-term, evidence-based, specialized interventions

   - Enhance systems through student support teams, partnerships, and collaborations
   - Alternative education programs
   - Priority population interventions (e.g., resource teacher instruction and family mobilization, programs for suicide prevention, teen parents, substance abusers, gang members, juvenile justice diversion programs, and other potential dropouts)

6. Intensive interventions

Tertiary Prevention[1]

Indicated Programs and Services[2]

   - System of care, placement guidance and assistance, case management, and resource coordination
   - Family preservation programs and services
   - Recovery and support programs
   - Dropout recovery and follow-up support
   - Services for severe-chronic psychosocial/mental/physical health problems

[1]Public Health Approach; [2]Institute of Medicine (IOM) Approach

FIGURE 2-1   From primary to tertiary prevention: A continuum of school community programs and services to address mental health concerns and problems of youth.
Source: Adapted from Center for Mental Health in Schools at UCLA. (n.d.). School–community partnerships: A guide. UCLA Department of Psychology School Mental Health Project. Retrieved from http://www.smhp.psych.ucla.edu

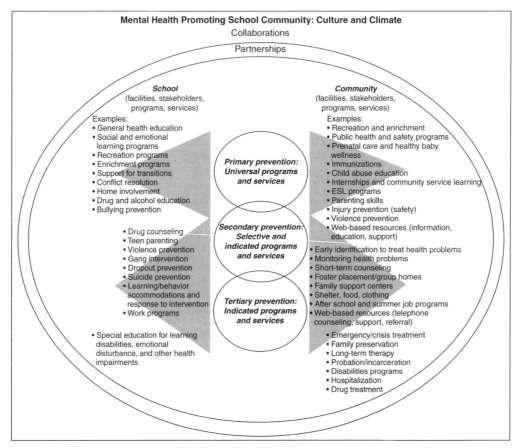

FIGURE 2-2 Mental health promoting school community: Culture and climate.
Source: Adapted from Center for Mental Health in Schools at UCLA. (n.d.). School–community partnerships: A guide. UCLA Department of Psychology School Mental Health Project. Retrieved from http://www.smhp.psych.ucla.edu

services to youth and their families. It contributes to a positive climate in the school community that is supportive to all youth. Most importantly, engaging youth adds their voices to the programs and services. It values and recognizes them as members of the school community.

Summary

You will be a champion and advocate for child and adolescent mental health. As a champion, you will know the setting, the mental health concerns, and the problems faced by children, adolescents, and their families. As an advocate,

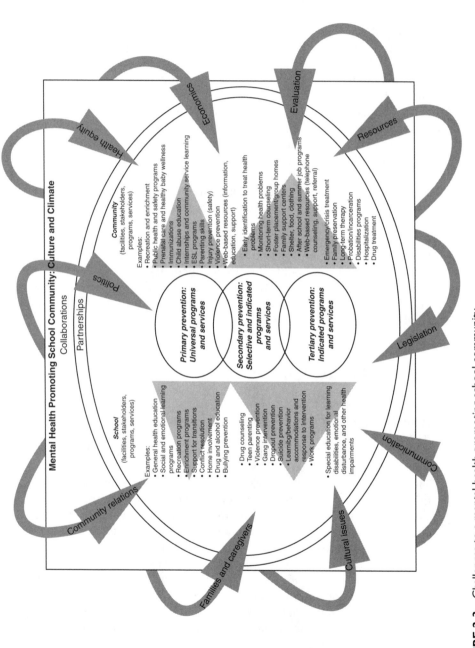

FIGURE 2-3 Challenges to a mental health promoting school community.
Source: Adapted from Center for Mental Health in Schools at UCLA. (n.d.). School–community partnerships: A guide. UCLA Department of Psychology School Mental Health Project. Retrieved from http://www.smhp.psych.ucla.edu

you will fight for resources, time, funding, and space for the program's operations. Throughout the text, we refer often to school community, culture, and climate. School community is the product of students, school staff, community professionals, parents, caregivers, families, residents, community organizations, public health agencies, government, hospitals, and businesses in a local community working to benefit young people. Schools are part of and reflective of their communities. School culture refers to a school's persona, which is made up of the attitudes of those within the school, as well as how people relate to each other and how they treat and feel about one another. School climate describes the quality of everyday life at the school and the way people feel inside the school, and how these factors affect learning and mental health. It is what students, parents, teachers, and other school staff experience within the school and how teachers engage students and parents in education and promoting mental health.

A mental health promoting school community with its programs and services is the product of the culture and climate of the school community. These school and community programs and service offerings combine and merge the Institute of Medicine prevention categories of universal, selective, and indicated with public health's primary, secondary, and tertiary prevention classifications. They reflect the merger of public health and medicine to promote the quality of life for all individuals and populations, regardless of their mental health status. Finally, adding the voice of young people is central to promoting the mental health of children and adolescents.

For Practice and Discussion

1. Reflect on the differences between being a "professional" (e.g., teacher, counselor, principal, social worker, nurse) and a "good person." Share your reflections.
2. Where in your life have you been a program champion? What did you do? What challenges did you face? What did you learn?
3. Think about the school you are attending. Who is part of your school community? What is the culture and climate of the school community? Identify three strengths of your school community. Identify whether they relate to climate or culture. If you could change one aspect of your school community, what would you change? Why make the change?
4. Discuss the challenges for a school community to plan and implement all or some of the programs and services listed in Figure 2-2. How do the challenges impact the school community values listed in Table 2-3?
5. How can you ensure that the voice of young people will be heard in the development and implementation of school community mental health programs and services?

Key Terms

References

Association of California School Administrators. (2010). School culture survey. Retrieved from http://www.acsa.org/MainMenuCategories/ProfessionalLearning/TrainingsandEvents/Creating-Academic-Optimism/Session-1/School-Culture-Survey.aspx

Center for Mental Health in Schools at UCLA. (n.d.). School–community partnerships: A guide. UCLA Department of Psychology School Mental Health Project. Retrieved from http://www.smhp.psych.ucla.edu

Fertman, C., Allensworth, D., & Auld, E. (2010). What are health promotion programs? In C. Fertman & D. Allensworth (Eds.), *Health promotion programs: From theory to practice* (pp. 3–28). San Francisco, CA: Jossey-Bass.

Gay Lesbian Straight Education Network (GLSEN). (2009). National school climate survey. Retrieved from http://www.glsen.org/binary-data/GLSEN_ATTACHMENTS/file/000/001/1675-2.pdf

KidsMatter Australian Primary School Mental Health Initiative. (2012). KidsMatter primary framework. Retrieved from http://www.kidsmatter.edu.au/primary/kidsmatter-overview/framework/

MindMatters. (2012). MindMatters Student Survey—Short Version. Retrieved from http://www.mindmatters.edu.au/verve/_resources/Student_Survey_Short_version.pdf

National Assembly on School-Based Health Care's School Mental Health. (2008). What students say about mental health. Retrieved from http://www.nasbhc.org/atf/cf/%7BB241D183-DA6F-443F-9588-3230D027D8DB%7D/MH_What%20Students%20Say.pdf

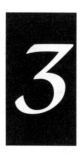

TEAMS, PARTNERSHIPS, AND COLLABORATIONS

In this chapter, we will:

✦ Define teams, partnerships, and collaborations

✦ Summarize how teams, partnerships, and collaborations promote child and adolescent mental health

✦ Explain how to build effective teams, partnerships, and collaborations

Scenario

It doesn't happen in every school. In fact, it wasn't until I transferred to this new school district where I took charge as school principal that I became part of a district with a history of a strong district-wide system of student support. One of the first things the superintendent had me do was participate in a training to assess the school district's capacity to address students' mental health needs. There were student support teams at each school to promote mental health, prevent mental illness by teaching life skills universally to all students, identify and intervene with those mental health issues that were barriers to learning and student achievement, and lastly, integrate and reinforce the lessons students learned during treatment. The district leadership envisioned a model where the wellness of all students is optimized.

Our student support teams are made up of teachers, the nurse, guidance counselors, social workers, the school psychologist, building and district *administrators, family members, and a community mental health organization representative. After a while, we began to see that teaming wasn't enough. We needed to look more strategically at our partnerships.*

We all came together to evaluate student and family needs, what school policies and practices were working in the schools, new practices and programs to consider implementing, program gaps, and staff support and training. Special attention was given to discussing the partnerships the school district had with local community mental health agencies, government services, community groups, and other school districts.

In one area, we couldn't figure out how to access the services the students needed. Finally, someone suggested we contact the state behavioral health office. You know, I found out that the state office was struggling with the same problem, except they had a plan. The State Department of Behavioral Health Services along with the Department of Education formed a collaboration to address the problem. They were working on legislation and changes in the state school code. I was surprised and pleased. The state child welfare office staff asked me for input and suggestions for other policy changes.

Source: Devon Smith, a principal in a suburban school district outside of Atlanta, Georgia

Defining Teams, Partnerships, and Collaborations

The terms *team*, *partnership*, and *collaboration* are used in many ways and have a variety of meanings to different people. This section provides the working definitions used in this text. One caution and potentially confusing issue is that the terms *partnership* and *collaboration* are commonly used interchangeably. We will show that these are, in fact, quite distinct terms. With all three terms, individuals and organizations work together to overcome challenges they cannot handle by themselves. They demonstrate the concept of synergy: the sum total of people's combined efforts will be greater than the effect each person would have working alone.

A **team** is a group of interdependent individuals who share responsibility for specific outcomes for their organization (e.g., school). The minimum defining features are shared responsibility and interdependence. Team members are interdependent if each depends on the others to carry out his or her role, to accomplish goals, or to create a product. For example, a team at a school addressing students' mental health concerns and problems might be composed of school staff (e.g., teachers, administrators, counselors, nurses) and community organization staff (e.g., mental health, drug and alcohol, juvenile justice, school-based probation). Each member brings expertise from their professional role and experience working with youth, shares the goal of helping and supporting children and adolescents, and works with other team members to create a plan of action and to identify **resources** and supports to address students' needs.

A **partnership** is a group of interdependent local organizations represented by individuals who share responsibility for specific outcomes across organizations at the local level. Similar to teams, the minimum defining features of a partnership are shared responsibility and interdependence. Partnership members use their organization's role and experience working with youth and their shared goal of helping and supporting children and adolescents to create resources and supports within and across a community to address students' needs. For example, local community partnerships among mental health agencies, drug and alcohol programs, human services and youth development organizations, faith-based programs, and schools develop and sustain a range of educational and health programs and services with multiple entry points and funding. The goal is to create an accessible, consumer-driven continuum of mental health practices and services.

A **collaboration** is a group of interdependent organizations represented by individuals who share responsibility for specific outcomes across a region or state(s) working at the governmental and public policy level. Similar to teams and partnerships, the minimum defining features are shared responsibility and interdependence. Collaboration members use their organization's role and experience working with youth and shared goal of helping and supporting children and adolescents to create resources and supports across a region or state(s) to address students' needs. For example, state-level departments of education, health, public welfare, and justice form a collaboration for planning, budgeting, and legislative actions to provide infrastructure to create and finance school-based mental health services.

Teams, partnerships, and collaborations arise as individuals and organizations (governmental, educational, nonprofits, community-based, and others) seek to overcome challenges they cannot meet alone. This shared goal (overcoming a challenge) defines the members of a team, partnership, or collaboration. In this text, we use the term *partnership* when discussing and describing local, community-level efforts. We use the term *collaboration* when explaining regional, state, and national efforts.

A Socio-ecological Approach to Promoting Child and Adolescent Mental Health

Teams, partnerships, and collaborations take a socio-ecological approach to promoting child and adolescent mental health (**Figure 3-1**). The **socio-ecological approach** considers all levels when addressing the mental health needs of children and adolescents. As we work with each level (i.e., children and adolescents, schools, community, etc.), we adapt practices to fit local needs and strengths. In this approach, the teams, partnerships, and collaborations are the links that unite the different levels to address students' mental health concerns and problems and to promote their mental health.

Teams occur mostly at the school building level, with the participation of families and youth from the building. At the school building level, local community human service agencies and programs are part of the school teams. Partnerships typically are formed at the school district level including all of the district buildings and joining with a broader range of community-wide agencies,

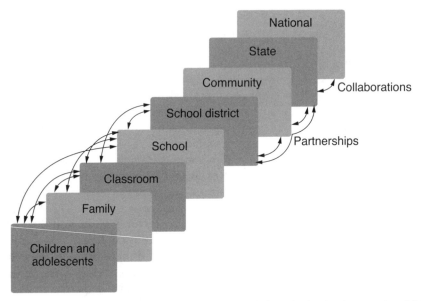

FIGURE 3-1   Teams, partnerships, and collaborations linking the levels of promoting child and adolescent mental health.

services, and programs. Health insurance providers, state government programs, and businesses often are partnership members. Collaborations reach higher to the national and state level to address broad public policies. Collaborations will seek input from many of the other levels (e.g., family, school districts, community), but the collaboration leadership tends to reside at the state or national level. All three together contribute to the mental health of children and adolescents.

School Teams

School teams are composed of school and community program staff, including school principals, assistant principals, resource specialists, psychologists, community outreach workers, social workers, teachers, and school counselors, who address students' mental health concerns and problems. They meet regularly to provide referrals, intervention, monitoring, and support. With the input of parents, they develop strategies to improve specific behaviors, and they seek additional resources and community services. According to Miller, Peterson, and Skilba (2002), there are a wide variety of teams in a school. Different from groups that are charged with a task, a team shares a common vision and mission. There is an emphasis on working together as a unit with evenly divided leadership, equal communication, and strong cohesion that result in task accomplishment.

Teams' effectiveness reflects the level of administrative support they receive, the availability of needed resources including sufficient time, the leadership of the team, and the focus, commitment, and motivation of team members. Team composition, size, membership, communication, and support from stakeholder groups (e.g., school and agency staff, community members, parents) also contribute to the team's effectiveness.

Miller et al. (2002) describe two types of teams: academic concerns teams and student support teams.

Academic Concerns Teams

Academic concerns teams deal with academic issues and operate mainly at the school with school staff. This type of team will frequently be driven by school curriculum, projects, and educational initiatives. For example, various grade-level and subject-area teams process information about student achievement and develop academic strategies to help students. Curriculum planning teams focus on how to improve student academic outcomes and achievement. School improvement teams are charged with meeting adequate yearly progress (AYP) and improving school climate. Often, multidisciplinary teams are formed to deal with the need for special education testing and placement. Finally, special education is rooted in a team approach that has as its core an Individualized Education Program (IEP), a legally binding document that spells out exactly what special education services a child will receive and why. It will include the child's classification, placement, services (such as a one-on-one aide) and therapies, academic and behavioral goals, a behavior plan if needed, the percentage of time in regular education, and progress reports from teachers and therapists. The IEP is planned at an IEP team meeting.

Student Support Teams

Student support teams are concerned with student behavioral health and school climate reflective of the system of care available within the school community. Expected members include staff from the school, community-based agencies and programs, government agencies, clergy, community members, and parents. Youth members may also be included on the teams. Student support teams go by many names (**Table 3-1**). Some have a broad focus and the mandate to address the mental health concerns and problems of children and adolescents. Others will focus on a specific concern such as bullying or safety. Regardless of their focus, as a member of a student support team, you can build the school community mental health promoting culture and climate.

Devon Smith, the principal in a suburban school district from the opening scenario, talks a lot about when he had an "aha moment" early in his teaching career related to addressing students' mental health concerns and problems. He was asked to serve on his school's student support team. After training,

TABLE 3-1   Student Support Teams Operating in Schools

❖ *School safety teams* (Stephens, 1995) focus on creating, implementing, practicing, and improving comprehensive safe school plans. School safety team plans generally include local police, fire, emergency management, and school district personnel that plan specific responses for a wide variety of natural disasters as well as safety concerns.

❖ *Crisis response teams* (Poland, 1999) are generally composed of school district personnel who work to prevent, respond to, and recover from acute crisis events, and facilitate the school communities' return to function.

❖ *Student assistance teams* (Fertman, 1999; Fertman, Tarasevich, & Hepler, 2003) are multidisciplinary trained teams that identify students' learning barriers and create plans to address these barriers. When the problem is beyond the scope of the school, teams connect students and families with community resources, and provide support during and after treatment (State of Pennsylvania Department of Education, 2002).

❖ *Positive behavioral support teams* (Sugai & Horner, 2001) are a three-tiered framework for decision making. Tier one teams address universal prevention practices in the school and classroom to prevent problem behavior in the school population. Tier two teams review discipline data by students, date, time, and location and review environmental as well as student-focused issues to create strategies that reduce the frequency of problem behavior in groups of students. Tier three teams address the individual needs of each student and create strategies to help reduce the intensity of problem behavior in that one student.

❖ *Bullying prevention teams* (Olweus, Limber, & Mihalic, 1999) are part of the Olweus Bullying Prevention Program, which is designed to improve peer relations and make schools safer, more positive places for students to learn and develop. A team is convened to address three goals: Reduce existing bullying problems among students, prevent new bullying problems, and achieve better peer relations at school.

❖ *Individual functional behavioral assessment teams* (Chandler, Dahlquist, Repp & Feltz, 1999) work to understand the antecedents, behaviors, and consequences of student behavior and create plans to reduce or extinguish negative behaviors through a series of prevention and positive rewards.

❖ *Safe and responsive schools planning teams* (Skilba, Peterson, Boone, & Fontinini, 2000) assess, plan, and implement efforts to address school violence prevention, discipline reform, and behavior improvement.

❖ *Learning support resource teams* (Adelman and Taylor, 2007) are key infrastructure teams that focus on school system-wide as well as community-wide resource mapping, continuous analysis, planning, development, evaluation, and advocacy for all students and the resources, programs, and systems to address barriers to learning and promote healthy development.

❖ *Coordinated school health teams* (Allensworth & Kolbe, 1987) are coalitions of individuals from within and outside the school community interested in improving the health of youth. The overall goal of this group should be to collaborate to create a healthy school environment where students are fit, healthy, and ready to learn.

he began to see that although he couldn't change a student's overwhelming depression, suicidal thinking, or substance abuse, he could finally talk about it with a multidisciplinary team of professionals and strategize ways to get the student help before a serious crisis emerged. This proactive approach appealed to Devon, and although he didn't see instant progress in these students, he knew that the school was now responding differently and in a more systematic way to their concerns.

Each school and community is unique in what they call their teams and how they staff them. You just cannot do it by yourself. As you work in schools and communities, one of your first tasks is to identify the student support teams working to promote young people's mental health and to join the effort. Being part of the teams, you benefit by being able to work smarter, not harder.

Student Support Teams   In this text, we view all teams, regardless of their name and particular priority population of children and adolescents and their families, as student support teams. For us, student support teams are all teams that build the school community mental health promoting culture and climate. They operate at every level of education (preschool, primary, secondary, postsecondary) and across all types of educational institutions (public, private, proprietary, religious, charter, online).

Entering a school, you will probably find a couple of support teams operating that address a particular student population. At some point in time, school communities reach team overload. There just is not enough time, energy, budget, and staff to have what can seem like endless team meetings. Eventually, teams in schools need to consolidate. It is working smarter in a time of increased economic pressures and decreased resources. You will need to know and honor the history of a school's student support team. This knowledge allows you to build on past successes and initiatives as well as to learn from prior challenges.

Student Support Teams Link to the Classroom   At the center of the student support team's work and the source of its greatest impact is its link to the classroom. Teams have direct contact with and support teachers (as well as other staff who teach). Classrooms reflect the school community's values, belief systems, norms, ideologies, rituals, and traditions, and they are shaped by the school community's political, social, cultural, and economic contexts (e.g., home, neighborhood, city, state, country). At the heart of the classroom are the teacher and students. Classrooms reflect this relationship. They reflect the individual teacher's style, organization, attitudes, morale, curricular and instructional practices, and expectations. Members of student support teams are allies and partners with classroom teams. Not every team member necessarily is involved with the classroom or at every other level in the socio-ecological model (Figure 3-1). Rather, members take on different roles. Depending on the particular team members' level of interests, time, and energy, involvement varies with students, classroom teachers, parents, partnerships, collaborations, and programs and services (primary, secondary, and tertiary). Key is that the team members have access to many points of influence in the lives of young people, one of them (but not the only one) being the classroom.

Partnerships: Schools, Community Organizations, and Many More

Partnerships at the local level reflect the commitment and investment of people and resources for the solution to local needs. Partnerships require specifically defined **roles and responsibilities**, and usually the commitment of resources (fiscal and otherwise) for the implementation of specific interventions, usually delineated in a formal document. Partnerships promoting the mental health of young people commonly occur at the county level, reflecting that many school districts encompass a county. For example, the Philadelphia School District and Philadelphia County are contiguous (geographically the same), as are the Los Angeles Unified School District and Los Angeles County.

Partnerships encompass a broad number of types of relationships. A partnership is "an undertaking to do something together . . . , a relationship that consists of shared and/or compatible objectives and an acknowledged distribution of specific roles and responsibilities among the participants which can be formal, contractual, or voluntary, between two or more parties" (*Partnership Resource Kit*, 1995). **Table 3-2** provides four **partnership models**. Donations and sponsorships are commonly associated with mental health promotion activities (e.g., family meals, supplies, materials, equipment). Cooperation means organizations may work together informally to achieve each organization's day-to-day goals, for example, through support or referrals. It is a relatively superficial level of interaction, as are interagency meetings and informal networking. Coordination is characterized by deliberate joint and often formalized relations for achieving shared or compatible goals. It involves establishing a common understanding of the services committed to and provided by each agency and by determining each agency's accountability and responsibility to specific groups.

The Santa Maria partnership (**Table 3-3**) is an example of a community partnership focused on coordination of programs and services to address the mental health concerns and problems of children and adolescents in the southwest community of Los Angeles, California.

Collaborations Work at the Regional, State, and National Level

By definition, expect collaborations to work on changes in practices and policies across a region, state, or states. State government agencies may align policies and regulations pertaining to the funding of programs and services. With the support of statewide advocacy agencies, legislative change can occur. Collaborations provide access to a broad scope of knowledge and expertise for program and service planning, implementation, and evaluation. Collaborations help schools implement and sustain a complex change process to address mental health issues systemically as part of a positive school climate to promote

TABLE 3-2 Models of Partnerships	
Donation One-time contributions (financial or non-financial) to support a program or service. Donors may expect public recognition or tax credits.	**Examples:** ❖ A restaurant donating food to a community wide violence prevention family activity event. ❖ Donating art supplies to a summer camp for children living in settings with few summer activities and recreational opportunities.
Sponsorship Giving financial support for a set time period or cycle of a program or providing a contribution for supporting a service program. Sponsors may expect public recognition in return for the support.	**Examples:** ❖ Local college provides office space or equipment for a prevention project. ❖ The local library provides a meeting space for family literacy participants.
Cooperation Organizational procedures, policies, and activities remain distinct and separate and are determined without reference to the procedures and policies of the other agencies. The organizations are autonomous, function independently in parallel fashion, and work toward the identified goals of their respective programs. It demonstrates a peaceful co-existence, but is neither genuinely interactive nor interdependent.	**Examples:** ❖ The governor creates by executive order a behavioral health cooperative partnership that will develop a coordinated, efficient state mental health system. This cooperative comprises Department of Corrections, Department of Health, Department of Welfare, Department of Juvenile Corrections, State Department of Education, Office of Drug Policy, and State Mental Health Planning Council.
Coordination A multidisciplinary approach in which professionals from different agencies confer, share decision making, and coordinate their service delivery for the purpose of achieving shared goals and improving interventions. Interagency coordination differs slightly from cooperation, but represents a more sophisticated level of interagency interaction. It is a process of engaging in various efforts that alter or facilitate the relationships of independent organizations, staffs, or resources.	**Examples:** ❖ Public health, social services, mental health, and school staff might hold case conferences to coordinate services for at-risk school children. ❖ At the county level members of school support team coordinators meet with county child and adolescent mental health, substance abuse, juvenile probation, behavioral health providers and managed care organizations to discuss emerging issues and create focused action plans.
Source: Adapted from Skage, S. (1996). *Building strong and effective community partnerships: A manual for family literacy workers.* Alberta: The Family Literacy Action Group of Alberta.	

academic achievement. Collaborations provide a sustainable infrastructure for partnerships and capacity to provide resources and training to school staff and community members.

In states such as California, New York, Texas, New Mexico, and Florida, it is common for the state department of mental health to take the lead in

---

TABLE 3-3   Santa Maria Community Child and Adolescent Mental Health Promotion Partnership

Santa Maria Community Child and Adolescent Mental Health Promotion Partnership partners and interacts with school and community agency staff; community members, including consumers, families, and businesses; and government, religious, and organizational representatives.

Santa Maria Community Child and Adolescent Mental Health Promotion Partnership serves as a forum for the identification and discussion of:

- ❖ Mental health needs of children and adolescents and their families
- ❖ Assets that promote mental health and competent young people
- ❖ Public and private sector policies related to mental health services and programs
- ❖ Education
- ❖ Events on a range of mental health–related topics

The Partnership was originally formed in 2008 to promote mental health in the county and increase the quality and accessibility of mental health services.

Mental health services include prevention and treatment services provided to children and adolescents. Recent initiatives have focused on children with severe and persistent mental illness, emotional disturbances, developmental disabilities, and substance abuse disorders.

The Partnership is open to anyone in the community who is interested. It is made up of a range of community members and representatives of organizations who are concerned about mental health, including those who receive mental health services, their families, and other partners:

Beach Latino Health Alliance	Santa Maria Community Drug and Alcohol Prevention Services
Santa Maria Hospital	Santa Maria Community Mental Health
Blue Cross, Blue Shield, Blue Care Network	Child Health Associates
Santa Maria City Services	Family Services and Advocacy
County Health Department	Community member
Southern Area School District Health Clinic	
Santa Maria Coordinated School Health Director	
County Health Department	
Drug and Alcohol Provider Association	
California State University	
Santa Maria Probation Office	
Community Prevention Partners	
Local Health Agency	
Wave Beach Hospital	
Crisis Team Intervention Services	

forming the collaborations (**Table 3-4**). These will be the most formal interorganizational relationships involving shared **authority** and responsibility for planning, implementation, and evaluation of a joint effort (Hord, 1986). **Regional collaborations** can also bring **autonomous organizations** together (**Table 3-5**) to fulfill a common mission that requires comprehensive planning and communication on many levels using shared rules, norms, and structures to act or decide on issues of concern (i.e., addressing child and adolescent mental health concerns and problems). The risk to each collaborating organization is greater because each member contributes its own resources and reputation (Mattessich, Murray-Close, & Monsey, 2001).

Collaborations require two or more agencies working together in all stages of program or service development; in other words, "joint planning, joint implementation, and joint evaluation" (New England Program in Teacher Education

---

TABLE 3-4   State Department of Mental Health Collaborations
The *New York State Office of Mental Health* collaborates with eight other state departments in The Children's Plan, a program designed to support the social and emotional wellness of children and their families, reduce barriers to care, promote child mental health, and provide resources to families. Services and resources are coordinated from departments including the State Education Department, Council on Children and Families, Office of Children and Family Services, and Office of Alcoholism and Substance Abuse Services. http://ccf.ny.gov/ChildPlan/index.cfm
The *Florida Department of Children and Family Child Mental Health Services'* system of care collaborates with families and caregivers, caseworkers, and community services providers to coordinate services from multiple agencies. These Family Service Planning Teams are headed by one designated individual who coordinates the collaboration of all involved organizations to help ensure that children with mental health and emotional problems are able to remain at home, succeed in school, and thrive in their communities. http://www.dcf.state.fl.us/programs/samh/mentalhealth/CMHsystem.shtml
The *New Mexico Behavioral Health Collaborative* is a collaborative created by the governor and the state legislature in 2004. The legislation allows several state agencies and resources involved in behavioral health prevention, treatment, and recovery to work as one in an effort to improve mental health and substance abuse services in New Mexico. This cabinet-level group represents 15 state agencies and the governor's office. http://www.bhc.state.nm.us
The *Texas Health and Human Services Commission* collaborates with parents, youth, and representatives from state organizations such as the Department of Family and Protective Services, Texas Youth Commission, and Department of Aging and Disability Services to create the Council on Children and Families. The goal of this program is to provide seamless, integrated health, education, justice, and human services to children and youth. http://www.hhsc.state.tx.us/about_hhsc/AdvisoryCommittees/Council.shtml

TABLE 3-5   Regional Collaborations

The *Pennsylvania Network for Student Assistance Services (PNSAS)* is a collaboration of the state departments of education, health, and public welfare for the statewide implementation of the Pennsylvania Student Assistance Program in all public and charter schools. School-based teams in collaboration with county liaisons provide support and referrals to students (and their families) with drug, alcohol, mental health, and other behavioral health issues that impede school success. Health and public welfare collaborate with county agencies to provide liaisons to school-based teams. Other collaborations exist (1) at the state, county, and/or local level to provide statewide training (Commonwealth Approved Training System), research-based practices, and technical assistance; and (2) with other agencies and professional organizations for health promotion activities.

http://www.sap.state.pa.us

The *Anoka County Children and Family Council* encourages the community agencies, individuals, school districts, shelters, police departments, and service providers that affect the lives of children and families in Anoka County, Minnesota, to work together. It does this by coordinating efforts to improve efficiency among agencies and by maintaining various grant programs that foster cooperation. It has developed and funded programs to address the needs of the families in its community, such as mental health, and the needs of newcomers for linguistically and culturally appropriate services. It is the council's position that prevention of crises provides a more stable and safe environment for children.

http://ww2.anokacounty.us/v4_collaboratives/accfc.aspx

The *Alameda County School Health Services Coalition's* mission is to bring education and health partners together to build communities of care that foster the academic success, health, and well-being of children, youth, and families in Alameda County, California. The School-Based Behavioral Health Initiative works with 140 schools across 12 school districts in Alameda County through diverse staffing models. Approximately 49% of these schools have achieved universal access to behavioral health services by weaving together resources and funding streams.

Through collaboration, the coalition members strive to achieve the following:

- ❖ Students are healthy—physically, socially, and emotionally.
- ❖ All students are given the chance and the expectation to succeed academically.
- ❖ Students are caring, competent, engaged, and prepared for college and career.
- ❖ Families actively support their children's education and healthy development.
- ❖ Schools are safe and healthy learning environments.
- ❖ Institutions effectively serve the needs of the whole child.
- ❖ Students live and learn in stable, safe, and supportive communities.

Defined as both a place and a set of partnerships between schools and communities that integrates academics, youth development, family support, health and social services, and community development and engagement, full service community schools improve student learning, build stronger families, and promote healthier communities.

http://acschoolhealth.org/SchoolBasedBehavioralHealthInitiative.htm

[1973] in Hord, 1986). There is a cooperative investment of resources (time, funding, and material), and therefore joint risk taking, sharing of authority, and benefits for all partners (*Partnership Resource Kit*, 1995). Collaboration connotes a more durable and pervasive relationship than a partnership (**Table 3-6**). Collaborations bring previously separated organizations into a new structure with full commitment to a common mission. Such relationships require comprehensive planning and well-defined communication channels operating on many levels. Authority is determined by the collaborative structure. Risk is much greater because each member of the collaboration contributes its own resources. Resources are pooled or jointly secured, and the products are shared.

TABLE 3-6 Elements of a Collaboration Among Organizations	
Vision and relationship	❖ Commitment of the organizations and their leaders to fully support their representatives. ❖ Common new vision and goals are created. ❖ One or more projects are undertaken for longer term results.
Structure, responsibility, and communications	❖ New organizational structure and/or clearly defined and interrelated roles that constitute a formal division of labor are created. ❖ More comprehensive planning is required that includes joint strategies and measuring success in terms of impact on the needs of those served. ❖ Beyond communication roles and channels for interaction, many "levels" of communication are created because clear information is a keystone of success.
Authority and accountability	❖ Authority is determined by the collaboration to balance ownership by the individual organizations with expediency to accomplish purpose. ❖ Leadership is dispersed and control is shared and mutual. ❖ Equal risk is shared by all organizations in the collaboration.
Resources and rewards	❖ Resources are pooled or jointly secured for a longer-term effort that is managed by the collaboration structure. ❖ Organizations share in the products; more is accomplished jointly than could have been individually.

Source: From Mattessich, P.W. & Monsey, B.R. (2000). *Collaboration: What makes it work,* p. 61. Fieldstone Alliance, an imprint of Turner Publishing Company. Use by permission.

Building Effective Student Support Teams

Student support teams that effectively address children and adolescents' mental health concerns don't just happen. They are the result of strategic effort and commitment from many people and organizations. They are all based on the concept of synergy: the sum total of a team's focused efforts will be greater than the effect each would have working alone. Members are interdependent and have shared responsibility for attaining a goal. Members are frank about the struggles and challenges they face. Teams do not always work well. There are conflicts and forces that derail the best intentions and plans. Effective teams share seven qualities (Fertman, 2004; Larson & LaFasto, 1989):

1. *Outcomes-oriented structure:* They establish measures that help to evaluate how they function and review effectiveness periodically through maintenance activities. Regular checkpoints, benchmarks, or short-term goals help to keep an organization moving forward. Likewise, periodic activities that build a common knowledge base or improve functioning further solidify the structure.

2. *Select highly skilled members:* Members are selected because of their diversity and skills. Team, partnership, and collaboration size is optimal. Members are either homogeneous and share similar experiences and views, or heterogeneous with different backgrounds and perspectives. Typically, more diversity produces better results. Sometimes the leader carefully selects members, or administrators choose the best people based on their professional expertise. Sometimes members recommend new members for approval.

3. *Commitment to vision and outcomes:* They are a team, partnership, or collaboration, not a group. Groups generally have finite tasks, and leadership isn't shared. Team, partnership, and collaboration members work with each other, disagree openly, and depend on the other's contributions. They have shared values and a sense of a mission. Usually, the shared vision or mission is reflected in that of the member's organization.

4. *High standards of excellence:* They have group norms, roles, responsibilities, and boundaries. Clearly defined roles and governance structure facilitate understanding of where one fits in. Teams, partnerships, and collaborations develop a culture that norms behaviors among the members.

5. *Leadership:* They have support from the highest levels of the organization. At each level (team, partnership, and collaboration), the leader(s) facilitates the process, making sure that information and knowledge are equally shared while providing for the needs of the members.

6. *Sufficient internal and external resources:* They have an infrastructure of support including clear policies and procedures, time, private space to meet, access to technology and files, and so on.

7. *Use experience and feedback to learn:* Ideally, they meet all goals and complete all assigned tasks, but that is not realistic. Frank discussion of hoped-for outcomes as well as what did or did not happen creates opportunities for learning and creative problem solving.

Team Logistics

Table 3-1 lists nine student support teams that you might find in a school building and throughout school districts. Typically school administrators at the building (e.g., principal, nurse, school counselor) and district level (e.g., assistant superintendent, pupil personnel director, school nursing services director) select team members from among pupil services (counselors), nursing staff, faculty (classroom, specialty), and support staff. Team management, leadership, and resource decisions are part of forming a team. Team leadership may rotate, with team members sharing tasks and responsibilities, or one individual may take the leadership responsibilities. For example, a school counselor, nurse, or assistant principal might be selected to supervise and direct the team. In some districts, the team leadership is from local community agencies. Team leadership responsibilities include information management (collecting student and family information), scheduling meetings, setting meeting agendas, meeting with families and caregivers, working with partnerships and collaborations, and serving on school curriculum review committees. The team leader at district level leads the mental health promoting school community initiative.

Additional team logistics to know are meeting times (e.g., before/after school, during the school day), meeting length (e.g., class period), and frequency (daily, weekly, bi-weekly). Finally, participation on a team (as well as partnership and collaboration) involves time-consuming work and responsibility. As part of any decision to be a team member, an individual needs to consider how his or her participation will fit into an already busy schedule and full list of activities and responsibilities. Participation and leadership roles may be included as part of job descriptions. Work schedules may be structured to reflect the participation (e.g., release time in the form of a reduced teaching or counseling load).

Team Dynamics

Dynamics are the unarticulated forces that exist "under the surface" that influence the way a team acts, interacts, and performs. Many factors affect team dynamics, such as personalities and skills of team members, how the team structures its work, and how team members relate to each other (Levi, L.J. 2010).

Dynamics relate to how team, partnership, and collaboration members accomplish assignments and how they relate to each other during task completion. Dynamics emerge from the way members communicate with each other and how decisions are made. In healthy teams, leadership and power are shared, although all members understand that the team leader may have to be the final arbiter and make the decision.

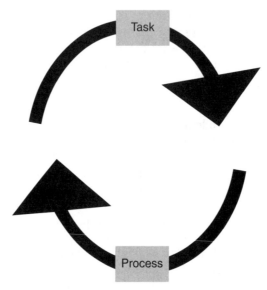

FIGURE 3-2 Team dynamics.

Two dynamics are constantly operating: task and process (**Figure 3-2**). Task dynamics deal with behaviors that accomplish the work that needs to be done and fulfills the goals and responsibilities. Process dynamics involve behaviors that help keep the team, partnership, or collaboration functioning, and foster good relationships. Some people naturally gravitate to task behaviors, whereas others are most comfortable with process behaviors.

Teamwork depends on both task and process behaviors occurring simultaneously. Task-oriented behaviors include initiating discussion, sharing information, clarifying the needs, summarizing dialogue and stating next steps, expediting process, and redirecting tangential discussions. Process-oriented behaviors include observing the actions and behaviors of members, harmonizing during disagreements, encouraging team members to speak, and compromising as necessary.

Managing Conflict

One important aspect of being a member of a team, partnership, or collaboration is **conflict management**. It is difficult to do. Many people are uncomfortable with conflict, but not dealing with it can paralyze your team. Consider five points to help better manage conflict (Segal & Smith, 2011):

1. *A conflict is more than just a disagreement.* It is a situation in which one or both parties perceive a threat (whether or not the threat is real).

2. *Conflicts continue to fester when ignored.* Because conflicts involve perceived threats to our well-being and survival, they stay with us until we face and resolve them.

3. *We respond to conflicts based on our perceptions of the situation, not necessarily an objective review of the facts.* Our perceptions are influenced by our life experiences, culture, values, and beliefs.

4. *Conflicts trigger strong emotions.* If you aren't comfortable with your emotions or able to manage them in times of stress, you won't be able to resolve conflict successfully.

5. *Conflicts are an opportunity for growth.* When you're able to resolve conflict in a relationship, it builds trust. You can feel secure knowing your relationship can survive challenges and disagreements.

The ability to successfully resolve conflict depends on one's ability to manage stress quickly while remaining alert and calm. By staying calm, you can accurately read and interpret verbal and nonverbal communication. You want to control your emotions and behavior. When you're in control of your emotions, you can communicate your needs without threatening, frightening, or punishing others. Pay attention to the feelings being expressed as well as the spoken words of others. Finally, be aware and respectful of differences. By avoiding disrespectful words and actions, you can resolve the problem faster.

Managing and resolving conflict requires the ability to quickly reduce stress and bring your emotions into balance. You can ensure that the process is as positive as possible by sticking to the following conflict resolution guidelines:

❖ *Listen for what is felt as well as said.* When we listen we connect more deeply to our own needs and emotions, and to those of other people. Listening in this way also strengthens us, informs us, and makes it easier for others to hear us.

❖ *Make conflict resolution the priority rather than winning or "being right."* Maintaining and strengthening the relationship, rather than "winning" the argument, should always be your first priority. Be respectful of the other person and his or her viewpoint.

❖ *Focus on the present.* If you're holding onto old hurts and resentments, your ability to see the reality of the current situation will be impaired. Rather than looking to the past and assigning blame, focus on what you can do in the here-and-now to solve the problem.

❖ *Pick your battles.* Conflicts can be draining, so it is important to consider whether the issue is really worthy of your time and energy. Maybe you don't want to surrender a parking space if you've been circling for 15 minutes. But if there are dozens of spots, arguing over a single space isn't worth it.

❖ *Be willing to forgive.* Resolving conflict is impossible if you're unwilling or unable to forgive. Resolution lies in releasing the urge to punish, which can never compensate for our losses and only adds to our injury by further depleting and draining our lives.

❖ *Know when to let something go.* If you can't come to an agreement, agree to disagree. It takes two people to keep an argument going. If a conflict is going nowhere, you can choose to disengage and move on.

Effective Partnerships and Collaborations That Work

Effective partnerships and collaborations consistently talk about and revisit six issues related to how the organizations interact and relate to each other (Fertman, 1992).

1. *Clear goals and realistic expectations:* Talk about what goals and expectations are for individuals and organizations. Be clear about why organizations are part of the partnership and collaboration. Talk about what each thinks they can contribute. Be specific about what problems, concerns, or issues are to be addressed. Define the priority population (i.e., primary, secondary, tertiary prevention). Gather available data for decision making and determining tasks. Remember to be realistic and respectful of demands made on everyone's time.

2. *Roles:* Overall, roles for effort need to be defined. Talk about what the structure will look like. How will leadership be shared? Define roles for each person and organization. Write down individual tasks and responsibilities. Be careful not to let one organization or individual take on the majority of tasks. Talk frankly about how to obtain the necessary information, and how to make decisions about what strategies and services are used. All members at the table must have an equal voice. Discuss the use of members' skills in different situations. Be aware that people and roles change with time and with each effort.

3. *Balance:* Working together implies that everyone contributes something. Participation does not always mean providing direct services. Often, what are needed are in-kind contributions, technical expertise, and access to desired resources and information. A second element of balance is efficient use of existing resources. Discuss how existing resources are being used to address the problem and whether there are any deficiencies in those resources. Also look for ways resources might overlap.

4. *Equality:* In the beginning stages of development, it is normal to have discussions full of minor conflicts as members begin to know and trust each other. Respect each other and work toward the best interests of the student, family, community, and school. No single job or task should overshadow the work of others or the goal that brought the different parties together. Attempts to work outside the process often create obstacles to future collaboration. Communication between and among members is very important and may avoid someone working outside the process simply because he or she "didn't know" or "wasn't told."

5. *Trust:* Establish ground rules for the process. Be candid about the risks and mutual benefits of working together. All organizations are justifiably concerned about possible damage to their reputations. Resolve conflicts that may arise among members. A mutual understanding of the risks as well as the benefits may help reduce some of the anxiety.

6. *Coordination:* To ensure plans progress as designed and goals are accomplished, a system must be established to coordinate the efforts. Once the system is in place, the challenge is to make it operational and keep it going. Helpful here is that the type of governance structure be defined and roles and duties assigned. Members need information and need to know who to go to for answers.

Summary

A team is a group of interdependent individuals who share responsibility for specific outcomes for their organization (i.e., school). A partnership is a group of interdependent local organizations represented by individuals who share responsibility for specific outcomes across organizations at the local level. Collaborations are groups of interdependent organizations represented by individuals who share responsibility for specific outcomes across a region or state(s) working at the governmental and public policy level. The minimum defining features of teams, partnerships, and collaborations are shared responsibility and interdependence. Teams, partnerships, and collaborations take a socio-ecological approach to promoting child and adolescent mental health.

Student support teams in schools address mental health concerns and problems and go by many names. Partnerships at the local level reflect the commitment and investment of people and resources for the solution of local needs. Partnerships promoting the mental health of young people commonly occur at the county level, reflecting that many school districts encompass a county. Collaborations work on changes in practices and policies across a region, state, or states. State government agencies may align policies and regulations pertaining to the funding of programs and services. With the support of statewide advocacy agencies, legislative change can occur. Collaborations provide access to a broad scope of knowledge and expertise for program and service planning, implementation, and evaluation.

Student support teams, partnerships, and collaborations that effectively address children's mental health concerns don't just happen. They are the result of strategic effort and commitment from many people and organizations. They are all based on the concept of synergy: the sum total of a team's, partnership's, and collaboration's focused efforts will be greater than the effect individuals would have working alone.

For Practice and Discussion

1. Most people were a member of at least a few different teams while growing up (e.g., community sports teams, summer camp teams, school academic teams, teams for class projects, high school and college sport teams). From your experience, what are positives and negatives of being on a team? How were the team members selected? Who were the leaders? What were the team's goals (what did it accomplish)? What was your role on the team?

TABLE 3-7 Team Member Self-Assessment					
Skills and Traits	Beginning 1	Developing 2	Accomplished 3	Exemplary 4	Score
Make Contributions					
Research and gather information	Do not collect any information that relates to the concern.	Collect very little information— some relates to the concern.	Collect some basic information—most relates to the concern.	Collect a great deal of information— all relates to the concern.	
Share information	Do not relay any information to teammates.	Relay very little information— some relates to the concern.	Relay some basic information—most relates to the concern.	Relay a great deal of information— all relates to the concern.	
Respect confidentiality	Not able to differentiate confidential information.	Able to differentiate confidential information but shares no information outside of team.	Able to differentiate confidential information from academic or behavioral strategies and sometimes generate appropriate action plans.	Grasp appropriate use of information without compromising confidentiality.	
Punctuality	Do not complete assigned tasks.	Complete tasks late.	Complete most tasks on time.	Always complete tasks on time.	
Take Initiative					
Fulfill responsibilities	Do not perform any duties of assigned team role.	Perform very few duties of assigned team role.	Perform nearly all duties of assigned team role.	Perform all duties of assigned team role.	
Participate appropriately	Do not speak during the team meeting.	Either give too little information or information that is irrelevant to concern.	Offer some information—most is relevant.	Offer a fair amount of important information— all is relevant.	

Complete assigned tasks	Always rely on others to do the work.	Rarely do the assigned work—often need reminding.	Usually do the assigned work—rarely need reminding.	Always do the assigned work without having to be reminded.	
Respect Opinions					
Listen to other teammates	Always talking—never allow anyone else to speak.	Usually doing most of the talking—rarely allow others to speak.	Listen, but sometimes talk too much.	Listen and speak a fair amount.	
Cooperate with teammates	Usually argue with teammates.	Sometimes argue.	Rarely argue.	Never argue with teammates.	
Utilize decision-making process	Usually want to have things own way.	Often side with friends instead of considering all views.	Usually consider all views.	Always help team to reach a fair decision.	

Select a team where you were a member and use **Table 3-7** to assess your personal team member skills. Compare and contrast your scores with your classmates'.

2. Tour a local school. During the tour, ask about the different school and community teams. Identify the purpose and membership of the teams. Collect information about team activities, programs, and services.

3. Do a Web search for mental health partnerships that serve children and adolescents in the local county. From the following list, identify the current members and their organizations. What are two other organizations that might strengthen and expand current services and programs?

   a. *Local and state public health officials and agencies,* such as boards of health, the state or local health department, human service agencies, environmental inspectors and agencies, workplace health and safety inspectors and agencies, and departments of public works

   b. *Health practitioners, administrators, and others who are part of the local public health system,* such as physicians, nurses, alternative medicine practitioners, hospital and clinic directors and administrators, mental health professionals, physical and massage therapists, and athletic trainers

   c. *First responders,* such as EMTs, paramedics, police, and firefighters

    d. *Local and state elected and appointed officials,* such as mayors, city or town council members, planners, county officials, and state/provincial or federal legislators

    e. *Human service organizations,* such as social service agencies, area agencies on aging, community health centers, senior meals and transportation services, food pantries and soup kitchens, Jewish Family Service, Catholic Charities, Diakon Lutheran Social Ministries, refugee and immigrant mutual aid organizations, support groups, and others

    f. *Community organizations,* such as service clubs (e.g., Lions, Rotary), the Chamber of Commerce, youth organizations, athletic clubs, or the YMCA

    g. *Schools,* including public schools, local colleges and universities, and other educational institutions

    h. *Faith communities,* such as Church World Services, ministeriums, community ministries for the homeless

    i. *Businesses,* such as grocery stores, pizza parlors, restaurants, fast food providers, office supply vendors, hardware and paint suppliers, florists, car washes, car dealerships

    j. *Community members*—people representing the diversity of ages and incomes, and the racial/ethnic mix in the community

4. The Philadelphia, Miami–Dade, and Los Angeles Unified School Districts are large school districts, contiguous with their counties (Philadelphia, Miami, and Los Angeles, respectively). Explore their Web sites to find and report on partnerships with the county departments of human services, family and children, health, and public safety. Look for partnerships that include parents, community members, community agencies, foundations, community colleges, universities, and business partners. Contact one of the partnership members and ask why they decided to form the partnership.

5. Do a Web search of your state government to identify collaborations between different state agencies and departments that address mental health services and programs for children and adolescents. Use the search terms *child adolescent mental health programs; drug and alcohol services; collaborations;* and *legislation.* Identify two and contact them for further information. Ask if you may attend their next meeting. Note the dynamics in action. Was it a productive meeting? Share the experience with the rest of the class.

6. The school administration is looking at the purpose and functions of existing teams and wondering about integrating several of them. Review Table 3-1 and select five teams. In your opinion, which teams have the same or similar functions? Should they be combined? Which teams should stand alone? Why or why not?

Key Terms

References

Adelman, H.S. & Taylor, L. (2007). Best practices in the use of learning support resource teams to enhance learning supports. In A. Thomas & J. Grimes (Eds.), *Best practices in school psychology V (Chapter 105 Vol 5, pp 1–17)*. Wakefield, UK: National Association of School Psychologists.

Allensworth D. D. & Kolbe L.J. (1987). The comprehensive school health program: Exploring an expanded concept. *Journal of School Health*, 57(10): 409–412.

Chandler, L.K., Dahlquist, C.M., Repp, A., & Feltz, C. (1999). The effects of team-based functional assessment on the behavior of students in classroom settings. *Exceptional Children*, 66(1): 101–121.

Fertman, C. (1992). Establishing a school–community agency collaboration. *NASSP Practitioner*, 19(1): 1–8.

Fertman, C. (1999). Power tools: Develop your SAP by using research and evaluation. *Student Assistance Journal*, 11(4): 22–27.

Fertman, C. (2004). Student assistance program practitioners talk about how to link students to behavioral health care. *Report on Emotional and Behavioral Disorders in Youth*, 4(4): 87–92.

Fertman, C., Tarasevich, S., & Hepler, N. (2003). *Retrospective analysis of the Pennsylvania student assistance program outcome data: Implications for practice and research*. Washington, DC: Center for Substance Abuse and Prevention.

Hord, S.M. (1986). A synthesis of research on organizational collaboration. *Educational Leadership*, 43(5): 22–26.

Larson, C.E., & LaFasto, F.M.J. (1989). *Teamwork: What must go right, what can go wrong*. Newberry Park, CA: Sage Publications, Inc.

Levi, L.J. (2010). *Group dynamics for teams*. Thousand Oaks, CA: Sage Publications, Inc.

Mattessich, P.W., & Monsey, B.R. (1993). *Collaboration: What makes it work*. St. Paul, MN: Amherst H. Wilder Foundation.

Mattessich, P., Murray-Close, M., & Monsey, B. (2001). *Collaboration: What makes it work* (2nd ed.). St. Paul, MN: Wilder.

Miller, C., Peterson, R., & Skilba, R. (2002). *Factors influencing the effectiveness of school-based behavior teams: An exploratory examination*. Lincoln, NE: Safe and Responsive Schools Project, University of Nebraska-Lincoln. Retrieved from http://www.unl.edu/srs/pdfs/teampaper.pdf

Olweus, D., Limber, S., & Mihalic, S. (1999). *Blueprints for violence prevention: Book nine: Bullying prevention program*. Boulder, CO: Center for the Study and Prevention of Violence.

Partnership resource kit. (1995). Ottawa: Government of Canada, Canadian Heritage.

Poland, S.M.J. (1999). *Coping with crisis: Lessons learned—A resource for schools, parents, and communities.* Longmont, CO: Sopris West.

Segal, J., & Smith, M. (2011). Conflict resolution skills. Retrieved from http://helpguide.org /mental/eq8_conflict_resolution.htm

Skilba, R., Peterson, R., Boone, K, & Fontinini, A. (2000). Preventing school violence: A practical guide to comprehensive planning. *Reaching Today's Youth,* 5(1): 58–62.

State of Pennsylvania Department of Education. (2002). Basic education circular 24 P.S. § 15-1547. Retrieved from http://www.education.state.pa.us/portal/server.pt/gateway/PTA RGS_6_2_50809_7503_507341_43/

Stephens, R.D. (1995). *Safe schools: A handbook for violence prevention.* Bloomington, IN: National Educational Service.

Sugai, G., & Horner, R. (2001). *School climate and discipline: Going to scale* (framing paper for the national summit on shared implementation of IDEA), 1–8. Eugene, OR: Center on Positive Behavioral Interventions and Supports, University of Oregon.

POLICY AND PROCEDURES

In this chapter, we will:

✦ Summarize the importance of school district mental health policies and procedures

✦ Discuss actions to support and create effective school district policies

✦ Identify tools to create effective policies and procedures

✦ Describe legal issues in mental health policies and procedures

✦ Explain codes of ethics, the guiding principles of professional activities

Scenarios

It had been 10 years since the last revision of the school district's policies and procedures, and the district knew that they were outdated. The school community had changed drastically in the last decade, and the policies and procedures no longer reflected the growing problems and needs of the community. Last year, the district completed a needs assessment that monitors health-risk behaviors that contribute to youth mental health concerns and problems: behaviors that contribute to unintentional injuries and violence, tobacco use, alcohol and other drug use, sexual risk behaviors, unhealthy dietary behaviors, and physical inactivity. From the assessment, they knew that they must update the district's suicide intervention and other mental health procedures, as well as its tobacco, bullying, and alcohol/drug policies. It had to create new procedures and consequences for weapons and violence violations. Recently students were bringing to school a new category of beverages—energy drinks and herb concoctions; although legal, their proliferation was a concern that perhaps needed to be addressed as part of the revised policies. I had to make the case for a committee to *be formed that included a school board member, the pupil services coordinator, a principal from each school, district drug and alcohol prevention team coordinators, parents, students, and community liaisons. Community resources and social support services had to be identified. The roles and responsibilities of central administration, each school's principals, student support team, and faculty needed to be identified to ensure the safety and welfare of the district's student body. I wanted to stress to the school board and the entire community that a major motivator for these revisions was prevention of mental, emotional, and behavioral problems. I explained that sound policy and procedures were designed to create a safe and secure school climate where life skills were taught, practiced, and reinforced. I knew from experience that attention to students' social and emotional learning and school climate increased academic achievement.*

Source: Kaye Simon, an assistant superintendent of a large suburban school district in Texas

As a community agency staff member who works in schools, I want to know as much as possible about the district policies and procedures. I never want to be caught in a situation where I am talking with a student in the counseling office, leading a small group, or presenting in a classroom, and something happens. It does not need to be anything major like a shooting or fire. I am always most concerned with student behavior— talking back, crying, bullying, and being oppositional. I want to know who to turn to, who to tell, and if I need to make a report. Also, as an agency person, I want my agency supervisor to do his or her best to prepare me and support me in a school district. I want them to know all the key people. I want to feel that he or she has my back if something does go wrong. I am not in the district alone. I am representing our agency; I am part of the team and larger partnership with the school district. I am also part of the system of care that exists in the community. Frequently I am the interface between systems. For me, the policies and procedures define just how much the school district (as well as community partner agencies and organizations) can and will do to help children and adolescents. Knowing school district policies and procedures makes me feel included, that I am not an outsider but part of the community with rights and responsibilities.

Source: Andres Reyes, a staff member of a community agency that serves the large suburban school district in Texas

The Importance of School District Mental Health Policies and Procedures

School district **policy** reflects the goals and ethos of the school community. It is part of the school district's overall strategy to promote student health and welfare, and is closely linked to the management of student behavior. The policies and **procedures** set the boundaries for how schools and communities operate and interact (**Figure 4-1**). They help everyone be clear about who is responsible and accountable for making sure schools and communities are working together to address young people's mental health concerns and problems.

School district mental health policy includes individual policies related to suicide, threats, harassment, crisis response, tobacco, and substance abuse. In this chapter, the term *behavioral health policies* will often be interchanged with *mental health policies,* reflecting the broad spectrum of social, psychological, psychiatric, substance abuse, and emotional concerns encompassed by the policies.

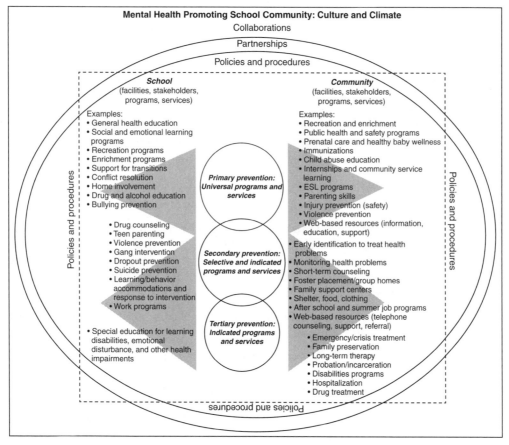

FIGURE 4-1   Mental health promoting school community framework.
Source: Adapted from Center for Mental Health in Schools at UCLA. (n.d.). School–community partnerships: A guide. UCLA Department of Psychology School Mental Health Project. Retrieved from http://www.smhp.psych.ucla.edu

The policy is school district board approved and enforced and reflects the school district's response to legal requirements (i.e., laws) and legislation. Every policy should have **procedural guidelines**, which are not necessarily board approved but describe a best practice or response to behavioral indicators of impairment, such as procedures for emergency crisis response to drug overdose, weapon possession, drug possession and distribution, and suicidal ideation.

Advantages of Effective School District Mental Health Policy

Effective policies are developed using a broad and thorough consultation process. They are based on laws that authorize the school board to take action. The policies must reflect good prevention science. In Kaye Simon's school district, mentioned in the opening scenario, everyone knew the need existed to revise the policies and procedures. However, she was charged with making the case for the revision. She argued that the district plays a pivotal role in the prevention of alcohol, tobacco, and other drug use, as well as mental health–related problems such as bullying, harassment, suicide, and the like, and that the policies and procedures would create an environment that fosters safety and success for all students by providing predictable structures and routines in the classroom, in the cafeteria, in the gym, on buses, at school activities (e.g., sports events, clubs, field trips), and during transitions. Finally, that by working as a committee, parents and the larger community would be engaged and informed of available mental health services and programs.

For the board and larger community, she listed eight advantages of the revised policies and procedures. The revised policies and procedures would:

1. Ensure compliance with current laws and regulations. Review of policies by the district solicitor prior to adoption will provide the authority for the policies and procedures developed as well as standardize and document the school community's agreed position on, and accepted procedure for, dealing with behavioral health–related incidents, concerns, and problems.

2. Demonstrate the responsiveness of the school community to issues of school and community concern.

3. Provide a planned and coordinated response to mental health concerns and problems (e.g., suicide, threats, harassment, crisis response, tobacco, and substance abuse). This ensures the efficient use of school community resources and promotes a better outcome for all parties involved. It should define confidentiality and provide for access to counseling and referral services where necessary.

4. Create and support a mental health promoting school district and building climate with set guidelines for students, staff, and visitors on what are acceptable and unacceptable behaviors on school premises.

5. Provide a step-by-step outline of actions to take when an incident occurs and incorporate appropriate and consistent disciplinary measures, if necessary. It would stipulate when parents and police are to be notified.

6. Clarify roles, rights, and responsibilities of all school community members in relation to mental health concerns and problems (e.g., suicide, threats, harassment, crisis response, tobacco, and substance abuse).

7. Ensure that school staff are not placed at risk by their actions through a clear statement of the school's legal and procedural responsibilities.

8. Clarify roles, rights, and responsibilities of all school staff in relation to mental health concerns and problems (e.g., suicide, threats, harassment, crisis response, tobacco, and substance abuse).

Actions that Support and Create Effective School District Policy

When working with a school district, you want to know what is included in its policies and procedures. You can find this information by asking two sets of questions. The first set of questions focuses on the scope of the policies (**Table 4-1**). The first question in this first set is critical: What are the mental health issues and concerns addressed? This question sets the agenda for the potential work of creating and revising school policies and procedures. You can expect substance use, suicide, harassment, bullying, and violent behavior will be addressed in the majority of school policies. Beyond those, you will encounter differences among districts; for example, you might expect differences related to sexual behavior, disordered eating, and gender identity.

The second set of questions helps you to know specific school district mental health procedures (**Table 4-2**). Within the umbrella of mental health policy, school districts have policy related to specific issues such as suspected use, abuse, and/or possession of a controlled or harmful substance. The need for such specificity was well stated by Andres Reyes in the opening scenario, wanting to know what actions he was required to take to respond to specific incidents. For example, a colleague walks into the boys' bathroom and immediately is hit in the face with the smell of marijuana and smoke coming from a stall. His first thought might be to turn around and walk back out the bathroom door; however, Andres knows that, according to the school district policies and procedures, the staff member would need to take two steps immediately. First, as a professional staff member working in a school building, he needs to inform his supervisor of his reasonable suspicion as well as the identity of the youth involved. Second, the staff member needs to follow the board-approved procedure for dealing with this issue, as detailed in school policy. Smoking marijuana is a district drug policy violation with both disciplinary consequences and mental health concerns.

TABLE 4-1   Questions to Determine the Scope of a District's Mental Health Policies

1. What are the mental health issues and concerns addressed?
2. How were staff, students, and parents involved in the development of the policies?
3. Do policies address problem prevention (before behaviors occur) and intervention (after behaviors occur)?
4. Because role models have a significant impact on students' behavior, do policies apply equally to school and community agency staff and students?
5. Do policies apply to school visitors?
6. Are staff members offered training to implement the policies? If so, when and how does it happen?
7. How are students, community members, and parents and caregivers informed about the policies?
8. How and when are the policies reviewed, and who will be responsible for this?
9. Have policies been reviewed by the district solicitor for legality and authority?

TABLE 4-2   Questions to Know About Specific District Mental Health Procedures

1. What support and counseling services will be made available to students experiencing the concern or problem, such as screening and mental health assessment?
2. What are the disciplinary consequences when a behavior violates the policy?
3. Does the procedure protect the health, safety, welfare, and confidentiality of the students while being consistent with the school's operation and ethos?
4. When and how will parents be informed about incidents, and who will be responsible for contacting them?
5. How are community organizations involved (roles) in implementing the procedure?
6. What are the referral and communication processes, and who will coordinate referrals to outside agencies?
7. Are the police and justice system involvement desired or required? What procedures are required for interviews and/or arrests of students or staff?

Structure of District Mental Health Policy

The following outline reflects successfully developed and implemented school mental health policies. Using the outline to review policies ensures that the policies are complete.

1. *Rationale:* The rationale may include
   ◆ The board's support of the aims of the policy
   ◆ Definitions of important terms in the policy

♦ A brief statement about the importance of the policy in relation to a comprehensive approach to mental health promotion in the school community
♦ A list of groups in the school community to which the policy applies
♦ A short description of how the policy has been developed
♦ A proposed date for the review of the policy

2. *Definitions:* These include important terms such as *tobacco, controlled substances, suicidal ideation, suicidal gesture,* and *tragic death.*

3. *Authority:* Legal citations that give the board authority to take action.

4. *Delegation of responsibility for prevention of unsafe and unlawful behavior:* A comprehensive approach to mental health promotion includes provision for

♦ Notification of all stakeholders by superintendent or designee and the development of procedures to implement policy
♦ Clearly stated school rules that define acceptable behavior for the total school community

5. *Procedural guidelines that outline the actions that are taken by staff once a policy is violated:* The procedures may or may not be board approved. Remember, good policies and procedures foster a safe climate for learning. Effective policies and procedures address prevention by

♦ Linking the school mental health policy with the goals and ethos of the school community and the overarching outcomes for the coordinated school health program
♦ Ensuring that mental health promotion practices (e.g., education, programs, and services) are allocated curriculum time and taught within a sequential, integrated K–12 program
♦ Ensuring that health and mental health promotion practices are adequately resourced, including the provision of regular, quality professional development for staff
♦ Regularly informing the school community of the aims of mental health promotion practices and the procedures for dealing with mental health concerns and problems
♦ Identifying roles and responsibilities of specific personnel in implementing, monitoring, and evaluating mental health promotion practices and procedures for dealing with mental health concerns and problems
♦ Establishing a schedule for the regular review of school mental health policy

6. *Intervention:* It is likely that, at some time, mental health concerns and problem incidents will occur on school premises or involve members of the school community and will require a response from the school. A school with a comprehensive mental health policy that addresses both intervention and

prevention will be well placed to respond to such incidents in a planned and coordinated manner. The intervention section of a school mental health policy may include

◆ Examples of behaviors that are unacceptable in the school community
◆ Details of assistance that will be provided for students and/or staff with mental health concerns and problems
◆ Details of assistance that will be offered to at-risk students and/or staff
◆ Procedures for dealing with mental health concerns, problems, or incidents

The school community requires specific action plans to address the immediate and long-term consequences of every mental health concern, problem, or incident. These plans should coordinate school and community resources. The safety and well-being of those involved is of the highest priority in the development of such plans. Other factors to consider are

◆ The roles and responsibilities of key personnel nominated in the plan; for example, the principal, deputy/assistant principal, school health nurse, and/or police officer
◆ The location of the incident; for example, on school premises or at an off-campus school function
◆ The rights and responsibilities of those involved in relation to being searched or questioned

7. *Identification of mental health concerns and problems:* Identifying mental health concerns and problems within school communities relies on the development of effective channels of communication. Timing and appropriateness need to be considered carefully, because if handled incorrectly they may impede further attempts to communicate about the issue.

Trying to establish a checklist of behaviors that may be consistent with mental health concerns and problems can be problematic, because changes in behaviors in students may be due to a range of causes. Furthermore, mental health concerns and problems of caregivers may also cause problems for young people. These problems, which include neglect, abuse, and exposure to undue risk, may go undetected if invasive and unreliable methods of identification are used. Although the identification of mental health concerns and problems can be difficult, staff should be aware that instances might arise in which such concerns and problems are revealed. These may include

◆ Students reporting or disclosing during health, mental health education, religious education, or other classes, or in the context of pastoral care programs
◆ The exploration of another issue; for example, truancy, declining academic performance, and sudden and uncharacteristic behavioral changes
◆ Peer reporting

- ◆ Parental or community concern; for example, complaints and police involvement
- ◆ The occurrence of a mental health or other related incident
- ◆ The presentation of physical symptoms, such as signs of intoxication

Schools should plan how most appropriately to deal with mental health concerns and problems, and the policy must provide staff with the necessary contacts so those involved can be adequately supported. Schools need to ensure that consistent messages are conveyed at all times, and this section of a school mental health policy should outline procedures for monitoring students who have, or may be at risk of, mental health concerns and problems.

8. *Assistance and referral:* Many schools are well placed to screen students and provide counseling in response to mental health concerns and problems; however, in some cases, more support will be needed than the school can provide. School staff should be alert to the need to seek assistance and, where necessary, refer cases to mental health counselors in the community. A list of appropriate community referral agencies can be included in this section.

Tools to Create Effective Policies and Procedures

School district mental health policy is representative of the beliefs and values of the school community and includes individual policies related to suicide, threats, harassment, crisis response, tobacco, and substance abuse. It is essential that all members of the school community have the opportunity to contribute to its development. The final document is more likely to be accepted and implemented effectively if the school community has been widely involved in its development, agrees with its content, and understands its purpose. A common practice is a school community–wide needs assessment of current community mental health concerns and problems among young people and the resources (e.g., agencies, programs, and services) that address these needs. In many communities, the school community partnership or the school district coordinated school health program staff develops and implements the needs assessment.

An accurate assessment views the community from multiple perspectives. It recognizes cultural, linguistic, ethnic, and economic diversity, as well as special needs. Information from diverse stakeholders including families, community members, and agency staff produces a more complete picture of the community. People's views vary regarding programs, agencies, services, and the relationships between agency staff and community members. People may also have different views on the issues strategies should address.

As part of a school **community assessment**, information is collected on youth health-risk and protective behaviors and on school community capacity. The information provides the foundation for the school policies and procedures. It also tells what is needed as well as the support, resources, and guidance that are available within any particular organization and system.

Tools to Collect Information on Youth Health-Risk and Protective Behaviors

The first type of information collected is on risk and protective factors (**Table 4-3**). **Risk factors** are any factors associated with the increased likelihood of a behavior that usually has negative consequences. Risk factors are characteristics of individuals, their family, school, and community environments that are associated with increases in alcohol and other drug use, delinquency, teen pregnancy, school dropout, and violence. Factors associated with reduced potential for mental health concerns and problems are called **protective factors**. Protective factors encompass family, social, psychological, and behavioral characteristics that can provide a buffer for the children and youth. These factors mitigate the effects of risk factors that are present in the child or youth's environment, but do not do so equally for all children. The risk and protective factors can be both internal and external. Internal factors are those within the child or individual; external factors are forces and experiences in the environment of the individual. Examples of internal factors include child temperament or social and emotional skill development; family conflict or domestic violence; and positive school climate. External factors include traumatic events, bullying, socioeconomic disadvantage, and family instability or breakup.

Most needs assessments begin by assembling and comparing information on risks and protective factors of youth already collected by various individual agencies, government offices, and school districts. Three widely used needs assessment tools for collecting information on youth risks behaviors are discussed in the following sections: the Youth Risk Behavior Surveillance System from the Centers for Disease Control and Prevention (CDC), Child and Adolescent Needs and Strengths (CANS), and Communities That Care Survey.

Youth Risk Behavior Surveillance System (YRBSS)   The **Youth Risk Behavior Surveillance System** (**YRBSS;** www.cdc.gov/HealthyYouth/yrbs/index.htm) was developed in 1990 to monitor priority health risk behaviors that contribute markedly to the leading causes of death, disability, and social problems among youth and adults in the United States. These behaviors, often established during childhood and early adolescence, include

- ❖ Tobacco use
- ❖ Unhealthy dietary behaviors
- ❖ Inadequate physical activity
- ❖ Alcohol and other drug use
- ❖ Sexual behaviors that contribute to unintended pregnancy and sexually transmitted diseases, including human immunodeficiency virus (HIV) infection
- ❖ Behaviors that contribute to unintentional injuries and violence.

In addition, the YRBSS monitors the prevalence of obesity and asthma.

The YRBSS includes national, state, territorial, tribal, and local school-based surveys of representative samples of ninth- through twelfth-grade students.

TABLE 4-3 Risk and Protective Factors Framework		
Domain	**Risk Factors**	**Protective Factors**
Child	Complications during birth and early infancy Difficult temperament (overly shy or aggressive) Poor social and emotional skills Pessimistic outlook on life Poor/inconsistent bonding with parents and caregivers	Prenatal and postnatal care Easy temperament Social and emotional skills Optimistic outlook on life Good attachment to parents or caregivers
Family	Family instability or breakup Overly harsh or inconsistent discipline style Parent/caregiver or sibling with serious illness, mental illness or substance abuse, or disability	Family harmony and stability Consistent (clear expectations, firm boundaries and limits) authoritative discipline style Support outside of the family: grandparents, aunts/uncles, churches, community organizations
School	Unsafe school climate Peer rejection and/or bullying Distrust and friction between family and school Persistent academic failure Poor attendance Few opportunities to contribute to the school community or develop interests outside of classroom	Positive school climate Anti-bullying and social-emotional learning Sense of belonging and connectedness between family and school Academic achievement Connection with at least one caring adult in school Opportunity for participation in a range of activities
Life events	Frequent, difficult school transitions Death of a family member Exposure to traumatic event(s) Experience of physical or sexual abuse	Transitional supports and plans Involvement with a caring adult Support available at critical times
Society	Discrimination Isolation Lack of access to support services Socioeconomic disadvantage High levels of neighborhood violence	Strong cultural identity and pride Participation in community networks Access to support services Economic security Community leadership and collaboration

Sources: Adapted from Arthur, M.W., Hawkins, J.D., Pollard, J.A., Catalano, R.F., & Baglioni, A.J. (2002). Measuring risk and protective factors for substance use, delinquency, and other adolescent problem behaviors: The communities that care youth survey. *Evaluation Review*, 26: 575–601; Hawkins, J.D., Catalano, R.F., & Miller, J.Y. (1992). Risk and protective factors for alcohol and other drug problems in adolescence and early adulthood: Implications for substance abuse prevention. *Psychological Bulletin*, 112: 64–105; and New Mexico Human Services Department. (2012). Risk and protective factor framework. Retrieved from http://www.hsd.state.nm.us/Synar/pdf/Hawkins%20and%20Catalano%20Risk%20and%20Protective%20Factor%20Framework.pdf

These surveys are conducted every 2 years, usually during the spring semester. The national survey, conducted by the CDC, provides data representative of ninth- through twelfth-grade students in public and private schools in the United States. The state, territorial, tribal, and local surveys, conducted by local, county, and state departments of health and education, provide data representative of public high school students in each jurisdiction.

Child and Adolescent Needs and Strengths (CANS)   According to the Child and Adolescent Needs and Strengths Executive Summary,

> The **Child and Adolescent Needs and Strengths** (**CANS;** www.praedfoundation
> .org/About%20the%20CANS.html) is a multi-purpose tool developed for chil-
> dren's services to support decision making, including level of care and service
> planning, to facilitate quality improvement initiatives, and to allow for the
> monitoring of outcomes of services. Versions of the CANS are currently used in
> 25 states in child welfare, mental health, juvenile justice, and early intervention
> applications. A comprehensive, multi-system version exists as well.
> The CANS was developed from a communication perspective so as to facilitate
> the linkage between the assessment process and the design of individualized
> service plans including the application of evidence-based practices. The CANS
> is easy to learn and is well-liked by parents, providers, and other partners in the
> services system because it is easy to understand and does not necessarily require
> scoring in order to be meaningful to an individual child and family. The way the
> CANS works is that each item suggests different pathways for service planning.
> There are four levels of each item with anchored definitions; however, these
> definitions are designed to translate into action levels (separate for needs and
> strengths).

Communities That Care (CTC)   A coalition-based community prevention operating system, **Communities That Care** (**CTC**) uses a public health approach to prevent youth problem behaviors including underage drinking, tobacco use, violence, delinquency, school dropout, and substance abuse. Ultimately, the beneficiaries of CTC are children and adolescents in the community. CTC helps decision makers in the community select and implement effective prevention policies, procedures, and programs to address the most pressing risks facing their youth. CTC guides the community coalition through an assessment and prioritization process that identifies the risk and protective factors most in need of attention, and links those priorities to prevention programs that are proven to work in addressing them.

CTC activities are planned and carried out by the CTC Community Board, a prevention coalition of community stakeholders who work together to promote positive youth outcomes. Board members participate in a series of six CTC training workshops in which they build their coalition and learn the skills needed to install the CTC system. The CTC is installed in a community through a five-phase process implemented over a 1- to 2-year period.

1. *Get started:* Assessing community readiness to undertake collaborative prevention efforts

2. *Get organized:* Getting a commitment to the CTC process from community leaders and forming a diverse and representative prevention coalition

3. *Develop a profile:* Using epidemiologic data to assess prevention needs

4. *Create a plan:* Choosing tested and effective prevention policies, practices, and programs based on assessment data

5. *Implement and evaluate:* Implementing the new strategies with fidelity, in a manner congruent with the programs' theory, content, and methods of delivery and evaluating progress over time

Having the most current and complete set of data possible gives communities the clearest possible picture of where their needs—and strengths—are. It is strongly suggested that communities use the Communities That Care Youth Survey for their risk and protection assessment in Phase Three: Develop a Community Profile.

The Communities That Care Youth Survey measures a comprehensive set of risk and protective factors among a community's adolescent population (students in grades 6 through 12), to identify problem behaviors and their prevalence rates. **Figure 4-2** shows a sample survey page. The survey provides a means to explain why these problem behaviors exist and what communities can do to prevent them. The surveys are completed by youth while at school. You need to obtain school district support, which may take time.

Tools to Assess School Community Capacity

The second type of information collected as part of a needs assessment is a capacity assessment (Gilmore & Campbell, 2005). A capacity assessment is a thorough and accurate assessment of the school community to determine what resources are available to address the mental health concerns and problems of children and adolescents—for example, mental health education curriculum, materials, technology (software packages, Web sites, and so on), staff, programs, funding, and services, as well as the service gaps and needs in these areas. A key element of a capacity assessment is the empowerment of potential program participants (e.g., children, adolescents, families) to mobilize forces to address and solve the health concerns and problems identified in the needs assessment. The following are three widely used assessments and resources to determine school community capacity.

School Health Index   The CDC has developed the **School Health Index (SHI;** www.cdc.gov/HealthyYouth/shi/). This self-assessment and planning guide will enable you to identify the strengths and weaknesses of your school's health and safety policies and programs, develop an action plan for improving student

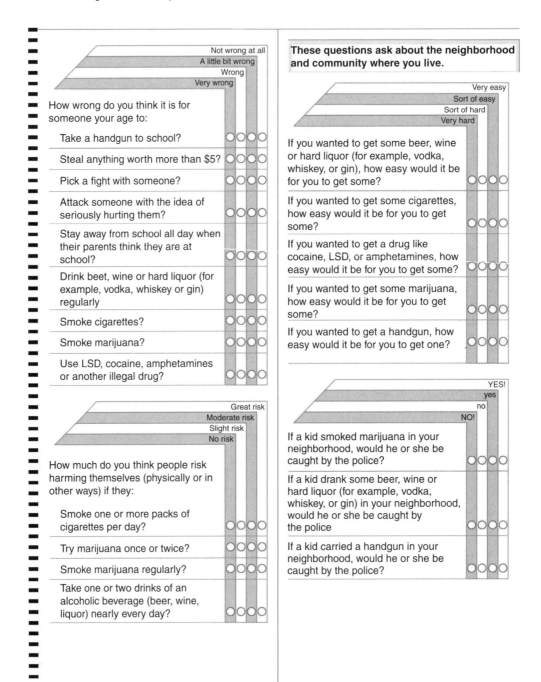

FIGURE 4-2 Sample page from Communities That Care Youth Survey.
Source: Substance Abuse and Mental Health Services Administration. (2004). Communities That Care Youth Survey. Retrieved from http://store.samhsa.gov/product/Communities-That-Care-Youth-Survey/CTC020

health, and involve teachers, parents, students, and the community in improving school policies and programs.

The SHI provides structure and direction to your school's efforts to improve health and safety policies and programs. First released in 2000, the SHI has been used by schools in nearly every state and in Canada. The SHI is designed for use at the local level; however, with appropriate adaptation it could be used at the district level as well, especially if the district has only a few schools and those schools have similar policies and programs. A school health team would lead the process, and it can reflect all eight areas of the CDC coordinated school health programs. The School Counseling, Psychological and Social Services component is most closely aligned with addressing students' mental health concerns and problems, although several sections assess policies and procedures for mental health risk behaviors (e.g., physical health—early sexual activity; school environment—violence).

The SHI is the school's self-assessment tool; it is not to be used to compare schools or evaluate the staff. There is no such thing as a passing grade on the SHI. The SHI scores only help personnel to understand a school's strengths and weaknesses and to develop an action plan for improving promotion and management of students' health and safety. The SHI uses a rating scale of 0–3 to determine whether a service or program is fully, partially, or not functioning in the school (see **Table 4-4**).

The SHI is available at no cost and can be completed in as little as 6 hours. Many of the improvements made after completing the SHI can be done with existing staff and resources. For those priority actions that do require new resources, SHI results can provide the information needed to stimulate school board and community support for school health programs and for funding requests.

The Guide to Community Preventive Services: Improving Adolescent Health   The **Guide to Community Preventive Services**: Improving Adolescent Health section (www.thecommunityguide.org/adolescenthealth/index.html) contains the U.S. Preventive Services Task Force (USPSTF) recommendations on the use of screening, counseling, and other preventive services that are typically delivered in primary care settings (i.e., community agencies and health clinics, schools, and community hospitals).

The interventions reviewed by the USPSTF and included in the clinical guide can provide support to community interventions because healthcare providers are typically the gatekeepers to health services. The community guide has a section dedicated to adolescents that provides information on policies and interventions on six types of adolescent health behavior that contribute to the leading causes of death and disability among youth: alcohol and drug use, injury and violence (including suicide), tobacco use, nutrition, physical activity, and sexual behaviors. **Table 4-5** contains a list of sample policies and interventions that, after a systematic review of available studies, provides strong or sufficient evidence that the intervention is effective. If an intervention is found to be effective, the community guide evaluates its economic efficiency (i.e., costs).

TABLE 4-4   School Health Index Sample Question to Assess Capacity Related to Students Who Are Victims or Perpetrators of Violence

Identify and refer students who are victims or perpetrators of violence

Instructions: Use the following rating scale: 3 = Yes, identifies and refers students to the most appropriate services; 2 = Identifies and refers students, but does not always refer them to the most appropriate services; I = Identifies students, but does not refer them to appropriate services; 0 = Does not identify students at risk, or the school does not have a counseling, psychological, or social services provider.

Does the school's counseling, psychological, or social services provider have a system for identifying students who are at risk of being victims or perpetrators of violence, and refer them to the most appropriate school-based or community-based services?

Indicators of students at risk of being victims or perpetrators of violence include

- ❖ Victims of child abuse or neglect
- ❖ Observers of violence at home, at school, or in community
- ❖ Victims of dating violence
- ❖ Victims of sexual assault
- ❖ Violent offenders
- ❖ Victims of bullying or harassment
- ❖ Suicide attempters
- ❖ Victims of other serious violence
- ❖ Those with special healthcare needs or mobility problems
- ❖ Survivors of serious unintentional impairments or injuries
- ❖ Those with learning or emotional disabilities
- ❖ Weapon carriers
- ❖ Users of alcohol or drugs (especially heavy users)
- ❖ Poor academic achievers

TABLE 4-5   Sample Guide to Clinical Preventive Services: Improving Adolescent Health Section Recommended Policies and Interventions

Improving caregivers' parenting skills: Person-to-person interventions
Preventing excessive alcohol consumption: Enhanced enforcement of laws prohibiting sales to minors
Reducing alcohol-impaired driving: Lower blood alcohol content laws for young or inexperienced drivers
Reducing alcohol-impaired driving: School-based instructional programs
Youth development behavioral interventions: Interventions coordinated with community service to reduce sexual risk behaviors in adolescents
Youth violence prevention: Therapeutic foster care to reduce violence for chronically delinquent juveniles
Youth violence prevention: School-based programs to reduce violence

State School Health Policy Database   According to the National Association of State Boards of Education,

> The **State School Health Policy Database** (nasbe.org/healthy_schools/hs/index .php) is a comprehensive set of laws and policies from 50 states on more than 40 school health topics. Originally begun in 1998, and maintained with support from the Division of Adolescent and School Health (DASH) of the Centers for Disease Control and Prevention (CDC), the policy database is designed to supplement information contained in CDC's School Health Policies and Programs Study (SHPPS).
>
> The database contains brief descriptions of laws, legal codes, rules, regulations, administrative orders, mandates, standards, resolutions, and other written means of exercising authority. While authoritative binding policies are the primary focus of the database, it also includes guidance documents and other non-binding materials that provide a more detailed picture of a state's school health policies and activities. Most of the collected laws and policies govern the education system, but health department, transportation, and social services policies are also included as appropriate. Hyperlinks to the full written policies are provided whenever possible.
>
> As part of a capacity assessment, the database is used to identify school health improvement strategies and policy language that is currently being used across the country. States' school health policies are part of the database organized into six broad categories:
>
> ◆ Curriculum and Instruction
> ◆ Staff
> ◆ Health Promoting Environment
> ◆ Student Services
> ◆ Accommodation
> ◆ Coordination/Implementation

Legal Issues

The two biggest legal concerns for children, adolescents, and families are protection of their confidentiality and privacy of educational and health information. Federal law provides protection for family and student rights during their involvement with the educational and social service systems.

Confidentiality

Confidentiality is an agreement not to disclose any information obtained when there is an expectation that the information will be kept private. Privacy is the control over the extent, timing, and circumstances of sharing oneself with others. Confidentiality is very important to establishing and maintaining a strong teacher–student relationship.

Students need safe places to explore the barriers that prevent them from learning. Some assurance of privacy is needed, or adolescents may avoid seeking the help that they need. Soler and Peters (1993) outline several reasons to protect the privacy of children and families. Potentially embarrassing information about a family or student, such as human immunodeficiency virus (HIV) status or mental health history, can create discrimination or judgment by school staff or other students, rendering teens vulnerable to mistreatment. Immigrant families in the country illegally may avoid working with student services or teachers for fear they will be reported to the Immigration and Naturalization Service (INS), who may take action against them.

Working in a school is different than working in a community agency setting where confidentiality is defined strictly with written releases of information describing the scope of what can be shared and with whom. The client–therapist relationship is the focus. In a school, we deal with minors required to be there and must not only build a connection with a student, but also balance and respect the rights of the parent to be "the guiding voice" in their child's life (Stone, 2003).

Confidentiality is a promise to keep personal information private unless there is potentially serious and foreseeable harm to a student. Working in schools requires that professionals protect the health, welfare, and safety of the child. The information must be shared, particularly when something damaging could happen in the future. Students are minors, and educators have a **duty to warn** parents when a danger exists. In addition, those in a position to help or protect the safety of the individual child, as well as others in a school, need to know.

Most states define school confidentiality in terms of need to know or what school personnel require to facilitate student learning, not what they *want* to know. Remember, we are working in an organization designed for academic instruction, and the rules are different than in a system designed exclusively for therapy. Confidentiality is much harder to maintain in a school because there are competing interests and few absolutes. In nearly all states, administration is entitled to information on students that is deemed need-to-know to optimize a student's learning (Stone, 2006).

Limits to confidentiality do exist. In working with students in schools, educators must talk about the exceptions to the promise of privacy because there are times when keeping information confidential can block helping a student or cause harm. Harm to self or others breaks all confidentiality deals. The American Psychological Association notes that confidentiality must be broken when a "clear danger to the person or to others" exists (1981). Usually students present one of three circumstances requiring the educator to break the confidentiality agreement:

- ❖ A threat to harm self
- ❖ A threat to harm another requires warning this person of the threat if it is credible
- ❖ Disclosure of any form of physical or sexual abuse and/or neglect requires reporting to civil authorities

As educators charged with optimizing student learning, we must communicate the limits to our own confidentiality. Suicide threats or ideation; child abuse; alcohol, tobacco, or other drug use on campus; or any violation of the law or school policy requires immediate reporting of the situation to an administrator.

This is usually followed by an appropriate referral. Remember, your primary job is to keep students safe.

When we are concerned about a child's safety, it may be necessary to share our concerns with a principal or with the student's parents. Try to speak to the student and include them in the process of choosing how and when to tell, and include them in the visit. However, if we cannot reach the student and there is immediate cause for concern, we must break confidentiality and make our report (Kessler, 2007). Always contact the parent because the "parents [have] legal and inherent rights to be the guiding voice in their children's lives" (American School Counselor Association [ASCA], 2011).

It is also important to inform students in developmentally appropriate ways of the limits to their working relationship. Explanations of confidentiality can concurrently be done in a global fashion, such as through classroom guidance lessons, the student handbook, school counseling brochures, or the school Web site.

When the student cannot or will not cooperate, educators may reveal the facts to prevent "serious and foreseeable harm to the student" (ASCA, 2011). This means if you do nothing, you foresee that something serious and harmful may occur. The younger or more developmentally challenged the child, the more quickly you should involve the parents. Although students need the assurance of privacy, it is best to balance that obligation with an understanding of parents'/guardians' legal and moral rights to be the guiding voice in their children's lives, especially in value-laden issues.

Privacy of Educational and Health Information

The **Family Educational Rights and Privacy Act (FERPA)** gives parents the right to access all records a school has on their children (U.S. Department of Education, 2011). With a few exceptions (such as a serious emergency), the school may not release student information outside of the school without consent of the parents. When the student reaches the age of majority, 18 years, those privacy rights transfer to the student. In cases where a student's safety is at risk (e.g., an abusive family situation), school staff must inform external authorities (e.g., child protective services).

Health information needs to be stored where confidentiality can be maintained but where the information can be utilized only by those who need it, for example, in response to an emergency. Schools should develop and use release forms that define the limits of information to be exchanged.

The **Health Insurance Portability and Accountability Act (HIPAA)** (www .hhs.gov/ocr/privacy/hipaa/administrative/combined/index.html) regulates healthcare providers sharing information with each other and with schools. Special considerations for school compliance with HIPAA often apply, for example, when confidential information is housed in school-based health centers. The school principal or the person creating the health record is usually the person responsible for this. For health information, the responsibility is often delegated to the school nurse. For mental health information, responsibility to protect student confidentiality is often assigned to the school nurse, school counselor, or school psychologist. Access to these files is restricted to specific individuals whose job it is to work with the student.

Ethical Considerations

Policies and procedures use codes of ethics or ethical standards to define the guiding principles of professional activities. In the past decade, increased public awareness of professional behavior, coupled with the passage of federal and state legislation controlling the helping professions, has underscored the importance of ethical concerns in service delivery. Stadler (1986) cites the Family Educational Rights and Privacy Act of 1974, state legislation requiring the reporting of child abuse, and *Tarasoff v. Regents of the University of California* (1976), which imposed a duty to warn potential victims, as examples of government action that directly affects the ethics of service provision.

Codes of Ethics

Professionals have responded to the dilemmas of service provision by developing codes of ethics or statements of ethical standards of behavior for the members of their profession. Codes of ethics or ethical standards reflect professional concerns and define the guiding principles of professional activities. As an aid to ethical decision making in dilemmas arising in service delivery, such standards or codes help clarify the professional's responsibilities to clients, the agency, and society. Typically, a **code of ethics** includes items that state the goals or aims of the profession, protect the client, provide guidance to professional behavior, and contribute to a professional identity for the helper. A complete understanding of a code of ethics or ethical standards requires knowledge of the code's strengths and purposes as well as its limitations.

The primary functions of a code of ethics or ethical standards are to establish guidelines for professional behavior and to assist members of the profession in establishing a professional identity (Corey, Corey, & Callanan, 1998; Welfel, 1998). Other purposes include providing criteria for evaluating the ethics of a professional's practice and serving as a benchmark in the enforcement of ethical standards (Kenyon, 1999).

Ethical codes do have limitations; they cannot cover every situation. They do, however, present a framework for ethical behavior, although their exact interpretation will depend on the situation to which they are being applied. As a result of this vagueness, codes may have a limited scope, and some codes of ethics will likely conflict with others regarding some standard of behavior. Such conflicts pose problems for professionals who are members of more than one professional organization.

Members who are bound by a code of ethics must be alert to the possibility that other forums may reach conclusions that differ from their code. Of course, this is especially critical when the other forum is a court of law or a legislative body.

Ethics and Professionals

A code of ethics is binding only to the members of the group or organization that adopts it. Several organizations in human services, such as the American Counseling Association, the National Association of Social Workers, and others in the fields of corrections, mental health, gerontology, and education, have issued codes of behavior expected of their membership (**Table 4-6**). Most codes of ethics stipulate that the worker's first responsibility is to enhance and protect the client's welfare. Codes also give guidance about the helper's responsibilities to employers, to colleagues in the profession and other fields, and to society in general.

Ethical codes adopted by a professional association are usually based on the premise that a profession polices itself. Members of helping professions are assumed to be responsible, sensitive persons who are accountable for their behavior and the behavior of their colleagues. Self-regulation involves two types of discipline: informal and formal. Informal discipline is seen in the subtle and not-so-subtle pressure that colleagues exert on one another in the form of consultations, client referrals, and informal and formal discussions. Formal discipline occurs when professional associations publicly criticize or censure their members—in extreme cases, barring them from membership.

Codes of Ethics and the Law

Laws are systems of rules created by elected representatives and enforced through the courts, either civil or criminal. A government entity usually can enforce compliance. **Ethics** are a system of rules created by a particular group or profession and apply only to the group or profession. Ethics may have dissenters, but they give guidance for reasonable behavior and decisions. Even when a professional association such as the American School Counselor Association unanimously agrees on an ethical standard, those who violate it are not subject to punishment from government.

TABLE 4-6   Professional Codes of Ethics

Counselors: American Counseling Association, www.counseling.org/Resources/CodeOfEthics/TP/Home/CT2.aspx

School counselors: American School Counselors Association, asca2.timberlakepublishing.com//files/EthicalStandards2010.pdf

Teachers: National Education Association, www.nea.org/home/30442.htm

School social workers: National Association of Social Workers, www.socialworkers.org/pubs/code/default.asp

School nurses: National Association of School Nurses, www.nasn.org/RoleCareer/CodeofEthics

School administrators: American Association of School Administrators, www.aasa.org/content.aspx?id=1390

The law is generally supportive of, or at least neutral toward, ethical codes and standards. It is supportive in that it enforces minimum standards for practitioners through licensing requirements and generally protects the confidentiality of statements and records provided by clients during service provision. It is neutral in that it allows each profession to police itself and govern the helper's relations with clients and fellow professionals. The law intervenes and overrides professional codes of ethics only when necessary to protect the public's health, safety, and welfare. There are specific instances when the legal system does not interfere with ethical standards; for example, an agency counselor who is a member of the American Counseling Association (ACA) may need to break confidentiality when the counselor believes there is a serious and foreseeable harm to the client (ACA, 2012). The general requirement that counselors keep information confidential does not apply when disclosure is required to protect clients or identified others from serious and foreseeable harm or when legal requirements demand that confidential information must be revealed.

The California Supreme Court's ruling in the case of *Tarasoff* (1976) legally supported a "duty to warn" possible victims of clients once counselors have this information. The court stated that

> when a therapist determines, or pursuant to the standards of his profession should determine, that his patient presents a serious danger of violence to another, he incurs an obligation to use reasonable care to protect the intended victim against such danger. The discharge of this duty may require the therapist to take one or more steps, depending on the nature of the case. Thus, it may call for him or her to warn the intended victim or others likely to apprise the victim of the danger, to notify the police, or to take whatever other steps are reasonably necessary under the circumstances. (p. 340)

Summary

School district policy reflects the goals and ethos of the school community. It is part of a school district's overall strategy to promote student health and welfare and to be closely linked to the management of student behavior. The policies and procedures set the boundaries for how schools and communities operate and interact. They help everyone be clear about who is responsible and accountable for making sure schools and communities are working together to address young people's mental health concerns and problems. Many tools and resources are available to school districts and community organizations regarding mental health policies and procedures. Policies and procedures respect the legal rights of children and their families. The two biggest legal concerns for children, adolescents, and families are protection of their confidentiality and privacy of educational and health information. Policies and procedures use codes of ethics or ethical standards to define the guiding principles of professional activities.

For Practice and Discussion

1. You are hired at a community agency as a school liaison to plan, implement, and evaluate the local school district mental health promotion and prevention programs and services. You have been given 30 days to prepare an action plan. As part of your initial work with the school district, what school policies and procedures do you want to review? What tools can help you learn more about the school mental health policies and procedures?
2. You are attending a partnership meeting, and during a coffee break, a colleague asks you about the current status of a young person participating in a mental health treatment program. How do you respond?
3. A parent telephones you upset that her daughter was sent home from school during the day for violation of the school drug policy. The parent demands to know the circumstances. What can you say? What are your options?
4. At a partnership meeting, a local agency is actively soliciting the members to refer children and adolescents to a new program. If the partnership members refer 25 new program participants, the agency will sponsor an outing to a local sporting event for partnership members. What are potential ethical issues with such an incentive? What are your options?
5. You are conducting community assessments as part of your work with a statewide collaboration to improve mental health program and service coordination. In the community assessment process, how can you use the Guide to Community Preventive Services and State School Health Policy Database?

Key Terms

Child and Adolescent Needs and
 Strengths (CANS)   74
Code of ethics   82
Communities That Care (CTC)   74
Community assessment   71
Confidentiality   79
Duty to warn   80
Ethics   83
Family Educational Rights and
 Privacy Act (FERPA)   81
Guide to Community Preventive
 Services   77
Health Insurance Portability and
 Accountability Act (HIPAA)   81

Laws   83
Policy   64
Procedural guidelines   66
Procedures   65
Protective factors   72
Risk factors   72
School Health Index (SHI)   75
State School Health Policy
 Database   79
Youth Risk Behavior Surveillance
 System (YRBSS)   72

References

American Counseling Association. (2012). American Counseling Association code of ethics. Retrieved from www.counseling.org/Resources/CodeOfEthics/TP/Home/CT2.aspx

American Psychological Association. (1981). *Ethical Principles of Psychologists*. Washington, DC: Author.

American School Counselor Association. (2011). American School Counselor Association. Ethical standards for school counselors. Retrieved from asca2.timberlakepublishing.com //files/EthicalStandards2010.pdf

Arthur, M.W., Hawkins, J.D., Pollard, J.A., Catalano, R.F., & Baglioni, A.J. (2002). Measuring risk and protective factors for substance use, delinquency, and other adolescent problem behaviors: The Communities That Care youth survey. *Evaluation Review*, 26: 575–601.

Corey, G., Corey, M.S., & Callanan, P. (1998). *Issues and Ethics in the Helping Professions*. Pacific Grove, CA: Brooks/Cole.

Gilmore, G.D., & Campbell, M.D. (2005). *Needs and Capacity Assessment Strategies for Health Education and Health Promotion*. Boston, MA: Jones & Bartlett.

Hawkins, J.D., Catalano, R.F., & Miller, J.Y. (1992). Risk and protective factors for alcohol and other drug problems in adolescence and early adulthood: Implications for substance abuse prevention. *Psychological Bulletin*, 112: 64–105.

Kenyon, P. (1999). *What Would You Do? An Ethical Case Workbook for Human Service Professionals*. Pacific Grove, CA: Brooks/Cole.

Kessler, R. (2007). Confidentiality. National Curriculum Integration Project. Retrieved from http://www.creducation.org/resources/Confidentiality.pdf

New Mexico Human Services Department. (2012). Risk and Protective Factor Framework. Retrieved from http://www.hsd.state.nm.us/Synar/pdf/Hawkins%20and%20Catalano%20 Risk%20and%20Protective%20Factor%20Framework.pdf

Soler, M.I., & Peters, C.M. (1993). *Who Should Know What? Confidentiality and Information Sharing in Service Integration* (Resource Brief No. 3). Falls Church, VA: National Center for Service Integration.

Stadler, H.A. (1986). Making hard choices: Clarifying controversial ethical issues. *Counseling and Human Development*, 19: 1–10.

Stone, C. (2003). Suicide: A duty owed. *ASCA School Counselor*. Retrieved from http://www .ascaschoolcounselor.org/article_content.asp?edition=91&section=140&article=780

Stone, C. (2006). In loco parentis, substantial interest, and qualified privilege. *ASCA School Counselor*. Retrieved from http://www.ascaschoolcounselor.org/article_content.asp?editi on=91&section=140&article=883

Substance Abuse and Mental Health Services Administration (SAMHSA). (2004). Communities That Care Youth Survey. Retrieved from http://store.samhsa.gov/shin/content//CTC020 /CTC020.pdf

Tarasoff v. Regents of the University of California. (1976). 17 Cal.3d 425, 131 Cal.Rptr. 14,551 P.2d 334.

U.S. Department of Education. (2011). Family Educational Rights and Privacy Act (FERPA) (20 U.S.C. § 1232g; 34 CFR Part 99). Retrieved from http://www2.ed.gov/policy/gen/guid/fpco /ferpa/index.html

Welfel, E.R. (1998). *Ethics in Counseling and Psychotherapy: Standards, Research, and Emerging Issues*. Pacific Grove, CA: Brooks/Cole.

REFERRALS AND OTHER WAYS TO CONNECT TO PROGRAMS AND SERVICES

In this chapter, we will:

✦ Discuss how children and adolescents connect to mental health programs and services

✦ Describe two types of connections

✦ Explain referral, crisis determination, and initial information collection

✦ Discuss parents' and caregivers' engagement and consent

✦ Identify how to communicate personal information

Scenario

I know my students struggle with lots of stress. It is part of their daily lives. It is not just school but families, economics, friends, and life in the community. Everyone is trying to do their best. For the general population of students, we have our health curriculum addressing risk and protective factors. We are considering teacher training in social emotional learning. For students we identify as having a concern, we have a variety of support groups and programs. For students with a serious mental health problem, we have school-based mental health counseling. We offer a lot of mental health programs and services beyond the school in the community through our school community partnerships at each school building in the district. Critical is getting our students connected into the system to take advantage of what our district and partnerships offer. Navigating the mental health system is difficult and challenging. We want to guide students and their families to the best resources in the school and community. We have 45 buildings across the district and we need to know what is happening in all of them. We can't have everyone doing their own thing. It would be chaotic. We have staff move between buildings. Likewise, families move, change, and enroll their children in different buildings. Consistency is important as students progress in their academic careers moving from elementary to secondary education buildings. Inconsistency and differences lead to confusion and potentially negative consequences. Students fall through the cracks. Each school community is unique, and differences can be expected, but we need some consistency across our schools and communities to get our students connected.

Source: Roberta Tyson, the district coordinator for student services in a southern California school district

How Children and Adolescents Connect to Mental Health Programs and Services

Most teenagers and children do not actively seek help for mental health concerns and problems for various reasons. They are content with the status quo of their lives, accepting (trusting) that the school community, through the existing structures, will somehow address and alleviate stress in their lives that might negatively impact their mental health. Unfortunately, not getting help for mental health concerns and problems can lead to a worsening of the condition, deterioration of physical and mental health, legal problems, school failure, behavior problems, substance abuse, and suicide. Talking with students, it is not unusual to learn that they believe their behavior, emotions, and mental status are normal, potentially resulting in a lifetime of disordered thinking that could be greatly improved with appropriate support and help.

Frequently students are not aware of feeling bad. They accept their situation not knowing there is an alternative. In other situations, they may believe that the particular concern will resolve on its own and do not understand that talking with someone might be beneficial. Many children and adolescents do not seek mental health care for financial reasons. A lack of family health insurance coverage, or coverage that leaves a large amount owed by the family, leads many to avoid seeking care. Also, students often are unaware of the free or discounted mental health services available to them in city, county, state, or private clinics and facilities.

Many students have poor access to mental healthcare services because they live in a rural community. Others cannot logistically get to services because of a lack of transportation or overwhelming work and home responsibilities.

For others, the range of available services might be limited, so depending on their particular need, services may or may not be available. In urban areas, clinics often have such long waiting lists that students and families give up on receiving care.

Finally, many young people and their family members feel a stigma exists regarding mental health programs and services, and that negative stereotypes could damage their school performance and relationships. Embarrassment and fear of what others may think prevents students from seeking or continuing the services they need.

Knowing that most teenagers and children do not actively seek help for mental health concerns and problems for various reasons means that you and your colleagues (fellow teachers, school counselors, school psychologists, nurses, principals, coaches, community mental health workers, community human service organizations, government programs, drug and alcohol agency staff members, and others) will need some way to connect students to the mental health systems. It is not easy or simple. The school community needs to have a clear and respectful way for the school and community professionals to get to know a child or adolescent, know the family, and talk with them about what might be possible. These conversations start through intentional action by school and community staff that engages young people in discussions about how to address problems and mental health concerns. Teams, partnerships, and collaborations encourage schools and community agencies to use two types of connection strategies to create these initial conversations (connections) with students and their families.

Connection Strategies: Structural and Formal

Two types of strategies connect children and adolescents to mental health programs and services: structural and formal (**Figure 5-1**). The strategies are clear and offer a user-friendly decision-making process for students, families, and staff.

Structural connection strategies are agreed upon and supported by the schools (and community organizations) and do not require parent permission to access and participate in mental health programs and services. Examples are health curriculum content, classroom programs by the school counselors, nursing services, and extracurricular activities (Figure 5-1). These are thought of as primary prevention addressing the developmental mental health needs of all students focused on promoting social and emotional health while proactively addressing mental health problems and concerns. Just by attending school or participating in a community organization activity young people get access and participate. Parents do not need to sign permission for their child to participate. If a parent has a concern about their child's participation in a particular activity, a note or telephone call to the school is typically sufficient to permit the child to do an alternative activity.

Formal connection strategies are agreed upon and supported by schools (and community organizations) and, depending on the state, may or may not require parent permission to participate in a process to match the needs of a child and family with existing school community resources (e.g., programs and services).

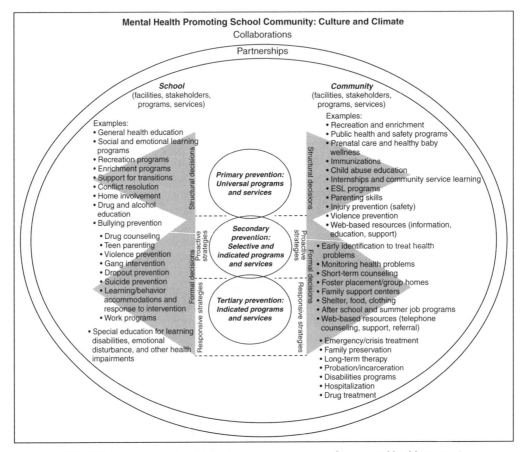

FIGURE 5-1   Structural and formal connection strategies for a mental health promoting school community.
Source: Adapted from Center for Mental Health in Schools at UCLA. (n.d.). School-community partnerships: A guide. UCLA Department of Psychology School Mental Health Project. Retrieved from http://www.smhp.psych.ucla.edu

The model for the formal connection strategies is the individual mental health concerns and problems intervention process approach. Use of student support teams to implement formal connection strategies tailored to individual school districts and communities is the best practice, although some school districts will delegate making formal connections (following the model) to a school social worker, counselor, or nurse. As part of the model, once a child or adolescent is referred to the student support team, the team will engage in a process to identify and clarify the needs of the child or adolescent—a clear and consistent process to collect and review information about a young person's mental health concern or problem. Examples of situations that require a formal strategy include participation in skill development groups for children from families experiencing stress from disruption, dysfunction, or chronic illness of a family member, and working with children experiencing severe stress due to depression, violence, or substance abuse (Figure 5-1). These are thought of as secondary and tertiary prevention (e.g., selected and indicated programs and services). Formal connection strategies are further delineated as proactive and reactive strategies. Participation in special education is another example where formal connection strategies are used. Often, student support teams with responsibilities for special education will include mental health programs and services as part of a student's Individualized Education Program.

Structural Connection Strategies

Structural connection strategies are the known and familiar school community staff, programs, and services. Walking into a school you expect a staffing pattern that includes many administrative, teaching, support, and operation positions. Building principal, school nurse, school counselor(s), teachers, secretarial, janitorial, food service, activity, and transportation positions are all required to operate a school. Each member of the school staff, through their daily carrying out of their job responsibilities, has the potential to directly (i.e., instruction, counseling, mentoring) or indirectly (i.e., role model, social support) help address students' mental health concerns and problems. Depending on the district size and economics, the positions might be full or part time, might be shared among buildings, and might have multiple individuals involved (e.g., assistant principals, school counselors). Some might be district-wide or assigned to particular buildings (e.g., school psychologist and school social workers). The key to maximizing the structural connections is to know all of the structural connections in a school community. **Table 5-1** is a sample inventory for identifying structural connections. It is expected that any individual who is part of a school community staff would describe as part of their professional training and job description the development of capable and competent young people. Further, that through their work they enhance protective factors and decrease risk factors found in the school community and families. As part of their professional responsibilities they are on the front line of working with youth and are constantly aware of being a gatekeeper into the mental health system.

An important action for teams, partnerships, and collaborations is for them to be clear about the structural connections at both the school community level and district wide. It is obvious that the teachers, administration, school guidance/counseling, and nursing staff are natural resources for students and families to talk with about promoting the mental health of children and adolescents. However, it is important to recognize that in a school community culture that promotes mental health, all staff are involved. To help you identify and know all of the structural connections in a school community, we recommend an inventory (map) of school building connections (Table 5-1). As part of the capacity assessment within a needs assessment, completing such an inventory is common.

TABLE 5-1 Structural School Community Connections Information Sheet	
Administrative Team: Principal, Assistant Principal(s) _____ _____ _____ _____	*Clerical/Secretarial/Support Staff* _____ _____ _____ _____
School Psychologist _____ Times at the school _____ • Provides assessment and testing of students for special services; counseling for students and parents; support services for teachers; prevention, crisis, conflict resolution, and program modification for special learning and/or behavioral needs	*Title I and Bilingual Coordinators* _____ _____ Times at the school _____ • Coordinate categorical programs; provide services to identified Title I students; implement Bilingual Master Plan (supervising the curriculum, testing, and so forth)
School Nurse _____ Times at the school _____ • Provides immunizations, follow-up, communicable disease control, vision and hearing screening and follow-up, health assessments and referrals, health counseling, and information for students and families	*Resource and Special Education Teachers* _____ _____ Times at the school _____ • Provide information on program modifications for students in regular classrooms as well as providing services for special education
Pupil Services and Attendance Officer(s) _____ _____ _____ Times at the school _____ • Provide a liaison between school and home to maximize school attendance, transition counseling for returnees, enhancing attendance improvement activities	*School Safety and Security (Police)* _____ _____ *Custodians (Name/Contact Number)* _____/_____ _____/_____ *Bus Monitors (Name/Contact Number)* _____/_____ _____/_____

Social Worker _____ Times at the school _____ • Assists in identifying at-risk students and provides follow-up counseling for students and parents; refers families for additional services if needed	*Student Activities Director and Club Sponsors (Name/Club)* _____/_____ _____/_____ _____/_____ _____/_____ _____/_____ _____/_____
Home and School Visitor: LSW _____ Times at school _____	*Athletic Director/Team Coaches* _____/_____ _____/_____ _____/_____
Counselors Times at the school _____ _____ _____ _____ _____ _____ _____ _____ • Provide general and special counseling/ guidance services; consult with parents and school staff *Before School and After School Program Coordinator* _____ Times at the school _____ • Coordinates before and after school programs	*Community Resources* • Provides school-linked or school-based activities and resources Who What they do When _____/_____/_____ _____/_____/_____ _____/_____/_____ _____/_____/_____ _____/_____/_____

There is no correct or magical mix of structural connections that a school and district can or should have. The particular school and school district mix reflects the students, faculty, staff, and families as well as the school community economics and social status. What is important is to know the inventory of structural connections of the school and school district—what programs and services students and families can access easily. As part of collecting this information, you also want to know the mental health promotion elements offered as part of the program and service.

Structural connections can turn into formal connections. For example, one common occurrence as part of a structural connection is when a student self-discloses (often innocently or inadvertently) a concern or problem.

The classroom curriculum and general primary prevention activities are designed to promote mental health and development of competent young individuals. At the same time, you want to be aware that these activities provide a venue for students to share information and concerns in what they perceive as a safe environment. Not that these activities are done specifically to identify children and adolescents struggling to address concerns and problems, but in the carrying out of the activities students share information. You need to be ready to respond.

Formal Connection Strategies

Formal connection strategies are rooted in the individual mental health concerns and problems intervention process approach. They are how a student makes an initial connection (i.e., how they are referred to the student support team). According to the model, the student support team uses formal connection strategies to identify the early indicators of problematic behaviors in children and adolescents as well as youth who are already demonstrating mental health concerns or problem behaviors. The formal connections in a school or district may be less known among students, faculty, staff, and families. Community members might have very limited knowledge of these formal connection strategies in schools. Distinguishing elements of the formal connection strategy are referral, initial information collection, and **crisis determination**. Teams, partnerships, and collaborations are active in the creation of these connections. They do not happen unless someone is willing to take leadership to work on the logistics and details necessary to create the connections. There are two types of formal connection strategies: proactive and responsive.

Proactive strategies identify the early indications of problem behaviors that, if left undetected, could create more serious issues. For example, children with poor emotional regulation skills may have problems in school with anger and sadness. The inability to cope constructively with anger and sadness are correlated with internalizing symptoms of depression, anxiety, and suicidality. The inability to cope positively with anger is significantly linked to externalizing symptoms of oppositional defiant disorder, substance abuse, and conduct disorders (Zeman, Shipman, & Suveg, 2002). The proactive strategy supports and guides staff (e.g., teachers, counselors, administrators) to take action to get the child or adolescent the support and resources needed to address a concern that otherwise left unaddressed might have negative consequences. There is no diagnosis or assessment by staff. Proactive strategies address concerns.

Responsive strategies are actions that link students presenting signs of internalizing and externalizing symptoms to higher levels of needed care, such as intensive therapy or medication management. Responsive strategies address problems. These students may benefit from proactive skill building; however, their problems impede their ability to cope with daily life. They require the concentrated efforts of the student support team to work with the student and family to determine the next best steps.

The Essential Elements of Formal Connections

Distinguishing elements of a formal connection strategy (both proactive and reactive strategies) are referral, crisis determination, initial information collection, and parent engagement and consent. To make the formal connection strategies work, to have a clear and consistent pathway for children and their families to know and follow into the mental health system, the teams, partnerships, and collaborations need to make sure that the referral, crisis determination, and initial information collection processes are defined and operating in the school community.

Referral Defined   The goal of the **referral** is to support students and their families in taking action to address a mental health concern and problem. As part of a formal connection, a referral is a process by which immediate student needs for care and supportive services are assessed and prioritized. Students (and their families) are provided with assistance in identifying and accessing the most appropriate services, such as setting up appointments and providing transportation. The student support teams play a critical role and are the first stop in this process. In the school community, the individual teacher, school counselor, parent, or school administrator refers a student to the team. The referral is a shifting and sharing of responsibility for dealing with a concern and problem from the individual teacher to the larger system in the school. The student support team can bring to bear more resources, support, and guidance through its network of partnerships and collaborations. The team helps move the individual from trying to resolve an issue alone to a more visible and strengths-based problem-solving process.

The term *referral* is widely used in the school community environment. On any given day, and for any number of reasons, students in schools are being sent (referred) to the nurse, counselor, and principal. Typically students do as they are instructed without question. It is also common that students themselves will initiate the referral with a request to attend a meeting, have a medical appointment, or participate in a school or community activity. Likewise, among their peers students are always telling their friends about music, food, activities, Web sites, and a whole host of items that are part of their daily lives. One prominent example of such referrals is posting something one likes on a friend's social networking site (e.g., Facebook). These referrals are freely given and received with little expectation that a person be obligated or required to follow through with some action to complete a specific task.

Nearly three-quarters of schools report that "social, interpersonal, or family problems" are the most frequent mental health issues for both male and female students. For males, aggression or disruptive behavior and behavior problems associated with neurological disorders are the second and third most frequent problems. For females, anxiety and adjustment issues are the second and third most frequent problems (Foster et al., 2005). The manifestation of these problems in the school setting is seen in academic performance and school behavior.

Referrals are made because someone has noticed something that is interfering with the child's academic achievement or school success. Repeated attempts by adults at school and at home to reach out and help the child have not worked. Remember that young people don't always have the words to tell adults what is going on inside of their heads. So, the feelings and thoughts come out through behavior patterns. The more serious the problem, the more frequent and intense the behaviors become. Most referrals come from school staff because of behaviors that the child has demonstrated during the school day. It is not unusual for teachers of art, drama, music, or physical education, who have the opportunity to see the student in a different context, make referrals. Also common are referrals from sponsors of afterschool events and bus drivers.

At times, staff will see a student or group of young people from the school using drugs, drunk, high, or engaging in other risky behavior at the shopping mall or another venue that is off the school campus. Staff can always choose to refer the child to see whether there are any consistent warning signs at school. A student with declining grades, increased disciplinary infractions, dropping out of an activity that they previously enjoyed, and chronic absences or tardiness needs more than education. We refer to school-based concerns that stem from off-campus activities as having a "nexus" or intersection between home and school life. A nexus must be observed before the school takes any action on the reports that come from evening or weekend off-campus activities.

Referrals commonly come from the teaching staff. They often see subtle changes early because they interact with the student every day. The staff member has tried to address these issues and is having very little impact. Prior involvement of the parents or other helping systems within the school is usually the norm before seeking additional support for the student.

Family members may be instrumental in the referral of a student for mental health services. Many times the family has knowledge of the involvement of their child in things that are deleterious to their health, safety, and welfare. A counselor may be working with a child and becomes aware that the child's involvement in substance abuse requires more intervention than the counselor can provide. Magistrates and probation officers support intervention efforts that have been court mandated. Staff from community agencies working within the district also refer students. In some districts, referral forms have been developed for the bus drivers.

Students may voluntarily request help with a mental health problem and are assured access to programs and services without penalty. The school's reputation for addressing students' mental health needs, the safety the student perceives in the process, and the approachability of school staff will play a role in the number of **student self-referrals**. Students are encouraged to seek the support of team members for issues that are barriers to learning and school success. If a student needs connection and an adult mentor, this type of support can be easily arranged. If, however, the mental health issues are serious, the team must involve the parents.

Key Referral Terms   When talking with school and community professionals as well as family members, three key terms and their definitions can help individuals look at students' behavior patterns in a focused way, and explain their concerns in objective language. These terms are *frequency, intensity,* and *duration.* To help you understand the importance of the terms, let's review the case of Jason, a tenth grader at a large New York City high school.

> Jason's father committed suicide last fall. It was a devastating event in Jason's life. At the time of the death the school counselor was in contact with Jason and his family. Some members of the school community attended the funeral. Previously, Jason did well in school. After his father's death, Jason seemed resilient but recently his grades have begun to slip and he was sleeping through most of his classes.

Frequency refers to how often you see a given action or cluster of behaviors. In Jason's case, the first period teacher first noticed he was sleeping in class. In the beginning, it was an occasional nodding off, but Jason was easily redirected. Then, it became harder to redirect him (i.e., wake him up) and keep him awake in class.

Intensity is the amount of disruption a child or adolescent experiences in her or his life. For example, Jason's sleeping in class caused him to miss essential information and skill development. His grades began to drop. Over a quarter (8 weeks) his grades dropped to Ds and Fs. Unable to adapt to the stressors in his life, Jason began staying home from school. Soon his mother called the school and reported he was up all night, sleeping all day, and wasn't bathing, eating, or coming out of his room. The intensity of Jason's mental health issues worsened over time to the point where he stopped functioning. In essence, he stopped doing all the things considered typical for an adolescent.

Duration is how long the behaviors have gone on. For Jason, it appears that he began having trouble remaining alert in class at the beginning of the first quarter, after his father's suicide. Over an 8-week period, all teachers were concerned about him and seeing similar issues; he was failing or close to failing in all of his courses; and eventually, he became so withdrawn that he stopped coming to school.

Referral Logistics and Form   Schools use a referral form to start and guide the referral process. Typically the forms are concise with the name of the student (with grade level and homeroom) and the name of the person making the referral (with contact information—telephone number and e-mail address). Generally, the form captures the objective verifiable information about academic, attendance, behavior/discipline, and/or health-related issues. These include:

❖ *Risk-taking behaviors:* History of run-away behaviors, stealing, vandalism, dropping out of an extracurricular activity

❖ *Declining academic performance:* Skipping class, cheating on tests, declining grades

❖ *Disciplinary infractions:* Sudden change in behavior—becoming increasingly shy/withdrawn or angry and belligerent, fighting, bullying, being dishonest, seeking constant reassurance

❖ *Attendance:* Tardy to school or class, frequent absenteeism, cutting class

❖ *Health:* Burn marks or evidence of other self-injury; eating too much or not enough; sleeping too much or not enough

The form is filled out as directed (**Figure 5-2**). It is given or emailed to a designated member of the student support team. Frequently, schools have the forms as online templates.

Crisis Determination   Referral forms are designed with an important student safety device. The first section (Figure 5-2) identifies students in an active crisis. If a child or adolescent is in active crisis, you want to immediately share the information with the building principal, social worker, or school counselor to implement the school's crisis response plans right away. Here are some crisis warning signs. Has this student:

❖ Been exposed to past traumatic event(s)?

❖ Expressed a desire to die?

❖ Made a suicidal threat/gesture?

❖ Shared suicidal ideas in writing?

❖ Given away prized possessions?

❖ Mentioned a recent death of a family member or close friend?

❖ Discussed having a weapon, narcotics, or other method

❖ Revealed or evidenced possession of alcohol, tobacco, or another drug?

❖ Discussed sexual assault or harassment?

❖ Threatened another person with serious harm?

❖ Talked about:

◆ Being homeless?

◆ Being abused now or in the past?

◆ Loss of a parent or loved one?

◆ Loss of a significant relationship?

◆ Separation/divorce of parents?

◆ Deployment or return of parent/caregiver

If the young person is not in active crisis, the student support team can proceed with identiying and clarifying the need. A member of the team may contact the person making the referral to ask three additional questions that are used to establish the referral is for a credible mental health concern and problem that needs to be addressed. In some situations a referral is made incorrectly. For example, a teacher may use a referral inappropriately for not completing a class assignment or not having a parent permission form signed for a class outing. The three clarifying questions are:

❖ Has the referral source (e.g., teacher, school aide, bus driver, coach, principal) talked with the student to attempt to resolve the issue?

❖ Has the child been referred to the school counselor, social worker, nurse, or disciplinarian?

❖ Are the parents/caregivers aware of the issue?

An acknowledgement is sent to the referring person to inform them of the team's actions (i.e., taking the referral under advisement and creating an appropriate plan for services). The referring person will be given information they will need to know to work with the child.

Initial Information Collection   **Initial information collection** is the act of collecting all objective and verifiable information that is available in the school. Figure 5-2 is a sample form used in several large urban school districts as a way to

---

CONFIDENTIAL: Do not leave this paper where others can see it

Date	
Student Name	_____ Days Absent
Completed by	_____ Days Tardy
Period/Time of Day	Course

1. Crisis Indicators: Has this student
- ☐ **expressed desire to die?**
- ☐ **made a suicide threat/gesture?**
- ☐ **shared suicidal ideas in writing?**
- ☐ **given away many possessions?**
- ☐ **mentioned a recent death of family member or close friend?**
- ☐ **talked about having a weapon?**
- ☐ **talked about or evidenced possession of drug/alcohol?**
- ☐ **discussed sexual assault/harassment?**
- ☐ **threatened another person with serious harm?**
- ☐ **talked about being homeless?**
- ☐ **talked about being abused now or in the past?**
- ☐ talked about loss of parent or loved one?
- ☐ talked about loss of significant relationship?
- ☐ talked about separation/divorce of parents?

NOTE: If you have checked one or more of the boldfaced items, please share this information immediately with your building principal, social worker, or school counselor.

2. Physical Symptoms
- ☐ Evidence of self-cutting
- ☐ Burn marks
- ☐ Has unexplained, frequent physical injuries
- ☐ Smells of alcohol/marijuana
- ☐ Glassy/bloodshot eyes
- ☐ Unsteady on feet
- ☐ Slurred speech
- ☐ Preoccupation with diet
- ☐ Frequent complaints of nausea/vomiting
- ☐ Sleeping/lethargy
- ☐ Noticeable change in weight
- ☐ Over- or underweight
- ☐ Poor hygiene

3. Risky Behaviors
- ☐ Expresses involvement with gangs
- ☐ Exhibits gang-related activity/clothing/colors/paraphernalia
- ☐ Talks of vandalism
- ☐ Steals or forcibly takes things from others
- ☐ History of running away
- ☐ Involved with juvenile justice system
- ☐ Dropped out of activity: sports, drama, extracurricular or after school activity

4. Home/Family Indicators
- ☐ Parent/guardian incarcerated
- ☐ Speaks of family addiction
- ☐ Speaks of family mental health issue
- ☐ Moves frequently between caretakers
- ☐ Foster care
- ☐ Parent divorcing/separating
- ☐ Parent/guardian deployed
- ☐ Parent/guardian lost job
- ☐ School transition

5. Academic Performance
- ☐ Skips class
- ☐ Cheating (copies others' academic work)
- ☐ Declining grades
- ☐ Has difficulty following classroom rules
- ☐ Disorganized materials and work space
- ☐ Does not turn in assignments given in class
- ☐ Does not turn in homework
- ☐ Does assignments carelessly
- ☐ Has difficulty participating in classroom activity/discussions
- ☐ Reluctant to ask for help
- ☐ Gives up easily
- ☐ Easily distracted

FIGURE 5-2   *(Continues)*

6. Interpersonal	8. Student Strengths
☐ Talks freely about drug use ☐ Wears drug/alcohol-related clothing ☐ Fighting ☐ Brings inappropriate materials to school (e.g. electronics, sexually explicit material, drugs, etc.) ☐ Constantly threatens or harasses ☐ Verbally abusive ☐ Frequently picked on by peers ☐ Frequently dishonest/untruthful ☐ Denies responsibility/blames others ☐ Caught cheating (games with friends/bending the rules) ☐ Argues with teacher ☐ Easily influenced by others ☐ Seeks constant reassurance ☐ Tends to interact with younger or older children ☐ Teases other students ☐ Isolates from peers ☐ Expresses hopelessness or helplessness ☐ Shy, withdrawn ☐ Appears sad ☐ States "I can't do it"	☐ Attentive ☐ Cooperative ☐ Shows interest in subject ☐ Works hard ☐ Strong grades ☐ Participates in class ☐ Works independently ☐ Works well in a group ☐ Well liked by others ☐ Creative ☐ Considerate of others ☐ Shows leadership skills ☐ Good attendance ☐ Appropriate sense of humor ☐ Organized ☐ Polite
7. Behavioral ☐ Sudden outbursts of anger ☐ Cries easily/frequently ☐ Sudden, dramatic change in behavior ☐ Hits/pushes other students ☐ Withdrawn/loner/submissive ☐ Has lost interest in preferred activities ☐ Frequently absent _____ (how many?) ☐ Frequently tardy _____ (how many?) ☐ Is not where he/she is to be during the school day ☐ Obscene language/gestures ☐ Constantly on the defensive ☐ Repeated requests to visit restroom, health office, counselor (circle which apply)	**9. Attempts to Resolve the Situation: Fill in appropriate dates to indicate steps you have taken to correct the behavior(s)** ☐ Student Observation Forms_____ ☐ Referral to Discipline_____ ☐ Referral to Social Worker_____ ☐ Referral to Counselor_____ ☐ Parent Conference_____ ☐ Student Conference_____ ☐ Referral to Principal_____ ☐ Telephoned Parent_____ ☐ Informal Hearing_____ ☐ Other_____
10. Comments (please use objective, verifiable statements)	

FIGURE 5-2 Referral/student information form: Individual teacher checklist.
Source: Courtesy of the School District of Pittsburgh, Office of Student Support Services–Student Assistance Program.

document a student's behavior and understand the intensity of his or her issues. Note that there are 10 sections of the form. The form is used to identify the student's strengths and assets, and acquire descriptive data on the problems observed by each staff member. A coherent picture begins to emerge that enables the student support team to decide on appropriate support. It is recommended that a referral log be maintained to allow for an accurate listing of students referred to the team and the disposition of the referral. Most student support teams use an Excel spreadsheet that is password protected and encrypted. Student information forms are not formal standardized mental screening instruments used to assess mental health risk and protective factors; rather, they are a consistent tool used by schools to gather objective observations from school staff on a student. There is value in having five teachers see that Jason's sleeping in class is an issue. When six of his teachers note his drop in grades, denying that a problem exists, and defensiveness, the school has verified through observable behavior that Jason is having difficulty in school, not just with one subject or at one time of day. This supports the team's work on behalf of the student.

Parents and Caregivers: Engagement and Consent

Parents and caregivers are part of the formal connection process. Their involvement varies depending on the programs in place in the school and board policy on how and when parents are notified. It also varies by state department of education policies and regulations.

Typically a member of the student support team will contact the parent/caregiver to explain the purpose of the team, the reason for the contact, referral, and initial information collection. This is an opportunity for the team and parents to begin collaborating and sharing all insights that may be relevant to the information contained in the referral form. Some school districts will require informed written **parental consent** before the process can continue. The parents also have the option of refusing the offer of help, doing nothing, or seeking assistance on their own.

It is important for all members of teams, partnerships, and collaborations to know how school districts and community organizations involve parents and caregivers so as to best shape the programs and services. As part of a formal connection process, written informed consent is the safest course of action for the school and community agency. Informed written consent outlines what services the parent/caregiver is authorizing. Consents are usually in effect for the current school year, but parents can withdraw consent at any time. Examples of services include, but are not limited to:

❖ Team-based problem solving

❖ Development of action plans

❖ Classroom behavioral support

❖ Skill development groups for anger management, conflict resolution, communication, or other life skills

❖ Recommendation for screening or assessment by a behavioral health professional to rule out substance abuse or another mental health issue

At times, parents and caregivers will refuse programs and services offered at the school. Often this is due to family concerns related to family privacy, stigma, and student confidentiality. Also, students may already be receiving services in the community outside of school, and parents view the school offerings as redundant and perhaps detrimental to the student's improvement. Schools document if a parent or caregiver refuses to participate. Parents and caregivers would sign a "refusal" form that documents that help was offered and they are not accepting the aid of the student support team at this time. The signed refusal of services does not relieve the district of its responsibility to do something to assist the child. The parents and caregivers can request the help of the team at some time in the future.

Many teams use a viewpoint checklist as a tool when initiating contact with a parent and caregiver (**Figure 5-3**). The **parent checklist** is concrete, positive, and strength-based with clear and reader-friendly language without educational and mental health jargon. It is in an easy-to-follow format and uses a language understood by the parents or caregivers. A team member typically contacts the parent/caregiver via a telephone call or maybe an e-mail. After the initial contact the form might be e-mailed, mailed, or even sent home with the child, depending on the parent's preference. A second tool that schools use is a brief **student support team flyer** to explain the student support team to parents, caregivers, and families (**Table 5-2**). The flyer can be included with other materials as well as shared in school-wide activities where families are present (e.g., school activities and athletic events).

Getting Ready for the Parent and Caregiver Conference   Team members will meet and talk with parents and caregivers. It can be daunting to invite them to a meeting and discuss problems. Remember that not everyone has had positive experiences with schools and educators. The goal in any **parent and caregiver conference** is to build a working relationship, if not a trusting one. Even if parents and caregivers are not convinced that their son or daughter needs the degree of assistance that the school does, it is best if the parent and caregiver know who to call if and when they are ready. Sometimes, a crisis brings the parent and caregiver to that readiness.

Set a time that is conducive to the parent and caregiver's schedule. It may be best to meet early in the morning before school, or later in the afternoon. Be as flexible as possible. Some parents and caregivers may not have transportation or be able to get public transit. In this case you could conduct a telephone conference, or perhaps a home-school visitor in the district can accompany several members of the team to meet the parent and caregiver in their home. Consider the following points when preparing for a meeting:

❖ *Optimize privacy:* Select a space that is private. Anticipate language or accessibility needs. Have an interpreter available (not a student).

❖ *Give a sense of what will be discussed:* Use the checklist (Figure 5-3) and ask that the parents and caregivers bring it with them.

❖ *Anticipate stress:* Remember that coming to school is stressful, particularly when there are mental health concerns to discuss. Some parents and caregivers report feeling anxious, angry, and/or overwhelmed by the experience. To ease their anxiety, use clear language free of educational jargon or psychobabble.

❖ *Be succinct:* There may be eight or nine key behaviors that are getting in the way of academic achievement. Prioritize them and select two or three that are the most serious and important to address.

❖ *Be specific:* Generally parents and caregivers have an idea about their child's academic achievement and progress. What they need are details. For example, be prepared to share in what subjects the child is currently failing or getting Ds in, and why. When discussing a behavior, share the behavior's frequency, intensity, and duration.

Dear Mr./Ms. *[Please type their names in AND customize it for each parent using the child's name and the parent's name]*

Welcome to our team! As a vital part of your child's team here at school, we want to gather some information from you about your child. **No one knows your child better than you do,** *and we ask you to work on this checklist so that we can get more information about the strengths and positive behaviors that you see in your child. Your insights are helpful to us as we work together to create plans to help promote his/her success at school. Please complete the following checklist and return in the attached envelope. If you prefer, please call me, and we can discuss these items over the telephone. Thanks so much for taking the time to help us.*

Thank you! [Type your name here] Telephone Number: _____-_____-_____

STRENGTHS *Please check all that apply to your child.*	**POSITIVE TRAITS AT HOME** *Please check all that describe your child's positive traits at home.*
❑ Is able to work independently ❑ Works well in a group ❑ Demonstrates desire/commitment to learn ❑ Demonstrates good logic/reasoning and decision making ❑ Exhibits leadership ❑ Is creative ❑ Accepts redirection/criticism easily ❑ Is considerate of others ❑ Good communication skills ❑ Cooperative ❑ Seems to value family support ❑ Possesses good interpersonal skills ❑ Demonstrates constructive use of time ❑ Helps others ❑ Strives to achieve his/her best ❑ Is connected to and likes school and staff ❑ Displays positive values (responsibility, honesty, equality, caring) ❑ Recognizes and respects appropriate boundaries and expectations ❑ Participates in extracurricular activities Other: _____ _____ _____	❑ Has a number of good friends ❑ Creative and imaginative in play ❑ Considerate of others ❑ Communicates well with adults, younger and older peers ❑ Appropriate sense of humor ❑ Organized ❑ Polite ❑ Cooperative ❑ Has a sense of hope for the future ❑ Shows interest in school and being successful ❑ Works hard ❑ Usually complies with family rules, curfews, routines, etc. ❑ Assists with household chores ❑ Participates in family activities, meals, etc. ❑ Shows care about appearance, health, etc. ❑ Demonstrates pride in self and possessions, keeps room reasonably neat ❑ Behavior is appropriate with peers and siblings ❑ Usually respectful toward parent(s)/caregiver(s), siblings, and others ❑ Deals with change easily Other: _____ _____

Listed below are several questions that will help us get to know your child better and be better able to help him/her to be more successful in school. Please take a few minutes to answer these questions.

- Other schools your child has attended _____
- Who lives in your household? _____
- Describe any recent changes at home that may be interfering with academic or behavioral progress _____
- What does your child tell you about school? _____
- Is your child currently receiving treatment from a physician or agency? _____Yes   _____No
- If yes, please explain _____

FIGURE 5-3   *(Continued)*

- Has your child had any outside evaluations for cognitive, emotional, or social reasons? ____Yes____No
- If yes, please explain _____
- What are your child's greatest personal strengths/interests? _____

Do you have concerns about...?
- Your child's academic progress?   _____Yes   _____No
  If yes, please explain _____
  _____
- Your child's behavior at home?   _____Yes   _____No
  If yes, please explain _____
  _____
- Your child's relationship with his/her peers?   _____Yes   _____No
  If yes, please explain _____
  _____
- Your child's emotional well-being?   _____Yes   _____No
  If yes, please explain _____
  _____
  _____

Parent/Caregiver Signature_____ Date_____

FIGURE 5-3 Parent/caregiver viewpoint checklist.

TABLE 5-2   Student Support Team Information Flyer for Parents, Caregivers, and Families

What is a student support team?
A student support team is a school-based team that meets regularly to discuss strategies and supports for students.

Who is on the student support team?
The student support team is composed of teachers, school counselor, nurse, vice principal, social worker, and professionals from community organizations.

When does a student's name get referred to the student support team?
When a student requires additional support or is having difficulty at school, the classroom teacher starts the problem-solving process. This should involve consultation with parents and other staff in the school, including the special education teacher and the in-school team. School staff may suggest academic accommodations or other strategies to support the student. When it is deemed that additional expertise should be involved in the problem-solving process, the student's name is referred to the student support team.

When your child's name is going to be referred to the student support team, this will be discussed with you and your consent to discuss your child will be requested. Parents are strongly encouraged to attend all student support team meetings and participate in making recommendations to determine the best way to support your child.

What is my role as a parent and caregiver?
You are an active participant in the student support team and are welcome to contribute to the discussion and ask questions.

What happens at a student support team meeting?

Student support team meetings are conducted in an informal atmosphere. One of the school staff will chair the meeting, introduce everyone present, and explain the purpose of the meeting. One of the team members will provide an overview of the situation to be discussed. Others, including you, are asked to provide information. You are encouraged to ask questions whenever you wish, and to join in the discussion.

At the end of the student support team meeting, there will likely be some agreed-upon recommendations. These may include, but are not limited to, the following:

❖ Suggested instructional strategies to support a student

❖ Suggested behavioral or social emotional supports for a student

❖ Recommendation that further testing or a formal assessment be completed

❖ Recommendation that an Individualized Education Program (IEP) be developed for a student

❖ Recommendations about community support options for a student/family

What happens after the student support team meeting?

After the student support team meeting, the recommendations are acted on. Recommendations of the student support team meeting are implemented, monitored over a period of time, and then evaluated. Information on the student's progress will be communicated between family and school.

❖ *Family structures differ:* In some situations, several meetings may be required to meet with sets of parents, stepparents, and caregivers.

❖ *Establish good ground rules:* Optimize time together by focusing on issues, not personalities, and keep the meeting on track.

Conducting the Conference   Select two or three team members so that you don't overwhelm the parents and caregivers. Establish roles (e.g., facilitator, information reviewer) and responsibilities for the meeting. Create an atmosphere of trust, open dialogue, and creative problem solving. All team members should be open and welcoming.

The facilitator meets and greets the parents and caregivers, introduces the other team members, and establishes the **parent or caregiver conference ground rules**. Also, the facilitator keeps the meeting moving, troubleshoots and promotes conflict resolution, and summarizes the content before bringing the meeting to a close.

The information reviewer outlines the two or three issues that concern the school and brought this group together. Before beginning the review, it is always best to start with a student's strengths.

Conduct the conference as follows:

❖ *Start with a warm welcome.* Thank the parent or caregiver for making time to meet. Be aware of what you say as well as how you say it. Convey empathy. Outline what will happen in the next 45 minutes or so. Describe the process that brought you together. Emphasize that this is a caring group of individuals and that this isn't a disciplinary action, but a helping mechanism.

❖ *Begin by discussing confidentiality.* Level with the parent or caregiver to assure them that all that you will discuss today is confidential. Only those who need to know specific things related to their work with the student will be told relevant information, such as strategies to work with the child better in class.

❖ *Ask, rather than tell.* After you have set the ground rules and discussed the school-based information, ask the parent or caregiver to share their concerns, observations, and expectations.

❖ *Use the parent's or caregiver's time efficiently.* Recognize that they have taken time from their day.

Communicating Personal Information

Communicating personal information continues to be an evolving area that is governed by law and regulation. Schools operate under the umbrella of health, safety, and welfare, so absolute confidentiality cannot be guaranteed. The question becomes how schools can guarantee the parents' and students' right to privacy while still providing what the school staff may need to work with the referred student and to protect other students and staff from harm.

Parents and Confidentiality

There are legal requirements that offer protection to students and parents regarding their mandatory participation in any helping program. Some of these are directly related to federal statutes. The Family Educational Rights and Privacy Act (FERPA) guarantees that parents have the right to inspect and review all educational records maintained by the school district. FERPA also requires that the school seek the written permission of the parents to release the information. Crisis situations are an exception to this rule. Also, directory information can be given to armed forces recruiters unless the parent opts out. In 2010, FERPA was amended again to allow districts and states to gather unidentified student information to evaluate the overall performance of the district.

Allowances are made in the statute for school employees who need to know. FERPA uses the term *legitimate educational interest.* This means that the team can share the information that may be needed to manage behavior or improve education, and no more.

Access to the written files is confidential. This means that a classroom teacher who is not on the team will not have the ability to view the files. The general professional standard is that access to these files is limited to the present team working with the student.

Schools must have a written policy of compliance with FERPA and must provide a copy to parents when requested. Information placed in a student assistance record must be objective and verifiable. This means all comments need to be observations rather than opinions. Teams look for verification of a cluster of behaviors from other school staff rather than using one teacher's subjective judgment.

Parents, as well as students who are emancipated, have the right to refuse services. Disclosures are guided by the need to know clause for school officials. When there is a need to involve someone other than school staff, informed written consent is required.

Professional training is required for teams to ensure compliance with state and federal laws protecting the privacy rights of parents and students. Schools must ensure that team members and others involved in the team process are knowledgeable about the laws and regulations governing students' and parents' right to privacy. We recommend the implementation of a regular schedule of professional development and legal updates. Stratified levels of training should be provided, based on the role and expertise required of the staff member.

Once the child reaches the age of majority (i.e., 18 years), the privacy rights enjoyed by the parents revert to the student. However, it is best practice to involve parents in school-focused issues as long as they are financially responsible for the young person. Some states have laws that allow students between 14 and 18 years of age to seek mental health or substance abuse treatment services without the consent of parents. It is always best for the school to refer the student to at least three agencies outside of the school if they want to pursue assistance in this manner.

Student Information: Parents and Caregivers

Many educators believe, and correctly so, that they work for the best interest of a child or adolescent. Yet, they work for principals, superintendents, and school boards as well. Parents and caregivers pay the taxes or tuition that support staff salaries. Beyond that, parents and caregivers are the primary decision makers in a child's life. The question of breaking a student's confidence and disclosing information about his or her health, welfare, or safety is always difficult. General best practice is the younger the child, the greater the responsibility is to parents and caregivers. According to Stone (2005), educators have the additional challenge of working in an organization designed to promote academic achievement. Students are required by law to be there, and the setting is designed for academic instruction rather than counseling. This increases the obligation to involve parents and caregivers when their child's health, welfare, or safety is in danger.

In summary, parents and caregivers have the right to see all files that the school maintains on students up to the age of 18. After 18, legally, the student has to give permission for the parents to see their school files. Best practice indicates that parents and caregivers be notified as part of any mental health intervention process and involved as part of the team. Written consent is optimal. Parents, caregivers, and students can refuse these services.

Student Information: Community Service Providers

Agency professionals often are part of a student support team. In order to attend meetings and have access to pertinent school files, agencies create a **letter of agreement (LOA)** with the school districts they serve. These documents outline the clinician's roles, responsibilities, and needs when in the school building.

Agency professionals are active participants on the team and bring a true multi-disciplinary focus to the teamwork.

When students need a screening or assessment, and the district refers the student to an in-school mental health treatment provider, the school must get written consent from the parent to release the student to the provider.

At times, children and teens need hospitalization to fully evaluate their condition and begin intensive treatment. Mental health records are confidential, and parents and caregivers cannot see them without student consent. At times, the treatment summary and recommendations are shared with the school. Once a file, in this case the treatment summary, becomes part of the school record, parents and caregivers can have access to it without the consent of the student, unless the child is age 18 or older.

Letters of agreement and releases of information are the policies and procedures that establish the roles and boundaries between the educational and human services domains. Laws for schools differ from the health and human services regulations that govern agency practice. When a treatment professional works on a school team, he or she follows all school laws, policies, and procedures, but also works within the constraints of his or her professional ethics.

A **release of information (ROI)** to other providers must be authorized by parents or caregivers. Schools generally deal with two types of ROIs. First, the parent or caregiver must sign a release of information for the school. This allows the school to give information about the student to select community providers for the purpose of complete assessment and treatment planning. Second, when working with a mental health clinician, it is a good but underused practice to ask parents and students to sign a release so that the professional can work with the school as part of the team and provide information so there is consistent progress toward treatment goals. As with consent, releases of information can be withdrawn at any time.

Summary

Two types of strategies connect children and adolescents to the mental health programs and services: structural and formal. The strategies are clear and offer user-friendly decision-making processes for students, families, and staff. Structural connection strategies are agreed upon and supported by the schools (and community organizations) and do not require parent or caregiver permission to access and participate in mental health programs and services. Formal connection strategies are agreed upon and supported by schools (and community organizations) and, depending on the state, may or may not require parent or caregiver permission to participate in a process to match the needs of a student and his or her family with existing mental health programs and services. Distinguishing elements of a formal connection strategy are referral, crisis determination, initial information collection, and parent or caregiver engagement and consent. Personal information about young people and their families is shared when making connections with mental programs and services. Schools operate under the umbrella of health, safety, and welfare, so absolute confidentiality cannot be guaranteed. The question becomes how schools can guarantee the parents', caregivers', and students' right to privacy while still providing what the staff may need to work with the referred student and to protect other students and staff from harm.

For Practice and Discussion

1. Most teenagers and children do not actively seek help for mental health concerns and problems for various reasons. What are some of the reasons? What would you say to a teenager when faced with their concerns?
2. Visit local schools to map the structural school community connections. Report how many you are able to identify and any differences that were found between schools (e.g., different districts, levels—elementary, middle, and high school).
3. You are working with Roberta Tyson, the district coordinator for student services from a southern California school district. Your job is to design a district-wide training including members of the school community mental health partnerships on the topic of referrals and initial information collection as part of connecting children and adolescents to mental health programs and services. The training is 90 minutes long. Prepare the training goals, learning objectives, outline, and activities.
4. You are a member of a student support team. You, along with a colleague, are going to meet with the parents of a middle school child who was referred to the team for concerns related to substance use. The parents have given consent for the child to work with the team. What are you going to do to prepare for the meeting? How might the preparation change for a high school or elementary school student? What if the mental health concern was for bullying, violence, or depression? How might this impact your preparation?
5. An eleventh-grade student does not want her parents to have access to her school records. The parents have a long history of involvement with their daughter. You are the team member working with the student and family. What do you recommend?

Key Terms

Crisis determination   94
Duration   97
Formal connection strategies   94
Frequency   97
Initial information collection   99
Intensity   97
Letter of agreement (LOA)   107
Parental consent   101
Parent and caregiver conference   102

Parent checklist   102
Parent or caregiver conference ground rules   105
Referral   95
Release of information (ROI)   108
Structural connection strategies   91
Student self-referral   96
Student support team flyer   102

References

Center for Mental Health in Schools at UCLA. (n.d.). *School-community partnerships: A guide.* Retrieved from http://www.smhp.psych.ucla.edu

Foster, S., Rollefson, M., Doksum, T., Noonan, D., Robinson, G., & Teich, J. (2005). *School Mental Health Services in the United States, 2002–2003* (DHHS pub. no. [SMA] 05-4068). Rockville, MD: Center for Mental Health Services, Substance Abuse, and Mental Health Services Administration. Retrieved from http://www.mentalhealth.samhsa.gov/media/ken/pdf/SMA05-4068/SMA05-4068.pdf

Stone, C. (2005). Cutting, eating disorders, and confidentiality. *ASCA School Counselor.* Retrieved from http://www.ascaschoolcounselor.org/article_content.asp?edition=91&section=140&article=800

Zeman, J., Shipman, K., & Suveg, C. (2002). Anger and sadness regulation: Predictions to internalizing and externalizing symptoms in children. *Journal of Child and Adolescent Psychiatry, 31*: 393–398.

SCHOOL COMMUNITY STAFF AND CHILD AND FAMILY PERSPECTIVES

In this chapter, we will:

✦ Illustrate two points of view regarding programs and services: school community staff and child and family

✦ Describe current school community mental health programs and services

✦ Discuss the school community staff point of view regarding programs and services

✦ Explain youth voice to engage and support children and adolescents

Scenarios

We have about 1300 students [in grades] 9–12. Over my years in the district, I have developed a lot of empathy for the students and parents facing mental health problems. For some families, it is the same old same old routine with their child. The parents are tired and burned out. They may have their own problems and concerns. The kids are problematic, scared (although they would never admit it), and sadly, lost. They experience problems without any clear or easy way to change. Some parents and families are blind and frozen in denial that the problem is as serious as it is. Other parents are caught off guard and willing to do anything, but just not sure what to do. One parent told me, "I was in a fog when we talked. I do not remember much of what you told me. That fog or denial was all that kept me from taking the bridge. It would take months until I could actually wrap my head around what was happening and find the strength to do what I needed to." Their kids too may be scared, but maybe not. It is hard to tell. In both situations, the teenagers as well as the parents and caregivers need to work hard and be resilient. Unfortunately, no matter how hard the teenager and the parent work, it may not be enough and so concerns and problems persist. I have also developed patience and empathy for administration and staff. Programs and services do not always happen as described, hoped for, or promised. There can be endless delays, miscommunications, as well as funding and staff changes. Do not get me wrong, many good programs and services work and help our kids and families. We have to be pragmatic when figuring out our strategies. It can be pretty complex and complicated. There can be a lot of hoops to jump through. It takes time; you have to be patient and persistent because there aren't very many instant solutions, which is hard.

Source: Rick Williams is a member of the Charleston, South Carolina, student support team at the James Island High School Charter School

I was a pretty motivated, bright, and determined young 15-year-old, but my folks would not support my goals of getting a college education and finding a good job. I had so many problems at home. I faced continual chaos and drama from my parents, and it was impossible for me to study, do my homework, and work with tutors. My grades were horrible. Finally, having no clue what to do, I ran away from home. I didn't know where to turn. Being on the streets, I got sad and scared, but I didn't stop going to school. I did not know what else to do. It has been one crazy journey with lots of bumps. Fortunately, I can talk to my parents now. I am living with an aunt. At school I meet weekly with a counselor and participate in a group run by the nurse for girls. I also got hooked up with some organizations in the community I never knew existed. My mom and dad probably didn't even know they were there. I'm glad I do now!

Source: Brionna, a student in a Berkeley Unified School District high school in California

Two Points of View: School Community Staff and Child and Family

The **school community staff point of view** is broad with knowledge and information on the range and diversity of available services and programs as well as the established procedures to participate in them (**Figure 6-1**). School community staff motivate and facilitate the **self-efficacy** of the child and family to participate and follow through with suggested services. Being a member of partnerships and collaborations, the school community staff may be able to draw upon guidance and resources (i.e., programs and services) across systems. For example, they may know about mental health services offered as part of juvenile justice programs

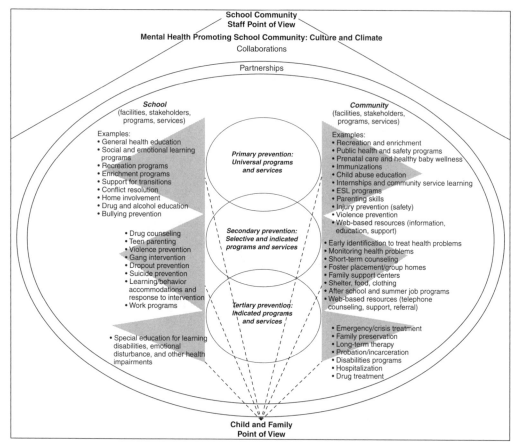

FIGURE 6-1 Two points of view of mental health programs and services.
Source: Adapted from Center for Mental Health in Schools at UCLA. (n.d.). School-community partnerships: A guide. UCLA Department of Psychology School Mental Health Project. Retrieved from http://www.smhp.psych.ucla.edu

or provided to foster families. At the same time, school community staff can become overwhelmed by the needs of the children, adolescents, and families being served. The support and synergy of the teams, partnerships, and collaborations are important to maintaining school community staffs' energy and commitment in the face of the challenges and struggles.

The **child and family point of view** focuses on the engagement and participation of the child or adolescent in need of services. Frequently, the child and family point of view of programs and services is narrow and concerned only with what is relevant to their particular mental health concern or problem (Figure 6-1). The general population of children, adolescents, and families will know about some of the primary prevention programs; however, they may not know or perceive them as primary prevention universal programs, but rather as school community programs and services in which their children participate. This is not to say they will not be aware of secondary and tertiary prevention programs and services, but rather they have not had cause to know and use them. Likewise, children, adolescents, and families addressing a mental health concern and problem will be focused on the programs and services relevant to them. They may or may not be aware of the student support teams, partnerships, and collaborations created to help. They probably will not know how to navigate the various options or know what exists across systems that might be available to them.

To familiarize you with generally available programs and services, the next section is a sample of mental health programs and services that exist in many school communities. Next discussed are the school community staff perceptions of the programs and services with a focus on engaging and supporting children and adolescents. Finally, youth voice is discussed as an approach to understanding their views of mental health programs and services.

Mental Health Programs and Services

Mental health programs and services are diverse and varied. Large urban districts such as the New York City Department of Education (1,042,277 students), Los Angeles Unified School District (667,251 students), Chicago Public Schools (413,694 students), and Miami–Dade County Public Schools (353,790 students) have complicated and complex networks of programs and services. The opposite is true for small school districts (districts of 2500 students or less) that educate a large percentage of all students. For example, California has the reputation of having many urban and suburban districts, but in fact, over 55 percent of California's districts serve fewer than 2500 students—80 percent of which serve fewer than 1500 students. Many of these districts are located in rural areas. The range of mental health programs and services found in small districts is far less complicated than in the large urban districts; however, the programs' diversity and their ability to address the mental health needs of youth may be restricted. Programs and services may be few with accessibility (distance) often being a barrier to receiving services. Listed and described in this section is a sample of mental health programs and services that exist in many school communities.

Classroom (Teacher) Strategies

School curriculum is the heart and soul of school. Classroom (teacher) strategies focus on the process of teaching and, in particular, student engagement. The primary concern for teachers is producing effective learning and ensuring that the student is truly engaged. This is especially important in preventing learning, behavioral, and emotional problems. Students expect to become engaged in an environment that both supports and challenges them to excel personally, socially, and academically. Teachers who make a difference in their students' lives share a number of characteristics, including being deeply interested in the students and in the material being taught, being adaptable to change, having high behavioral and academic expectations for students, and relating to students on their level. Teacher strategies are one of the areas where information is collected by the student support team. As part of the planning and recommendations, teacher strategies might be recommended.

Social and Emotional Learning

Social and emotional learning (SEL) is the process of developing fundamental social and emotional competencies in children. SEL programs are based on the understanding that many different kinds of problem behaviors are caused by the same or similar risk factors, and the best learning emerges from supportive relationships that make learning both challenging and meaningful. Effective SEL programs work to develop five core social and emotional competencies in students: self-awareness, social awareness, self-management, relationship skills, and responsible decision making.

Recent studies support that students who participate in school-based SEL programs improve significantly with respect to the following (Durlak J.A., Weissberg R.P., Dymnicki A.B., Taylor R.D., Schellinger K.B., 2011):

❖ Social and emotional skills

❖ Attitudes about themselves, others, and school

❖ Social and classroom behavior

❖ Conduct problems, such as classroom misbehavior and aggression

❖ Emotional distress, such as stress and depression

❖ Achievement test scores and school grades, including an 11-percentile-point gain in academic achievement

These positive results do not come at the expense of performance in core academic skills, but rather enhance academic achievement.

Special Education

Special education is defined as specially designed instruction and the related services needed by the student to benefit from that instruction. As part of special education, teachers adapt the content (what is taught), methodology (the process used to teach), or delivery of the curriculum to take account of the student's learning needs and to ensure that the student has access to the general curriculum provided to children without disabilities. The driving forces in special education are the student's Individualized Education Program (IEP) and the opportunity for students to make meaningful progress toward their IEP goals. The IEP spells out exactly what special education services a student will receive and why, and includes eligibility classification (learning disabled, emotionally disturbed, etc.), placement, services, academic and behavioral goals, a behavior plan if needed, percentage of time in regular education, and progress reports from teachers and therapists. **Table 6-1** lists special education services that might be found in a school.

TABLE 6-1 School Special Education Services	
Consultant teacher services	Provide direct and/or indirect services to students with disabilities enrolled full time in regular education classes, including career and technical education.
Related services	Supportive services required to help a student with a disability to benefit from special education. Such services include speech pathology and audiology, psychological services, physical and occupational therapy, recreation, early identification and assessment of disabilities in children, counseling and rehabilitation counseling services, and medical services for diagnostic or evaluation purposes. This category also includes transportation, school health services, social work services, and parent counseling and training.
Resource room	A separate special education classroom in a regular school building where some students with educational disabilities, such as specific learning disabilities, receive direct, specialized instruction and academic remediation and assistance with homework and related assignments as individuals or in small groups. These classrooms are staffed by special education teachers and sometimes paraprofessionals. The number of students in a resource room at a specific time varies by state, but generally consists of at most five students per teacher.
Collaborative support service/ team-taught classes	Provide special education in regular education classrooms. Today, more special education students are taught in regular classrooms, and collaboration is increasing. Collaboration helps to ensure children with learning disabilities get a free, appropriate public education, including specialized instruction, in a regular classroom.
Special classes	Classes consisting of students with disabilities who have been grouped together because of similar individual needs for the purpose of being provided a special education program. Such students receive their primary instruction within the special education classroom. Students may be in special classes for only part of the day or for certain subjects.
Continuum of placements	Settings that have students with disabilities who may or may not be with typically developing peers. They may be placed in a separate school or a residential school.
Home or hospital instruction	Student receives instruction at home or in a hospital program.

Crisis Response Plans

Escalating levels of violence in schools, natural disasters, and other crises are some of the most difficult and confounding issues educators face today. School districts' **crisis response plans** focus on four key areas at both the district and school level: prevention/mitigation, preparedness, response, and recovery. Emergency plans include community and first responders and address responses to the multitude of hazards that can impact a school and its related activities. They help educators provide a safe, thriving environment in which students can learn and staff can work. School emergency planning and practice help school staff know how to lead their students through a crisis situation. It is especially important for schools to have written protocols and action steps (i.e., a checklist) to respond to students in crisis at the school and classroom level. Knowing how to respond during a crisis will help everyone involved to remain calm, understand their roles, and act as safely and efficiently as possible. Many districts and their schools have crisis response teams composed of staff that are specially trained.

From toxic spills to a student medical emergency, crisis planning and practice provide school and district personnel with concrete actions they can take immediately. This requires planning and practice with community responders from the district level down to the individual school. Families trust schools to keep their children safe during the day and expect school staff to be properly equipped to handle emergencies when they do occur. By working with teachers, principals, and staff, parents/guardians can provide resources and assistance to support their school's emergency preparedness. If it is determined that a student is in crisis, the crisis response plan immediately becomes operational until such time as the crisis has passed. At that time, the student may once again be referred to the support team for case management or follow-up and support.

School Counselors, Mental Health Counselors, Social Workers, and Psychologists

School counselors, **mental health counselors**, **social workers**, and **psychologists** employed by the school or school district frequently offer curriculum-based programs and classroom guidance to enhance social and emotional functioning, focusing on a variety of mental health and life skills topics such as anger management, prevention of violence and bullying, conflict resolution, problem solving, resisting peer pressure, communication skills, substance abuse prevention, and character education. They may provide counseling and support in individual or small group counseling sessions, as well as in support groups designed to assist with specific issues such as social skills, self-esteem, and depression stemming from issues such as divorce or bereavement.

School Nurse

The role of the **school nurse** encompasses both health and educational goals. Students today may face family crises, homelessness, immigration, poverty, and violence, which increase both their physical and mental health needs. School nurses perform a critical role within the school health program by addressing the major health problems experienced by children. This role includes providing preventive and screening services, health education, assistance with decision making about health, and immunization against preventable diseases. In addition, school nurses may provide interventions for acute and chronic illness, injuries and emergencies, communicable diseases, obesity, substance use and abuse, adolescent pregnancy, mental health, dental disease, nutrition, and sexually transmitted infections.

Evidence-Based Programs

Evidence-based programs can be conceptualized as the delivery of optimal care through integration of current best scientific evidence, clinical expertise and experience, and preferences of individuals, families, organizations, and communities. Evidence-based health promotion interventions identify the priority populations that benefited from the intervention and the conditions under which the intervention works, and may indicate the change mechanisms that account for their effects. A defining characteristic of evidence-based interventions is the use of health theory in both developing the intervention approach and evaluating the intervention.

Response to Intervention

Response to Intervention (RtI) is a general education framework integrating assessment and intervention within a multi-level prevention system to maximize student achievement and to reduce academic problems. With RtI, schools use academic data to identify students at risk for poor learning outcomes, monitor student progress, provide evidence-based interventions and adjust the intensity and nature of those interventions depending on a student's responsiveness, and identify students with learning disabilities or other disabilities. Some in the field have designed positive behavioral interventions using the RtI framework.

Positive Behavioral Interventions and Supports

Improving student academic and behavior outcomes is about ensuring all students have access to the most effective and accurately implemented instructional and behavioral practices and interventions possible. **Positive Behavioral Interventions and Supports (PBIS)**, sometimes referred to as School-wide Positive Interventions and Supports (SWPBIS), is a systems approach that creates a positive social environment and provides behavioral supports needed to promote a climate conducive to learning for all students. PBIS is not a prepackaged curriculum or program. It is a decision-making framework that guides selection, integration, and implementation of the best evidence-based academic and behavioral practices to improve all students' academic and behavioral outcomes. The concept is to evaluate and devise unique support systems that meet the cultural and programmatic needs of each school. The approach is grounded in recent advances in applied behavior analysis, instructional design, mental health, and education reform. PBIS uses three tiers of support as seen in **Figure 6-2**:

1. **Primary Prevention Practices**: Provides proactive support for students in all locations at all times.

2. **Secondary Prevention Practices**: Targets students at risk for behavioral problems and educational failure.

3. **Tertiary Prevention Practices**: Provides intensive support for students with chronic patterns of problem behavior.

PBIS is a school-wide system that can be developed at the elementary, middle, and/or high school level.

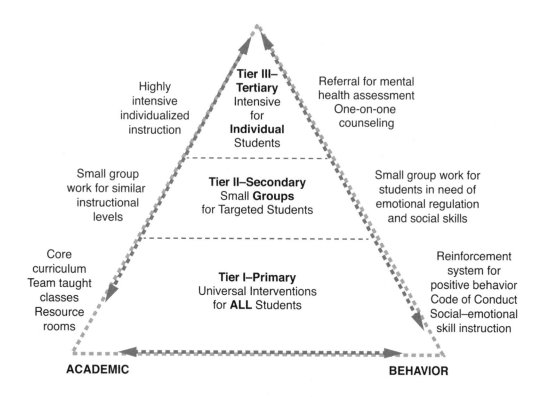

FIGURE 6-2   Examples of practices in schools implementing RtI and PBIS.

PBIS is a school-wide or district-wide system of positive behavioral support, which includes the following components:

a. An agreed-upon and common approach to discipline
b. A positive statement of purpose
c. A small number of positively stated expectations for all students and staff
d. Procedures for teaching these expectations to students
e. A continuum of procedures for encouraging displays and maintenance of these expectations
f. A continuum of procedures for discouraging displays of rule-violating behavior
g. Procedures for monitoring and evaluating the effectiveness of the discipline system on a regular and frequent basis

Evaluation is an integral part of PBIS. Specifically designed tools are available to monitor the degree of implementation of the three tiers of PBIS, as well as the extent to which implementation is associated with improved school safety and improved student outcomes.

Community Mental Health Agencies and Programs

County agencies are planning for the integration of children's services and are asking local schools for their input. This process takes time and requires effort, but results in the reduction of duplicated services and faster delivery. Mental health agencies and programs based in the community provide services in a number of categories (**Table 6-2**). Some are done on site at the school, whereas others are done in the community. These services reflect the process of families, youth, teachers, counselors, nurses, community members, clergy, child-care workers, principals, public officials, and lawyers coming together to identify gaps in services, advocate for funding, champion the need, and design, implement, and staff the programs and services. Schools and communities work to develop and engage as many of these programs and services as possible to address the mental health concerns and problems of the students.

Alternative Education Programs

Alternative education programs are generally those educational programs that address the needs of a particular student population. They can be enrichment programs such as those found in magnet schools, or they can be developed to support students at risk. Here, we are concerned with the latter, and then only those related to students enrolled in public schools, although they may be in other physical placements. School districts create and employ alternative education programs to deal with students whose challenges include oppositional disruptive behavior, multiple suspensions, and aggression (Lange & Sletten, 1995). Other issues such as learning difficulties, teen pregnancy, drug and alcohol

TABLE 6-2	Traditional and Innovative Mental Health Programs and Services in Schools and Communities	
Type	**Service**	**Program Characteristics**
Child Find and screening	Screenings	❖ Required pediatrician and EPSDT (Early Periodic Screening, Diagnosis, and Treatment) ❖ On-site (e.g., school, community center, workplace) mental health screening and information ❖ Child Find is a continuous process of public awareness activities, screening, and evaluation designed to *locate, identify, and refer as early as possible* all young children with disabilities and their families who are in need of Early Intervention Program (Part C) or Preschool Special Education (Part B/619) services of the Individuals with Disabilities Education Act (IDEA)
	Consultation and education services	❖ Policy and procedure review and development ❖ Mental health education and program planning, implementation, and evaluation ❖ Staff training ❖ Parent education and information
Pediatric interventions		❖ Screening, assessment, and medication by primary care provider ❖ Vaccinations and preventative care
Mental health	Case management	❖ Individual case support and management
	Emergency services	❖ Crisis situation intervention to aid and advise ❖ Emergency numbers operate 24 hours a day
	Supportive counseling	❖ Traditional outpatient counseling ❖ Individual, group, family, and couple formats
	School-based mental health treatment	❖ Satellite outpatient office in school ❖ Therapeutic classroom
	Home-based services (mobile therapy)	❖ Delivered primarily in family's home; also available in other community settings ❖ Committed to family preservation and reunification ❖ "Ecological" perspective and involve working with the community ❖ Flexible service delivery hours to meet needs of families ❖ Multifaceted services: education, counseling, skill training, etc.

(Continues)

TABLE 6-2	Traditional and Innovative Mental Health Programs and Services in Schools and Communities *(Continued)*	
Type	**Service**	**Program Characteristics**
	Day treatment models in schools	❖ Educational assessment and planning ❖ Special schools that provide full-day educational programs ❖ On-site mental health services linked to in-home services for families and full-time residential schools
	Day treatment (partial hospitalization)	❖ Falls in the middle of the continuum of care, between inpatient and outpatient ❖ Setting varies from hospital-based to school-based ❖ Considered most intensive of long-term, nonresidential mental health services available to children ❖ Can include special education, counseling, vocational education, crisis intervention, recreational, etc.
	High-fidelity wrap-around process	❖ A family and a mental health team develop, implement, and fine-tune a plan of care that is individualized to achieve positive outcomes for the family
	Family therapy	❖ Counseling in which members of a family are treated ❖ Members of the family counseled to encourage all members to partake in open communication and healing
	Residential treatment	❖ Extended treatment in restricted setting ❖ Multifaceted services: education, counseling, skill training, etc.
	Inpatient psychiatric care	❖ Short-term (typically less than 2 weeks) care in psychiatric hospital due to crisis ❖ Emergency room service, crisis support ❖ Evaluation and treatment recommendation
Substance use disorder	Prevention	❖ Evidence-based education programs to develop knowledge, life skills, and healthy attitudes about ATOD use ❖ Early identification of internal and environmental risks including fetal alcohol/drug spectrum disorders (FASDs) and targeted intervention services

		❖ Early identification and intervention with youth risk behaviors (DUI, school policy violations) providing appropriate level of care, education with targeted curriculum, and student support programs
	Intervention	❖ Screening, brief intervention, and referral to treatment (SBIRT) ❖ Primary care centers, hospital emergency rooms, trauma centers, and other community settings provide opportunities for early intervention with at-risk substance users before more severe consequences occur
	Treatment	❖ Outpatient addiction treatment programs ❖ Partial hospital or day treatment programs ❖ Free-standing residential addiction treatment centers ❖ Long-term residential treatment or extended care programs ❖ Therapeutic communities ❖ Adolescent- and teen-focused treatment programs ❖ Online or "e-therapy" ❖ Medication-assisted therapies
	Support groups and aftercare	❖ Alcoholics Anonymous (AA), Narcotics Anonymous (NA), and other 12-step-like programs ❖ Al-Anon holds regular meetings for spouses and other significant adults in an alcoholic's life; Alateen is geared to children of alcoholics
Child welfare	Family-based treatment	❖ Multidimensional family therapy (MDFT)
	Therapeutic foster care	❖ Least restrictive form of care among residential services ❖ Provides treatment for troubled children within private homes of trained families ❖ Combines family-based care with specialized treatment
	Respite services	❖ Provided both in child's home and in out-of-home settings by trained respite providers

(Continues)

Type	Service	Program Characteristics
TABLE 6-2 Traditional and Innovative Mental Health Programs and Services in Schools and Communities (*Continued*)		
	Group homes for specific populations	❖ Created for children and adolescents who cannot function in the family setting, but do not require institutional or residential care ❖ Child is maintained in the community and continues to be involved in community life up to his or her best ability ❖ Typically limited to eight or fewer residents
	Independent living	❖ Residential programs helping young adults ages 18 to 25 successfully achieve independence ❖ Assist youth in planning for education and career, and working to resolve personal and family problems
Juvenile justice: corrections	School-based probation/juvenile corrections	❖ Designed for youth on probation for minor offenses or youth who have been adjudicated through the courts ❖ Some corrections programs are wilderness-type programs; others are secured residential programs ❖ Some youth may be placed in adult institutions. ❖ Balanced and restorative justice (BARJ)
Community- and faith-based supports	Alternative activities	❖ Mental health promotion activities focused on social competency and support
	Faith-based programs	❖ Individual, group, family, and couples counseling based on religious principles ❖ Addresses spiritual concerns ❖ Prayer is an integral part of the programs
	Self-help groups	❖ Community-based peer and social support ❖ Assistance for seeking help and referral (NAMI) ❖ Sense of belonging
	Complementary and alternative medicine	❖ Body–mind focus ❖ Holistic approaches focused on stress management and wellness

Key: ATOD = alcohol, tobacco, and other drugs; DUI = driving under the influence; NAMI = National Alliance on Mental Illness

issues, juvenile justice involvement, truancy, or weapons possession are also found in alternative education programs. Placements and type of program vary, but most are characterized by the following:

- ❖ Safe and caring school climate
- ❖ Mutual respect between teachers and students
- ❖ Student, parent, and community involvement in program development
- ❖ Individualized student support (counseling, groups, therapy)
- ❖ Individualized and small group instruction and teams; independent learning
- ❖ Alternative settings
- ❖ Flexibility
- ❖ Freedom from some rules and regulations that apply to districts and other schools
- ❖ Review of student progress on a regular basis
- ❖ Evaluation of program implementation
- ❖ Content that is meaningful and relates to students' lives

Child Welfare System

The **child welfare system** is a group of services designed to promote the well-being of children by ensuring safety, achieving permanency, and strengthening families to care for their children successfully. Although the primary responsibility for child welfare services rests with the states, the federal government plays a major role in supporting states in the delivery of services through funding of programs and legislative initiatives such as the Child Abuse Prevention and Treatment Act (CAPTA).

Most families first become involved with their local child welfare system because of a report of suspected child abuse or neglect (sometimes called child maltreatment). Child maltreatment is defined by CAPTA as serious harm (neglect, physical abuse, sexual abuse, and emotional abuse or neglect) caused to children by parents or primary caregivers, such as extended family members or babysitters. Child maltreatment also can include harm that a caregiver allows to happen or does not prevent from happening to a child. In general, child welfare agencies do not intervene in cases of harm to children caused by acquaintances or strangers. These cases are the responsibility of law enforcement. It is important to remember that each state has its own laws that define abuse and neglect, state the reporting obligations of individuals, and describe required state and local child protective services agency interventions. For state-by-state information about civil laws related to child abuse and neglect, visit the Child Welfare Information Gateway website at www.childwelfare.gov/systemwide/laws_policies/state (Child Welfare Information Gateway, 2011).

Family Resource Centers

Family resource centers are sometimes called family support centers, family centers, parent–child resource centers, family resource schools, or parent education centers. Family resource centers serve diverse populations and are located in a variety of community settings, including churches, school buildings, hospitals, housing projects, restored buildings, and new structures. Family resource centers promote both the strengthening of families through formal and informal support and the restoration of a strong sense of community. They provide caring, affordable, and high quality health care and supportive services to everyone, with a special commitment to uninsured, low income, and medically underserved persons. Services may include:

❖ Health care

❖ Drop-in centers

❖ Home visiting

❖ Job training

❖ Substance abuse prevention

❖ Violence prevention

❖ Services for children with special needs

❖ Parent skill training needs

❖ Mental health or family counseling

❖ Child care

❖ Literacy

❖ Respite and crisis care services

❖ Assistance with basic economic needs

❖ Housing

Justice System

Justice system involvement in schools strives to improve the academic and career and technical training of youth who are involved in the juvenile justice system. Officers can also work in a preventative way with the general student population. Two examples of justice system school involvement are **school resource officers** (**SROs**) and **school-based probation officers** (**SBPOs**). School resource officer programs help to bridge the gap between police officers and young people through law-related education, student counseling, and law enforcement in the schools. School-based probation officers work directly with students under court supervision so that they are able to continue going to school.

Parent Engagement

Critical to promoting the mental health of students is **parent engagement**. Parents are recognized as allies to schools, and their roles include acting as decision makers and participating on community interagency teams to help design, implement, and evaluate services and curriculum for their children (Osher & Osher, 2002).

Community Coalitions

Community coalitions are a popular strategy found in many schools and communities to promote mental health among students and families. Typically, coalitions consist of a broad range of organizations and individuals (e.g., parents, teachers, administrators, community members, business leaders, social service organization staff, governmental leaders) who share a commitment to a particular issue. The coalition is both part of the school and part of the larger community. Davies (1991) notes that the schools most successful at creating coalitions will likely be the ones where the need is more broadly recognized and where substantial numbers of teachers, staff, parents, and other community members can agree on the nature of the problems and needs to be addressed.

School Community Staff Point of View of Programs and Services

Members of teams, partnerships, and collaborations have the big picture of the school community mental health programs and services. They are concerned with three issues. First, that programs and services in the school community are constantly changing. Second is having current information on the programs and services. Third is to help children and adolescents follow through on recommendations to participate in the programs and services.

Implementation Process

All of the programs and services in the school and community, even the school curriculum, are in a constant and continual cycle of implementation. Every year there are new teachers, retiring and transferring teachers, new community organization staff, staff getting promotions or leading new projects, and staff on family or medical leave dealing with personal concerns. To help understand the flux that programs and services experience, regardless of whether they operate in schools, community organizations, hospitals, government offices, or public health agencies, Fixsen et al (2005) proposed a six-phase implementation cycle. The cycle can help staff gauge the capacity of programs and services to meet the needs of the youth and families recommended to them.

1. *Exploration and adoption* is program planning, including needs assessments and programmatic decisions about mission, goals, objectives, interventions, outcomes, policies, and procedures. Achieving acceptance and support for the program in the setting is part of this stage. Frequently in schools and communities you will hear about new legislation and funding for an initiative to work with a particular group of youth. There can be a lot of excitement about the possibilities; however, the reality of the funding and staffing and the eventual program and service capacity will be unknown.

2. *Program and service installation* focuses on the structural supports necessary to initiate a program or service. The funding is usually available. Now the need will be for personnel and supportive policy as well as creating referral mechanisms, reporting frameworks, and outcome expectations. Often in this phase we find out that we need to realign current staff, hire and train

new staff members, secure appropriate space, or purchase needed technology (for example, cell phones or computers). These activities and their associated start-up costs are necessary first steps in beginning a new program in any setting.

3. *Initial implementation* means operating a program or service for the first time with the children, adolescents, and their families. No amount of planning and discussion can account for all the complexities involved when staff members run a program with the program participants; there are too many unknowns until a program has been operating for some period of time. During initial implementation, the compelling forces of fear of change, inertia, and investment in the status quo combine with the inherently difficult and complex work of implementing something new at a time when the program is struggling to begin and when confidence in the decision to do the program is being tested. Learning from this initial experience, and in particular from unanticipated consequences (both good and bad), is important to meeting the students' needs. Surprises and challenges may change the trajectory of the program, but hopefully will not derail its work to address youth's mental health needs. The strength of many programs can be traced to what is learned during the initial implementation about program participants' needs, critical staff skills, program policies and procedures, and the match between the program interventions and participant needs.

4. *Full operation* occurs when a program is operating with a full staffing complement and the full participation of children and adolescents. All of the realities of doing business are impinging on the newly implemented program. Once an implemented program and service is fully operational, referrals are flowing according to the agreed-on inclusion or exclusion criteria, practitioners are carrying out the evidence-based practice or program with proficiency and skill, managers and administrators are supporting and facilitating the new practices, and the setting has adapted to the presence of the program. In this phase of the cycle, the anticipated benefits are realized as the program staff members become skillful and the procedures and processes become routine.

5. *Innovation* happens over time as staff, stakeholders, and participants learn what works with the children, adolescents, and families they serve. Changes in staff, feedback from evaluations, and new conditions present opportunities to refine and expand the program. Ensuring cultural competence of the program is an important part of program innovation.

6. *Sustainability* is about long-term program operation. Skilled practitioners and other well-trained staff leave and must be replaced with other skilled practitioners and well-trained staff. Leaders, funding streams, and program requirements change. New social problems arise; partners come and go. External systems change with some frequency; political alliances are only

temporary; and champions move on to other causes. In spite of all these changes, program staff, stakeholders, and participants adjust without losing the functional components of the program or letting the program die from a lack of essential financial and stakeholder support. The goal during this phase is the long-term survival and continued effectiveness of the implementation site in the context of a changing environment.

Current Information on the Programs and Services

Having current information on programs and services is critical to being responsive to the needs of children, adolescents, families, and caregivers. Staff want and need to know what is happening in the school and community to make effective use of all mental health programs and services. Critical is for staff to take time to consider how to stay updated and current. They have to consider what is available and what might work best in an age of emerging technologies that includes smartphones, Facebook, Google Groups, apps, computer notebooks, and tablets that provide endless options. Having the information on a hard drive on an office computer may provide security, but would be difficult to access when attending a meeting in a location other than the office.

Building a personal **information network** is recommended. Consider summary information such as a description of the curricula, programs, and services; phone number and address; e-mail address; URLs for websites; and a contact person. Collect information from colleagues, children, adolescents, families, and caregivers; handbooks of agencies; newspapers; professional meetings; the phone book; the Web; and any community service directories produced by other agencies. The Internet has increased access to information about many mental health agencies, and e-mail and shared databases have facilitated communication between programs and services.

Building an information network also involves knowing and having personal contact with many school community professionals to help navigate the many programs and services. Being active with partnerships and collaborations is one of the best methods to establish communication with colleagues. It helps build credibility as a serious professional interested in building and maintaining networks among colleagues on the teams, partnerships, and collaborations. Furthermore, it creates social support among staff and a shared history of working together to solve problems and deal with difficult situations and challenges.

Motivate and Facilitate Child and Family Self-Efficacy to Participate and Follow Through

Across primary, secondary, and tertiary prevention programs as a member of a team, partnership, or collaboration, one of the most important staff roles is to motivate and facilitate children, adolescents, parents, caregivers, and family members' self-efficacy to participate and follow through on plans and recommendations. In this role, staff are facilitators, making connections and creating a pathway for a person to link to needed mental health programs and services. Although this is true for all children, adolescents, and families, it is particularly important for those youth and their families who are moving through the individual mental health concerns and problems intervention process approach.

The concept of self-efficacy is a construct of social cognitive theory developed by Albert Bandura (2004). It is a person's confidence in his or her ability to pursue a behavior (take a specific action, perform a specific task). Working across the prevention programs as a member of your teams, partnerships, and collaborations, you are going to want people to take an action. According to Bandura (2004), self-efficacy is behavior-specific and in the present. It is not about the past or future. Self-efficacy plays a central role in behavior change and mental health. Bandura (2004) notes that, unless people believe that they can produce the desired change by their own efforts, there will be very little incentive to put in that effort. In your member role as a facilitator, you will work with people to develop their ability and confidence to take actions that create a mental health promoting culture and climate for others as well as for themselves.

A number of strategies are used to build self-efficacy. For example, working with young people to participate and follow through on their recommendation. If there are a lot of steps to making the recommended connections, break them down into practical and doable steps. Recruit role models (i.e., peer helpers) and mentors who can work with you to demonstrate what to say (i.e., role play). Talk with the child or teenager using persuasion and reassurance that he or she has the ability to take action. Finally, recognize that taking action is stressful. Work with the child or teenager on how to manage and reduce the stress he or she might be feeling.

Youth Voice to Engage and Support Children and Adolescents

The child and family point of view is filtered through many lenses. The three most prominent are child, parent (family), and culture. In this section we will focus on how to understand children and adolescents' point of view of mental health programs and services for the purpose of their engagement and participation. We want to hear their voices, understand their point of view, and get their input to shape and direct the programs and services.

Adding the voice of young people is central to promoting the mental health of children and adolescents. It is important to know how adults in the school community make all youth feel supported. We want to know young people's perceptions of how adults respond to youth with mental health concerns and problems. It is how we can engage youth and support their participation in mental health programs and services, regardless of their particular concern and problem. One approach to understanding the point of view of children and adolescents is youth voice.

Youth Voice

Youth voice refers to the distinct ideas, opinions, attitudes, knowledge, and actions of young people as a collective body. The term *youth voice* often groups together a diversity of perspectives and experiences, regardless of backgrounds, identities, and cultural differences. It is frequently associated with the successful application of a variety of youth development activities, including service learning, youth research, and leadership training. Engaging youth voice is an essential element of effective organizational development among school community mental health programs and services.

Fletcher and Vavrus (2006) proposed a five-step process to engage young people to share their voice. Working at each level of prevention programs and services you can implement the process both with groups of youth and individually. If we want youth to participate we need their feedback on what works.

❖ *Step 1: Listen to young people:* Successfully engaging young people in social change inherently requires listening to children and youth. Personal assumptions, organizational barriers, and cultural expectations are often obstacles to listening to young people. One-to-one conversations, group discussions, youth action research, youth-created media, or artistic expression can be successful avenues.

❖ *Step 2: Validate young people:* When children and youth speak, it is not enough to just nod your head. However, validating young people does not mean automatically agreeing with what is said, either. It is important to offer young people sincere comments, criticism, and feedback. Disagreeing with children and youth lets young people know that you actually heard what was said, thought about it, and that you have your own knowledge or opinion that you think is important to share with them and that you feel they are entitled to because they shared their perspectives. Young people must know that democracy is not about autonomous authority, and that a chorus of people, including young people but not exclusive to young people, is responsible for what happens throughout our communities.

❖ *Step 3: Authorize young people:* Young people are repeatedly condemned, denied, or abandoned every day because of the identities they possess. Democracy inherently requires *ability*, which comes in the form of experience and knowledge. Authorizing young people means going beyond historical expectations for children and youth by actively providing the training, creating the positions, and allowing the space they need in order to affect change.

❖ *Step 4: Mobilize young people:* Transitioning from passive participants to active change agents and leaders requires young people actually taking action to create change. Mobilizing children and youth with authority allows them to affect cultural, systemic, and personal transformation in their own lives and the lives of others. It also encourages adults to actively acknowledge young people as partners throughout society.

❖ *Step 5: Reflect about young people:* Social change led by and with young people is not and cannot be a vacuous event that affects only young people or the immediate situation. Children, youth, and adults should take responsibility for learning from social change by engaging in conscious critical reflection that examines assumptions, reactions, outcomes, and change. Young people and adults can also work together to identify how to sustain and expand the cycle of youth engagement by applying what is learned through reflection to the first step of the cycle.

Whether we are working at the primary, secondary, or tertiary prevention level, youth (and families) appreciate and participate when asked to help define the effectiveness of different programs and services intended to reduce negative peer behaviors, along with the harmful impact that often accompanies those behaviors. Mitra (2004) found that high school students who were given opportunities to voice their opinions regarding school community programs and services made gains in three characteristics associated with positive youth development: agency, belongingness, and competence. When students felt their ideas were heard, they increased their ability to articulate opinions to others, constructed new identities as change makers, and developed a greater sense of leadership (agency). Opportunities for youth to develop positive forms of identification led to improved interactions with teachers, increased attachment to school, and willingness to develop relationships with caring adults (belongingness). As students worked with teachers to develop leadership skills, they also developed problem solving, facilitation, and public speaking skills (competence). Oldfather (1995) found that enhancing student voice in the school community gave disconnected youth a sense of ownership and helped them to reconnect to their school community. Student voice opportunities helped young people to gain a stronger sense of their own abilities and build student awareness so they could make changes in their school community for themselves and others. Nixon and Davis (2010) worked with youth to compile and document effective interventions to help adults and youth reduce bullying and harassment in their own school community.

One of the most powerful strategies at the local level to gain youth voice and perspective is **PhotoVoice** (Wang, 1999). PhotoVoice is a method mostly used in the field of community development, public health, and education, which combines photography with grassroots social action. Youth already post photos and videos through social media such as Facebook, Twitter, Instagram, and text messaging to represent their lives. With PhotoVoice, youth are asked to represent their community, school, family, or point of view by taking photographs and videos, discussing them together, developing narratives to go with their photos and videos, and conducting outreach or other action. PhotoVoice as a strategy of youth voice attempts to bring the perspectives of children and adolescents to impact education and social services available in the school community. PhotoVoice is a powerful approach to engage youth (Community Tool Box, 2013):

1. *The rewards of taking photographs are immediate.* A camera, especially a digital one, produces nearly instant results, thereby encouraging participants to continue.

2. *Photography is fun and creative.* Often, survival is the main focus of people living in difficult circumstances. The opportunity to create art can be a powerful and fulfilling experience, and can lead to viewing oneself in a different and more positive light. In addition, for many people, it opens the door to talent they didn't know they had.

3. *Taking photographs or videos of familiar scenes and people can change participants' perceptions about their social and physical environment.* When they're forced to think about how they want to picture the scenes they're recording, participants themselves may start to see those scenes differently and to think about alternatives in new ways.

4. *Basic photography is easy to learn and accessible to almost everyone.* Anyone who can see and hold a camera, from children as young as four or five, to people with disabilities, to seniors, can take pictures. They may not be artistically excellent, but they will tell a story. Even those who can't see or hold a camera can participate with the help of someone who can, by indicating what they want pictured.

5. *"A picture is worth a thousand words."* Seeing what someone else sees is more powerful than being told about it. Effective advocacy conveys a need for change, and photos or videos can almost always make a far better case than words alone.

6. *Images can be understood regardless of language, culture, or other factors.*

7. *Policy makers can't deny reality when it's staring them in the face.* It is often easy for policy makers to assume—or to claim—that anyone with a need or problem is exaggerating it. When faced with photos or videos of actual conditions, they have to acknowledge reality.

Involve young people in the partnerships and collaborations. Adding youth voice can be a powerful force on the legislation and public policy that shape and fund the school community mental health programs and services. State youth advisory councils, community youth mapping, and youth-run grant programs are three examples of such efforts.

Create and Support State Youth Advisory Councils   To ensure the voices of youth are heard and play a meaningful role in shaping youth policy, state policymakers can pass legislation to create statewide youth advisory bodies, such as youth councils, that work with legislators, executives, and state children's cabinets. Quality state-level youth advisory structures institutionalize youth voice in the policy-making process. Maine's Legislative Youth Advisory Council, for example, allows its youth members to conduct public hearings, draft legislation, and make recommendations on proposals being considered by the legislature. The council is co-chaired by a member of the state legislature and a young person, and members of the state's children's cabinet regularly attend the Youth Advisory Council meetings.

Involve Youth in Local Mapping and Planning Efforts   To better understand the resources available to youth in their communities and to ensure that community development reflects the needs of youth, state policy makers can support involving youth in local community mapping and municipal/state planning efforts. State policy makers can facilitate and fund community youth mapping, a process developed by the AED Center for Youth Development and Policy Research that enables youth to evaluate and analyze local resources and develop recommendations for future funding, development, and policy. The Texas Workforce Commission Youth Program Initiative offers training and resources to local communities to facilitate their youth-led processes of mapping services for youth. In addition, state policy makers can require the inclusion of youth in local planning processes. In 2004, Louisiana passed the Children and Youth Planning Boards Act, which mandated that local jurisdictions create children and youth planning boards to assist in the assessment, alignment, coordination, and measurement of all available services and programs that address the needs of children and youth.

Establish/Support Youth-Run Grant Programs   States can create and support youth-run grant programs that enable young people to create funding priorities and criteria, design and review applications, award funds to youth projects, and monitor and report on implementation of proposals. Such involvement amplifies youth priorities and their implementation while allowing youth to deeply engage in policy, planning, and decision making with their peers. The Arizona Governor's Youth Commission, for example, is composed of youth commissioners from across the state, and is responsible for administering grants for youth-driven projects, such as the Alcohol Retailer Mapping in Proximity to Youth Mini-Grant.

Summary

Mental health programs and services are diverse and varied and can be viewed from two points of view. The school community staff point of view is broad with knowledge and information on the range and diversity of available services and programs as well as the established procedures to participate in them. Members of teams, partnerships, and collaborations have the big picture of the school community's mental health programs and services. They are concerned with three issues: programs and services in the school community are constantly changing; having current information on the programs and services; and helping children and adolescents follow through on recommendations to participate in the programs and services. The child and family point of view focuses on the engagement and participation of the child or adolescent in need of services. Frequently, the child and family point of view of programs and services is narrow and concerned only with those programs or services relevant to their particular mental health concern or problem. Part of the child and family point of view focuses on understanding the perceptions of children and adolescents to engage and support their participation in primary, secondary, or tertiary programs and services, regardless of particular concerns and problems. One approach to understanding the point of view of children and adolescents is youth voice.

For Practice and Discussion

1. Contact a local school district to arrange a time to visit and talk with a building administrator, school nurse, teacher, or guidance staff. Using **Table 6-3**, identify mental health programs and services that are fully in place, partially in place, under development, or not in place. Share your findings in class. Compare and contrast differences between districts that were visited.
2. You have been asked by the administration to describe the phases to expect when implementing a new student and family prevention program. Focus particularly on the reasons for the different phases and what course corrections you might suggest to keep the project on target. Give ideas for building the sustainability of the project after the initial funding is gone.
3. Take a mental health concern, such as substance abuse or crisis, and outline how you would help fellow student support team members and school staff stay current on issues, contacts, programs, and available community services.

TABLE 6-3   Mental Health Programs and Services

	Fully in Place	Partially in Place	Under Development	Not in Place
1. Classroom (teacher) strategies				
2. Social and emotional learning				
3. Special education				
4. Crisis response plans				
5. School counselors, mental health counselors, social workers, and psychologists				
6. School nurse				
7. Evidence-based programs				
8. Positive behavioral interventions and supports				
9. Response to intervention				
10. Community mental health agencies and programs				
11. Alternative education programs				
12. Child welfare system				
13. Family resource centers				
14. Justice system				
15. Parent engagement				
16. Community coalitions				

4. Bandura's work indicates that people need to believe that they can produce the desired change by their own efforts, or there will be very little incentive to put in the effort. In your own words, define self-efficacy. Brainstorm strategies for helping children and their families build self-efficacy and follow through on recommendations.

5. In your own words, explain why including the voice of students is critical to the success of any prevention program or service. Propose a PhotoVoice project to engage young people and share their voice.

Key Terms

Alternative education   120
Child and family point of view   113
Child welfare system   125
Community coalitions   126
Crisis response plans   117
Evidence-based programs   118
Family resource centers   126
Information network   129
Justice system   126
Mental health counselors   117
Parent engagement   126
PhotoVoice   132
Positive Behavioral Interventions and Supports (PBIS)   118
Psychologists   117

Response to Intervention (RtI)   118
School-based probation officer (SBPO)   126
School community staff point of view   112
School counselors   117
School nurse   117
School resource officer (SRO)   126
Self-efficacy   112
Social and emotional learning (SEL)   115
Social workers   117
Special education   115
Youth voice   131

References

Bandura, A. (2004). Health promotion by social cognitive means. *Health Education and Behavior*, 31: 143–164.

Center for Mental Health in Schools at UCLA. (n.d.). School-community partnerships: A guide. UCLA Department of Psychology School Mental Health Project. Retrieved from http://www.smhp.psych.ucla.edu

Child Welfare Information Gateway. (2011). State statutes search. Retrieved from http://www.childwelfare.gov/systemwide/laws_policies/state/

Community Tool Box, (2013). Implementing PhotoVoice in your community. University of Kansas. Retrieved from http://ctb.ku.edu/en/tablecontents/chapter3_section20_main.aspx

Davies, D. (1991). Schools reaching out: Family, school, and community partnerships for student success. *Phi Delta Kappan*, 72: 376–382.

Durlak J.A., Weissberg R.P., Dymnicki A.B., Taylor R.D., Schellinger K.B. (2011). The impact of enhancing students' social and emotional learning: a meta-analysis of school-based universal interventions. *Child Development*, 82(1): 405–32.

Fixsen, D.L., Naoom, S.F., Blase, K.A., Friedman, R.M., & Wallace, F. (2005). *Implementation Research: A Synthesis of the Literature*. Tampa, FL: University of South Florida, Louis de la Parte Florida Mental Health Institute, National Implementation Research Network (FMHI Publication #231).

Fletcher, A., & Vavrus, J. (2006). *The Guide to Social Change Led by and with Young People.* Olympia, WA: CommonAction. Retrieved from http://www.freechild.org/publications.htm

Lange, C., & Sletten, S. (1995). Characteristics of alternative schools and programs serving at-risk students (Research Report No. 16). Minneapolis, MN: University of Minnesota Enrollment Options for Students with Disabilities Project.

Mitra, D. (2004). The significance of students: Can increasing "student voice" in schools lead to gains in youth development? *Teachers College Record, 106*(4): 651–688.

Nixon, C., & Davis, S. (2010). Youth Voice Project. Retrieved from http://www.youthvoiceproject.com

Oldfather, P. (1995). Songs "come back most to them": Students' experiences as researchers. *Theory into Practice, 34*(2): 131.

Osher, T., & Osher, D. (2002). The paradigm shift to true collaboration with families. *Journal of Child and Family Studies, 11*(1): 47–60.

Wang, C. (1999). PhotoVoice: A participatory action research strategy applied to women's health. *Journal of Women's Health, 8*(2), 185–192.

PROGRAM AND SERVICE DECISIONS

In this chapter, we will:

◆ Discuss mental health program and service decisions

◆ Explain school district decisions and decision making

◆ Describe family decisions and decision making

Scenario

As a member of the school community mental health partnership, I have a seat on the school district curriculum and program committee. We review and recommend the school curriculum K–12. We review the health curriculum. We also review all of the subject areas in elementary through high school, including special education programs. I get to give input into not only content, scope, and sequence, but also instructional philosophy and methods. At one point in my career, I was a member of a student support team. Working one on one with students and their families, I was in there supporting, cajoling, and struggling to help make decisions about how to address a young person's mental health concerns and problems.

Source: Valerie Keener-Anderson, executive director of the Santa Maria Community Child and Adolescent Mental Health Promotion Partnership

Mental Health Program and Service Decisions

Decisions about mental health programs and services are made at two levels: **structural decisions** and **formal decisions** (**Figure 7-1**). These decisions flow from structural and formal connections regarding how to make the initial connection for children and adolescents to mental health programs and services. The structural and formal decisions are about the programs and services children and adolescents are being offered. These decisions are critical to the health and well-being of children and adolescents. They determine to a large extent what support, schools, and resources children and adolescents will be able to access and utilize.

Similar to structural connections, structural decisions are made for primary prevention programs and services. Similar to formal connections, formal decisions are made for secondary and tertiary prevention programs and services.

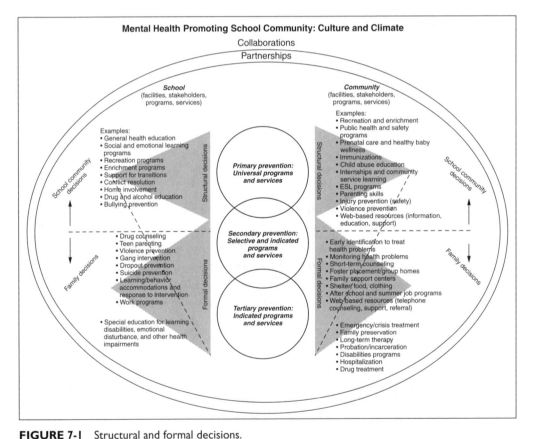

FIGURE 7-1   Structural and formal decisions.
Source: Adapted from Center for Mental Health in Schools at UCLA. (n.d.). School-community partnerships: A guide. UCLA Department of Psychology School Mental Health Project. Retrieved from http://www.smhp.psych.ucla.edu

Likewise, the model for the formal decisions is the individual mental health concerns and problems intervention process approach.

There are two big differences between structural and formal connections versus decisions. First, structural decisions may also be made for secondary and tertiary prevention programs. We will talk more about this later in the chapter. Second, structural decisions relate to the school community infrastructure. The school district staff are the decision makers. For the formal decisions, the children, adolescents, and families are deciding how to address mental health concerns and problems.

School District Mental Health Program and Service Decisions

School district mental health program and service decisions are structural decisions reflecting school district policies for mental health programs and services that do not require parent permission for students to access and participate in. Examples are health curriculum content, classroom programs, school counselors, nursing services, and extracurricular activities. These are thought of as primary prevention, addressing the developmental mental health needs of all students and focused on promoting social and emotional health while proactively addressing mental health problems and concerns. Just by attending school or participating in a community organization activity, young people get access and participate. Parents do not need to sign permission for their child to participate. And if a parent had a concern about their child's participation in a particular activity, a note or telephone call to the school is typically sufficient to permit the child to do an alternative activity.

Secondary prevention programs in some situations may also be decided upon within the infrastructure of schools. The family may still need to decide whether a child can participate, but the structural decision is not about the child but rather whether a particular program or service will be offered in the school community. Examples of such programs and services are school-based counseling programs that address developmental concerns, family relationships, anger management, conflict resolution, personal relationships, and stress management. These small groups have a curriculum that the counselor/facilitator uses to focus the group on skill building.

Structural decisions related to tertiary prevention programs focus on the mix of programs and services available in the school community. Likewise, input can be sought on which and how programs and services are offered as well as funding, staffing, locations, service hours, and approaches.

Complex Decision Making

School district mental health program and service decisions are complex. School districts have complicated structures and many different types of jobs. **Figure 7-2** shows a large district organizational chart that illustrates such complexity. Districts have a school board that maintains authority over the school district operation. In addition to choosing and hiring a superintendent (in most, but not all,

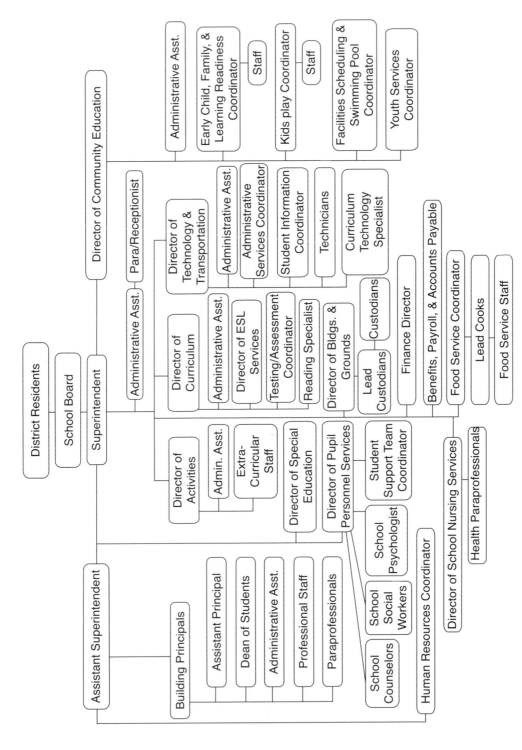

FIGURE 7-2   School leadership.

school districts), school board members make decisions about the school district's budget, curriculum, and policies within the framework established by state laws and policies. School boards are composed of five to eight community members who are elected by fellow residents in the district to serve 4-year terms. Some school districts elect a board representative from designated regions of the district, whereas others allow residents from any part of the district to serve. There are cases where school boards are appointed by and respond to another municipal authority (e.g., School District of Philadelphia) or where state legislatures delegate authority to other entities.

School district superintendents provide leadership to all schools within a school district and to district administrators. Superintendents serve as chief executive officers of their district and are charged with managing personnel, providing educational leadership, developing operating procedures based on policy, and acting as a district spokesperson. In most school districts in the United States, the superintendent is appointed by the district school board. In some school districts in Florida, Alabama, and Mississippi, the superintendent is elected by school district residents (National School Boards Association, 2013).

A school district will often employ assistant superintendents who support the work of the superintendent and focus on a particular element of the school district, such as curriculum and instruction. Other school support personnel who work in administration may include directors of activities, community education, special education, technology, communications, and school health. Staff who work with the superintendent, responsible for school operations across all of the school buildings, are referred to as central office administrative staff (or just central office staff). Staff in school buildings are building staff.

School buildings are led by a school principal. The principal supervises instruction and discipline; enforces rules, policies, and laws; supervises and evaluates teachers; and represents the school to parents and the community. Many schools have assistant principals who support the work of the principal (Bogden, 2003).

Looking at Figure 7-2, the individuals most involved with the mental health program and service *decisions* are the school board members, superintendents, central office, and building-level staff. Those responsible for initiating, designing, and implementing the program would be those central office administrators that are directly responsible for overseeing the process that occurs in local schools. Particularly involved would be individuals in the districts with titles such as directors of curriculum, special education, pupil personnel, school health, early childhood and family programs, school activities, and community education, as well as assistant superintendent (who supervises building principals for secondary or primary education). These individuals will be influential in the approval of all school health (including mental health) curricula, programs, and services (primary, secondary, and tertiary prevention). Likewise, the building principals and building-level administrators and staff, as well as faculty who implement programs and services, are important. For secondary and tertiary prevention program decisions, information often will be sought on financial, liability, and legal issues.

School District Curriculum Decisions

School districts make decisions on primary and secondary prevention programs that involve curriculum-based instruction and group activities. A school curriculum is a written plan of study that establishes objectives and expectations for students for each grade level and subject area. The curriculum defines the standards that students are expected to know by the end of the school year, including the global ideas and supporting concepts, and the skills students are expected to be able to perform related to each standard. It will also explain how students will be evaluated on each standard to demonstrate a comprehensive understanding of the global idea and supporting concepts. The curriculum may include just standards and performance indicators, leaving the plan of how the material is taught up to individual teachers, or it can include a detailed plan that covers exactly how teachers will deliver material to the students (Telljohann, Symons, Pateman, & Seabert, 2012). A well-written, thorough curriculum ensures that teachers are armed with the proper materials and that all students in the same grade-level subject course throughout the district are learning the same material and meeting the same objectives.

When deciding upon school health curricula, school administrators often use the National Health Education Standards as well as state and local curriculum standards as a guide to determine what and how the district's students will learn. A well-written, thorough health education curriculum will include learning outcomes and objectives that contribute to health promotion, health literacy, and healthy behaviors; planned progression that leads to achieving objectives; continuity between lessons and experiences that reinforce the importance of adopting and maintaining healthy behaviors; supplemental materials that correspond with and reinforce learning objectives; and strategies for assessing student achievement. Because many health education curricula have been proven to be ineffective, the **Health Education Curriculum Analysis Tool (HECAT)** (www.cdc.gov /HealthyYouth/HECAT/) is often used to aid in developing appropriate and effective health education curriculum (Telljohann et al., 2012). **Figure 7-3** shows a sample HECAT scoring sheet for a middle school curriculum covering alcohol and other drugs (Centers for Disease Control and Prevention [CDC], 2011). Educators can customize the HECAT to address the needs of their community, as well as to meet curriculum requirements set by their school district and state (CDC, 2011).

School curriculum is under continual review, and schools may use a number of strategies for designing and implementing curriculum changes. Teachers from each high school and middle school department and elementary grade level might meet periodically to discuss the current curriculum and suggest changes. A teacher may find that a particular technique no longer resonates with the students and wants to make a modification, or a teacher might have a concern about students in one grade level not being prepared to meet the standards of the following grade level. Large school districts may employ content coaches or instructional teacher leaders in specific subject areas who observe classes, work closely with teachers, and make curriculum suggestions to the central office.

Standard 1   Students will comprehend concepts related to health promotion and disease prevention.

After implementation of this curriculum, by grade 8, students will be able to:

ALCOHOL AND OTHER DRUGS **(Check all that are given attention in the curriculum)**

☐ Explain the dangers of alcohol and experimenting with other drugs, including inhalants.
☐ Differentiate between proper use and abuse of over-the-counter medicines.
☐ Differentiate between proper use and abuse of prescription medicines.
☐ Summarize the negative consequences of using alcohol and other drugs.
☐ Describe the relationship between using alcohol and other drugs and other health risks, such as unintentional injuries, violence, suicide, sexual risk behaviors, and tobacco use.
☐ Determine reasons why people choose to use or not to use alcohol and other drugs.
☐ Describe situations that could lead to the use of alcohol and other drugs.
☐ Describe how mental and emotional health can affect alcohol or other drug-use behaviors.
☐ Explain why using alcohol or other substances is an unhealthy way to manage stress.
☐ Discuss the harmful effects of using weight loss pills.
☐ Describe the health risks of using performance-enhancing drugs.
☐ Explain the dangers of drug dependence and addiction.
☐ Explain the risks associated with using alcohol or other drugs and driving a motor vehicle.
☐ Explain school policies and community laws about alcohol and other drugs.
☐ Determine the benefits of being alcohol and drug free.
☐ Describe positive alternatives to using alcohol and other drugs.
☐ Describe the relationship of alcohol and other drug use to the major causes of death and disease in the United States.
☐ Explain the relationship between intravenous drug use and transmission of blood-borne diseases, such as HIV and hepatitis.
Additional Concepts
☐ _____

CONCEPT COVERAGE SCORING: Complete the score based on the criteria listed below.

The curriculum addresses: **CONCEPT COVERAGE SCORE**
4 = all of the concepts. (100%)
3 = most of the concepts. (67–99%) ──────────► ☐
2 = some of the concepts. (34–66%)
1 = a few of the concepts. (1–33%)
0 = none of the concepts. (0%)

TRANSFER THIS SCORE TO THE HEALTH INFORMATION/CONCEPTS **LINE OF THE** OVERALL SUMMARY FORM **(CHAP. 3).**

Reminder: The HECAT is designed to guide the analysis of curricula for local use. Users are encouraged to add, delete, or revise concepts to reflect community needs and to meet the curriculum requirements of the school district.

HECAT: Promoting an Alcohol and Other Drug-Free Lifestyle
AOD - 5

FIGURE 7-3 Sample HECAT.
Source: Reproduced from Centers for Disease Control and Prevention. (2011). Health education curriculum analysis tool. Division of Adolescent and School Health. Retrieved from http://www.cdc.gov /HealthyYouth/HECAT/

Curriculum changes can come about from outside the school. A teacher might hear about a new method being used in another school, for example, and work with school administration to see how it might work in their school. Suggestions might be made by parents, community members, and board members. If a school administrator thinks such a suggestion has merit, they might involve principals, other administrators, and teachers in a research and development process to see about making such changes.

Students help shape curriculum. For example, if students are not registering for particular electives, school administrators will look into the reasons behind the lack of interest. If a technology course is outdated, school staff will need to find out what they could offer that is more current and that students are interested in.

For new courses, a principal or curriculum director or coordinator might work with teachers to develop a course outline that includes performance indicators for assessment. When writing the initial curriculum, teachers and curriculum coordinators should keep in mind that what is planned might not always work in the classroom. Students might not meet performance indicators as hoped, or they might not respond to a particular lesson in the way the teacher imagined.

During the first year of teaching the course, teachers will discover which ideas they thought would work are successful and which are not. Teachers should take notes during the school year about their modifications, and then work with the principal or curriculum coordinators to formalize their changes into the written curriculum. Curriculum can always be improved upon, and most schools will review and change curriculum annually. **Figure 7-4** shows the difference between the planned curriculum process and the reality of implementing and changing curriculum.

Evidence-Based Mental Health Programs

When making decisions related to primary and secondary prevention programs, school districts often will limit their considerations to evidence-based programs. These integrate current best scientific evidence, clinical expertise, and experience, as well as the preferences of individuals, families, organizations, and communities. They provide school community staff with programs that are critically appraised and that incorporate scientific evidence into practice. **Evidence-based mental health programs** identify the priority populations that would benefit from the program and the conditions under which the program works, and may indicate the change mechanisms that account for program effects. The programs include various tested strategies that target different diseases or behaviors. A defining characteristic of evidence-based programs is their use of health theory in both developing the program content (activities, curriculum, and tasks) and evaluation (measures, outcomes). Numerous mental health promotion programs have been initiated and evaluated and found to be effective.

Two key sources of evidence-based mental health promotion programs have been developed by the federal government. The first is the **National Registry of Evidence-Based Programs and Practices (NREPP)**, which was

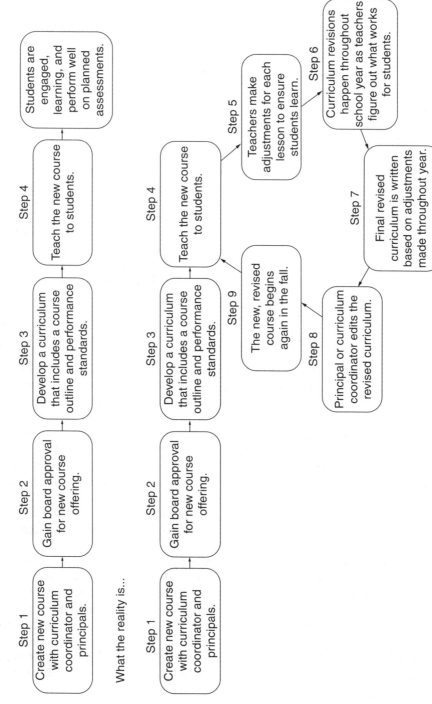

What the plan is…

Step 1
Create new course with curriculum coordinator and principals.

Step 2
Gain board approval for new course offering.

Step 3
Develop a curriculum that includes a course outline and performance standards.

Step 4
Teach the new course to students.

Students are engaged, learning, and perform well on planned assessments.

What the reality is…

Step 1
Create new course with curriculum coordinator and principals.

Step 2
Gain board approval for new course offering.

Step 3
Develop a curriculum that includes a course outline and performance standards.

Step 4
Teach the new course to students.

Step 5
Teachers make adjustments for each lesson to ensure students learn.

Step 6
Curriculum revisions happen throughout school year as teachers figure out what works for students.

Step 7
Final revised curriculum is written based on adjustments made throughout year.

Step 8
Principal or curriculum coordinator edits the revised curriculum.

Step 9
The new, revised course begins again in the fall.

FIGURE 7-4   Planning versus the reality of curriculum planning and implementation.

developed and is maintained by the Substance Abuse and Mental Health
Services Administration (SAMHSA) in the U.S. Department of Health and
Human Services. NREPP (www.nrepp.samhsa.gov) is a searchable database of
interventions for the prevention and treatment of mental and substance use
disorders. NREPP uses a voluntary, self-nominating system in which program
developers elect to participate. Programs undergo an expert peer review process. If accepted, the reviews are posted online for consumers to consider in
their decisions to use a program. There will always be some programs that are
not submitted to NREPP, and not all that are submitted are reviewed and
accepted. Nevertheless, new program summaries are continually being added
to the site.

The second federal source of evidence-based mental health promotion programs, **Research-Tested Intervention Programs (RTIPs)**, was developed and is
maintained by the National Cancer Institute. RTIPs (http://rtips.cancer.gov
/rtips/index.do) is linked to the Guide to Community Preventive Services (www
.thecommunityguide.org/index.html), a resource from the Centers for Disease
Control and Prevention that evaluates the effectiveness of broad intervention
categories through systematic research reviews. RTIPs is a database of actual
programs and products that individuals, groups, and organizations can access
and use.

Family Decisions and Decision Making

Formal decisions are made by families and caregivers about their child's participation in secondary and tertiary prevention mental health programs and
services. These are children and adolescents with an identified mental health
concern or problem. These children and adolescents were referred to the student support team and determined not to be in crisis (i.e., sexual abuse, neglect,
suicidal, violence), and initial information has been collected. The parents and
caregivers have been contacted and have signed any required consent forms to
permit their child's participation in the process. The parents and caregivers also
have received information on the student support team. The support team members (and you as a support team member) are set to get the child or teenager as
well as their families to participate—to use the available secondary and tertiary
prevention programs and services.

It is common and expected that student support teams will have to deal with
a range of mental health concerns and problems. A percentage of children will be
in need of special education programs and directed into the district special education process. A percentage of the children and adolescents will present with
both learning and behavior concerns. With these students the teams will initiate classroom-based strategies to address learning and behavior challenges. The
team will also work with students who have physical health problems that may
require that mental health concerns and problems be addressed. These students

might already have **individualized healthcare plans** completed by the school nurse (Silkworth, Arnold, Harrigan, & Zaiger, 2005). We will discuss individualized healthcare plans later in this section.

Many children and adolescents will not be eligible for or in need of special education, will not need learning support, and will not have an individualized healthcare plan. Rather, the students will present concerns related to substance use, anxiety, depression, sleep disorders, school phobia, violence, bullying, aggression, grief and loss, homelessness, family changes (divorce), sexual gender and identity issues (lesbian, gay, bisexual, and transgender [LGBT] youth), disordered eating, relationship problems, disruptive behavioral issues, or attention deficit disorders. The ultimate outcome of the team addressing the concern and problem is the child and family being linked to mental health services. The plans recommended through the process range from classroom instruction support to a mental health screening, which in turn can lead to a number of different outcomes such as counseling, alternative education placement, partial hospitalization, day treatment, and family counseling.

Following the individual mental health concerns and problems intervention process approach, teams will take a number of actions. The team collects additional information and clarifies the young person's mental health need, consults with the child or adolescent and their family and caregiver, formulates goals and plans, and if needed, has the student (with parent/caregiver approval) participate in a mental health screening. Use of student support teams to implement formal decision strategies tailored to individual school districts and communities is the best practice, although some school districts will delegate making formal decisions (following the model) to a school social worker, counselor, or nurse.

Depending on the resources and size of the district, as well as its philosophy, some student support teams are internally coordinated by a school employee (usually a school counselor or school social worker). Other districts may choose to contract with a staff member from a local community agency to coordinate and lead the student support team. Regardless of who employs the facilitator, the role is a crucial one. The coordinator collaborates with the team to accomplish the following tasks:

- ❖ Obtain referrals
- ❖ Organize the gathering of objective information about the student's academic, behavioral, attendance, and health status
- ❖ Engage the student and the parent in the process
- ❖ Obtain necessary consents
- ❖ Facilitate action planning, case management, follow-up, and support

The coordinator is also charged with holding a larger vision for the team, providing needed updates and maintenance to the team while preparing information and materials for team meetings, and monitoring both process and outcome evaluation for the program. The coordinator compiles all of the collected information into a single form (**Figure 7-5**) to show the status of the various team tasks (e.g., collecting information, clarifying need), as well as their completion dates and the team member responsible for each. Recommendations by program and service type are also listed. The form allows teams members to know the current status of a student and aid in the decision-making process.

Collect Information and Clarify Needs

As the team works through the process to collect information and clarify needs, it can have contact with lots of people. **Table 7-1** presents the types of information schools generally access to put together a complete picture of the student's problem. There are various sources for different types of information; for example, the school administrator is a resource for school attendance, discipline, and policy violations, whereas teachers and pupil services personnel give information about class attendance and academic performance. Any particular information source can vary by school and school district.

Teams use a variety of forms and checklists to gather objective data about students' academic, behavior, attendance, and health-related issues that act as a barrier to learning and school success. **Tables 7-2**, **7-3**, **7-4**, **7-5**, and **7-6** are sample checklists and information forms that teams use to inform planning and decision making. Information about what the classroom teacher has attempted is described in Table 7-2. Tables 7-3, 7-4, and 7-5 are a sample of information forms used at the secondary level in school districts as part of their student support teams. Table 7-6 shows an individualized healthcare plan form. These forms most likely would have been introduced to teachers and school community staff as part of an in-service training related to the student support team operation. Some resistance from staff to complete the forms can be expected due to staff being busy. However, for the most part, teachers as well as other staff appreciate the additional support. As part of training, and when the forms are distributed to the school community, it is essential to take the opportunity to restate the crisis warning signs (**Figure 7-6**) and required actions if present (e.g., Do *not* promise confidentiality; thank the student for trusting you, and accompany the student to the counselor, nurse, social worker, or principal and stay with them).

Classroom teachers often see changes in their students before parents, administrators, and counselors. Therefore, teachers are asked about their prior (if any) actions and activities related to the child or adolescent. They are asked about their interactions with family; referrals to counselors, social workers, and nurse; and specific interventions (e.g., changed seat, behavior management, time-outs, peer tutoring) to help the child be successful. Teachers document the strategies that worked and did not work. Table 7-2 outlines a variety of teacher-led interventions that are available to all students and are usually considered primary prevention interventions. This information aids the student support team

Student Support Team Planning and Recommendation Documentation and Process		
Name	Grade	Date
School building	Team staff member	
Task	Completion date	Staff member
Collect information		
Clarify need		
Student consultation		
Family consultation		
Goals		
Plan		

Recommendations

Primary Prevention/Universal Programs and Services

Academic and career planning	
Social connection and skills	
Anti-bullying and conflict resolution	
Transition planning	
Study habits	
Guidance curriculum series	
Special education	

Secondary Prevention/Selective Programs and Services

School mentoring	
Peer programs	
Individual counseling	
Small group counseling	
Consultation with parents, school staff, administrators, and community agencies	

Tertiary Prevention/Indicated Programs and Services

Mental health screening	
Dropout prevention/outreach	
Self-advocacy	
Community referrals (agency -)	

FIGURE 7-5 Student support team form to document the planning and recommendation process.

Information Type	School Administrator	Teachers	School Nurse	Parent	Pupil Services Personnel
TABLE 7-1 Information Sources to Support Goals, Plans, and Recommendations					
School Attendance Information	X				
Discipline Information	X				
Student-Initiated Requests	X				
Inappropriate Behavior	X				
Policy Violation	X				
Class Attendance Information		X			X
Strengths and Resiliency Factors		X	X		X
Academic Performance Information		X			X
Disruptive Behavior or Illicit Activities		X	X		X
Atypical Behavior		X	X		X
Physical Attributes		X	X		X
Home/School/ Family Indicators		X			X
Health Room Visit Information			X		
Temperament Issues				X	
School Problems				X	
Friends/ Relationships				X	
Physical Health				X	
Legal/Financial				X	

TABLE 7-2   Middle and High School Prior Interventions Checklist

Student Name and Grade: _____

Referring Teacher: _____ **Date:** _____

Please indicate the types of interventions you have tried prior to referral by placing an *x* in front of the strategies you have implemented.

_____ Student conference

_____ Set specific goals with student

_____ Student contract

_____ Spoke with parent on the telephone   Phone No. _____ Date: _____

_____ Emailed the parent _____ times   Describe situation: _____

_____ Held conference with parent at school

_____ Sent notices home regarding behavior/schoolwork

_____ Referred to counselor, social worker, principal, nurse (please circle)

_____ Initiated RtI (academic) interventions at Tier 1/Tier 2

_____ Suggested parent interventions (Specify _____)

_____ Checked cumulative folder

_____ Built on student's successes

_____ Identified student's strengths

_____ Provided extra attention to student

_____ Referred for ELL/ELS service

Environmental	Behavioral
_____ Changed group	_____ Behavior management system
_____ Changed seating	_____ Oral vs. written tests
_____ Ignored behavior	_____ Used self-monitoring
_____ Provided additional time to complete	_____ Assigned student after school detention
_____ Consulted with colleagues/team	

Organizational	Academic Accommodations
_____ Used graphic organizers	_____ Adjusted content level
_____ Used organizational charts	_____ Adjusted amount of work
_____ Utilized time-out area	_____ Provided additional individual assistance
_____ Guided practice	_____ Peer tutoring / _____ Adult tutoring
_____ Restated directions	

Key: RtI = Response to Intervention; ELL = English Language Learner; ELS = English Language Service/School

TABLE 7-3   Classroom Teacher Information Form

Middle/High School Student Support Indicators of Concern Data Form
Please check all the following indicators of concern for this student.

Student's Name: _____   Today's Date: _____

Gender: _____ Grade Level: _____ Subject: _____

Your Name: _____

Remember that crisis indicators (harm/threats to harm self or others, traumatic event, or recent loss) must be referred immediately to a counselor, social worker, nurse, or principal.

Behaviors: Check all that apply

_____ Disorganized

_____ Forgetful

_____ Defiant of rules

_____ Fails to accept responsibility

_____ Blames others

_____ Uses attention-getting behaviors

_____ Appears agitated, hyperactive, or nervous

_____ Regular daydreaming

_____ Isolated or withdrawn

_____ Mood swings

_____ Sexually preoccupied

_____ Cheats on assignments

_____ Inappropriate language

_____ Cries inappropriately

_____ Bullies others

_____ Demonstrates aggressive behavior

_____ Steals others' belongings

_____ Dishonest or lies to teacher and others

_____ Vandalizes others' property

_____ Overly concerned about achievement

_____ Overly sensitive to criticism

_____ Talks about personal substance use, depression, gang-related activity, sexual issues, harassment, or homelessness

_____ Multiple office discipline referrals

_____ Other:_____

Academic: Check all that apply

_____ Drop in grades

_____ Inconsistent work

_____ Lack of motivation

_____ Appears to have problems with reading class material

_____ Incomplete homework

_____ Incomplete classwork

_____ Failing quiz grades

_____ Compulsive overachiever

_____ Change in participation

_____ Does not follow directions

_____ Gives up easily

_____ Other:_____

Development assets: Check all that apply

_____ Self-motivated

_____ Demonstrates the following:

    _____ restraint

    _____ honesty

    _____ responsibility

    _____ regard for self

    _____ regard for others

    _____ sense of purpose

    _____ patience for others

_____ Tolerates change

_____ Expresses positive view of future

_____ Engages in school activities

_____ Has creative outlets

Physical concerns: Check all that apply	Developmental assets (continued)
_____ Frequent absences due to illness	_____ Reads for pleasure
_____ Frequently fatigued	_____ Asks for assistance
_____ Sleeping in class	_____ Other: _____
_____ Hygiene problems	_____ Expressed a positive relationship with
_____ Frequent physical complaints	staff member _____
_____ Slurred speech	_____ Other: _____
_____ Overly concerned about body image	
_____ Evidence of multiple cuts or skin abrasions	**Parent contact and results**
_____ Requests passes to see school nurse	_____ Number of phone calls to parents/ guardians
_____ Talks about physical issues that raise concern	_____ Number of letters sent to parents/ guardians
Other: _____	Dates of parent conferences:
_____	_____
	_____
	_____

as plans and recommendations are formulated. The team can then build focused plans to address the child's needs.

All of a student's teachers would be asked to provide information (Table 7-3) to document the observable strengths and challenges that student exhibits in different settings and times during the school day. It is important to educate teachers on crisis indicators that may warrant a student's immediate referral to the counselor, social worker, nurse, or principal. The team also needs to collect as much data as possible about the student.

Many districts have school-based student health clinics that are regularly staffed by certified nurse practitioners, registered nurses, licensed professional nurses, and/or nurse's aides. These professionals see students free from the disciplinary and academic judgments of teachers. Student support teams need to have one of these health professionals working consistently with the team. Often, nurses are not in schools full-time, but their information is important to the planning process and is needed to inform decision making. Table 7-4 is a sample form used to obtain this essential information.

Administrators, counselors, and social workers have unique roles that give them opportunities to work with students, parents, and teachers and thus have a perspective that informs **goal setting** and decision making. School administrators have contact with students and parents for a variety of reasons. Often disciplinary issues emerge, particularly policy violations, and it is important for administrators to offer assistance to students and parents with significant

---

TABLE 7-4   Student Support Team Child/Adolescent Health Indicator Report

Student: _____ **Grade/Team:** _____

Nurse/Health Professional: _____ **Date:** _____

Please provide appropriate health information on the above student to the Student Support Team.

Do you have any concerns about this student's physical or mental health? Please explain.

_____

_____

Previous Health History
Known health problems:

_____

_____

Long-term medications that may impact school performance:

_____

_____

Physical Appearance (i.e., personal hygiene, dress, odor of smoke, etc.): Please supply any additional information that would be helpful to the Student Support Team in working with this student.

_____

_____

Visits to Nurse: Please supply any information about this student's visits to the health office that would be of value to the Student Support Team in working with this student.

_____

_____

Other Pertinent Information:

_____

---

disciplinary infractions. Administrative involvement in the support team is critical. Yet, sometimes crisis events emerge that prevent the administrator from attending meetings consistently. Counselors and social workers offer crucial information as well. Often these professionals keep standardized test scores, Individualized Education Programs (IEPs), and 504 plans, while also providing

TABLE 7-5   School Administration, Social Work, and Guidance Staff Information Form

To: _____

From: Student Support Team Program

Student: _____ Date: _____

Information about your contact with the above-named student will help the Student Support Team understand him or her and develop effective educational and behavioral strategies. Please complete the following and submit.

To: _____ By: _____

1. Approximately how many times has this student been referred to your office during this school year for behavioral or other reasons? _____
2. Approximately how many times have the parents/guardians been contacted by your office regarding concerns about this student? _____
3. Briefly describe your indicators of concern (behavior, academic, health, attendance) about this student.
4. List any/all policy violations, the date, and disposition
5. List dates and reasons for in-school suspension.
6. List dates and reasons for out-of-school suspension.
7. What additional concerns do you have about this student?
8. What strategies have you tried with this student that have been successful?
9. What strategies have you tried with this student that the student has not responded to?

Guidance Support Group Title I Reading	IEP ELL/ESL
Reading scores (Dibels, etc.) Math scores State standardized testing scores Psychological testing	Grade repeated Attendance (days absent)
Previous schools	Outside agencies involved

Key: IEP = Individualized Education Program; ELL = English Language Learner; ESL = English as a Second Language

social and emotional skill development and career planning. They also have insights into students' adjustment and other issues and offer specialized information that can help create a successful action plan.

A final example of information that is collected is the comprehensive individualized healthcare plan form completed by the school nurse (Table 7-6). The information that is already collected by the nurse is used for a student with a physical health problem (and referred to the team by the nurse) who is identified as needing to address a mental concern or problem.

TABLE 7-6   Sample Individualized Health Plan Completed by Nurse

Individualized Health Plan	
Child's Name: Address:	Healthcare Provider: Provider's Phone: Individual Health Plan Written By:
Parents/Guardians/Caregivers: Parent/Guardian/Caregiver: Phone – home: Phone – cell: Phone – work: Email: Email:	School: Teacher: Counselor: Grade: Date: Review:

Concern and problem statement:

Assessment Data	Nursing Diagnosis	Goals	Nursing Interventions	Expected Outcomes

Suicide threat/gesture Physical or sexual abuse Suicide note (including poetry or cyber posting) Has given away many possessions	Expressed desire to die Exposure to traumatic event Talks about loss of parent or loved one Talks about loss of significant relationship Recent death of family member or friend

FIGURE 7-6   Crisis warning signs.

Child and Family Decide on Program and Service Goals

For children and adolescents with an identified mental health concern and problem, families are the decision makers. Helpful in the decision-making process is to set goals that are:

❖ *Clear:* It is easy to understand the expected result/outcome.

❖ *Written clearly:* Simple wording is used, without confusing middle steps and jargon.

❖ *Realistic:* The goals are based in reality and are relevant to the situation.

❖ *Specific:* Actions to be taken are specified in clear terms with benchmarks.

❖ *Owned:* Students, family members, and caregivers take responsibility for implementation.

The student information collected is used to set goals. Goal setting with a student and family is not easy. Initially, it may be easier to work with children, adolescents, and families by defining the issue/concern, how it is affecting the individual/family, what the family would like to see happen and how they think change could happen, and by when they think it could happen. Ask what the most important concern to address is. Then work together to further clarify what is realistic given the resources available. Also talk about small steps and changes as well as intermediate steps on the way to reaching the goal. Work to build consensus among the family members (children, parents, caregivers). Building consensus is important to the ultimate success of the goal.

Many models and strategies for goal setting are available. One widely used model is **SMART goals**: specific, measurable, attainable, realistic, and time delineated. SMART goals were originally developed for the business world; however, this model for setting goals has been adapted for use in many areas where goal setting is needed, and can be used once you have come to a consensus about the problem or issue you are addressing to further define the goals.

One such adaptation, SMARTER goals, adds two additional goals appropriate for our work: ethical and resourced (**Table 7-7**).

Corey (2012) notes that rarely does a person begin by requesting assistance in achieving specific behavioral changes. Instead of saying "I want to be able to talk to teachers without getting nervous," the student is likely to say "I am shy." In other words, a personal characteristic has been described rather than the ways in which the characteristic is expressed. It then becomes the counselor's job to help the student describe those ways in which the characteristic is expressed and, consequently, could be expressed differently.

Taking nonspecific concerns and translating them into specific goal statements is no easy task for the team member, who must understand the nature of the student's problem and the conditions under which it occurs before the translation can begin.

What can you expect of yourself and your students and families in terms of setting specific goals? First, the goals that are set can never be more specific than your understanding and your student's understanding of the problem. This

	TABLE 7-7 SMARTER Goals		
Name:			
Goal:			
Date:			
Reason this goal is important to me:			
Step	**Mnemonic**		**Description**
I	Specific Exactly what is it you want to accomplish? Good goal statements explain what, why, who, where, and when. If your goal statement is vague, you will find it hard to achieve because it will be hard to define success.		
2	Measurable You must be able to track progress and measure the result of your goal. Good goal statements answer the question how much or how many. How will I know when I achieve my goal?		
3	Agreed The goal must be relevant to and agreed upon by all parties; examples include student, family, teachers, counselors, community agencies, etc.		
4	Realistic The goal should be stretching, but realistic and relevant to you and your situation. Ensure the actions you need to take to achieve your goal are things you can do and control. Is this goal achievable?		
5	Time-Bound Goals must have a deadline. A good goal statement will answer the question: When will I achieve my goal? Without deadlines, it's easy to put goals off and leave them to die. As well as a deadline, it's a good idea to set some short-term milestones along the way to help you measure progress.		
6	Ethical Goals must sit comfortably within your moral compass. Most people resist acting unethically. Set goals that meet a high ethical standard.		
7	Resourced You will need to commit enough resources to achieve your goal. This may include time, money, information sources, or support from friends and colleagues. You may need to make sacrifices to achieve your goal.		

Source: Adapted from Haughey, D. (n.d.). SMART goals. Retrieved from http://www.projectsmart.co.uk/smart-goals.html

means that at the outset of counseling, goals are likely to be nonspecific and nonbehavioral. But nonspecific goals are better than no goals at all.

Corey (2012) describes these nonspecific or general goals as intermediate mental states, but he emphasizes that one cannot assume such goals will free up students to change their overt behavior. The point is that intermediate mental states are temporary, a first step along the way. At the earliest possible time, the counselor must strive to help the student identify more concrete objectives.

As you and your student explore the nature of a particular problem, the type of goal(s) appropriate to the problem should become increasingly apparent. This clarification will permit both of you to move in the direction of identifying specific behaviors that, if changed, would alter the problem in a positive way. These specific behaviors can then be formulated into goal statements; as you discuss the student's problems in *more* detail, gradually you can add the circumstances in which to perform the behaviors and how much or how often the target behaviors might be altered.

Child and Family Decide on Plans and Recommendations

The goals set by the child and family are the foundation for the plan and recommendations (**Table 7-8**). The team, with the student and parents, lists the goals and their priorities. (Rank them 1 to 4, with 1 being most important.) For each goal, you then establish what will occur (goal) and who will implement the goal. When will this occur? How will it be measured? How will you know when it is completed? Finally, who is going to monitor the progress (or lack of progress)?

Often, as part of the planning process, behavior contracts are used. Behavior contracts can provide the means to improve student behavior. They describe the desired behavior, establish the criteria for success, and lay out both the consequences and rewards for behavior (**Table 7-9**). Behavior contracts are fairly straightforward and can be used for most behaviors. There is room for only one or two behaviors; more than two behaviors may only confuse the student and dissipate the effort you need to place on identifying the replacement behavior and praising it. After each goal, there is a place for a threshold. Here you define when the goal has been met in a way that merits reinforcement. For example, if your goal is to eliminate calling out, you may want a threshold of two or fewer instances per subject or class. In these contracts, rewards come first, but consequences also need to be spelled out. The contract has a review date; it makes the teacher and students accountable. Make it clear that a contract does not need to last forever.

Mental Health Screening

A **mental health screening** is a relatively brief process designed to identify children and adolescents who are at risk of having disorders that warrant immediate attention, intervention, or more comprehensive review. Identifying the need for further assessment is the primary purpose of screening. Mental health screening instruments are never used to diagnose a child, but instead, to inform parents,

TABLE 7-8   Student Support Team Planning Form

Prioritize concerns identifying those as most critical or immediate needs:

_____ short/long term

_____ short/long term

_____ short/long term

Create specific targets for intervention (maximum effect, foundational skills and needs):

Priority Level _____   _____

Priority Level _____   _____

Priority Level _____   _____

Priority Level _____   _____

Established goals for this student that are specific and measurable:

Goal: What Will Occur	Who Will Implement	When This Will Occur	Measurement Indicator/ Benchmarks	Monitoring Schedule

What is the dosage/level necessary for progress to occur?

What resources, instruction, or coaching needs to occur to implement the plan?

TABLE 7-9   Student Support Behavior Contract

Date: _____

This is what is happening that needs to change:

_____

_____

_____

This is what will be happening after that change:

_____

_____

_____

This is what I need to be doing to make that happen:

_____

_____

_____

_____

My checkup day and time is _____. If I have complied with my contract, my
positive consequences will be:

_____

_____

_____

_____

_____

Student's name: _____

Adult's name (school/agency personnel): _____

Parent/Caregiver's name: _____

---

caregivers, and those working with families of concerns needing further assessment. If further assessment is required, then the child or adolescent would have a mental health diagnostic assessment.

Confusion about the term *mental health screening* exists in many schools and communities. The term is often used to describe a checkup as part of a public health approach to the early identification and treatment of behavioral health problems. The mental health checkups are "universal"—that is, they are given to all the children and adolescents in a grade, school, or community activity. Children and adolescents who may be at risk of an illness are not singled out. The checkups are not a diagnosis, but a tool to identify possible symptoms of a larger problem. An example is the Ages & Stages Questionnaire (ASQ) system for young children, which is quick and easy to use. The ASQ was designed to be completed by parents. It is used in programs such as early care and education, early Head Start and Head Start, early intervention for developmental monitoring, and offices of children, youth, and families. The ASQ screens developmental domains including communication, gross motor, fine motor, personal-social and problem solving, and social and emotional competence (e.g., self-regulation, compliance, communication, autonomy, affect, and interaction with people). For older children and adolescents, the Child and Adolescent Needs and Strengths (CANS) is widely used. Both require training to administer correctly.

Well-established screening programs such as ASQ strongly recommend active parental consent for any screening in schools and community settings. Weist et al. (2007) recommend careful and thorough preparation for implementation of any such screening, which would be done as a primary prevention service and would require support from the entire school community.

If further assessment is required, then the child or adolescent would have a **mental health diagnostic assessment**. A diagnostic assessment is a more comprehensive, expensive, time-consuming examination of the psychosocial needs and problems identified during the initial mental health screening. It is concerned with consequences and behaviors related to serious life stressors (**Table 7-10**) in the life of a child or adolescent and their families. Although the student support teams are the primary source of objective information about a child, research-based, reliable, and valid instruments are available and used in school communities to screen for more clinical issues. These instruments can help licensed mental health professionals determine whether the child would benefit from further assessment and evaluation. Student support teams do not screen, but do link students and families with the appropriate professionals in the school or community to provide this service.

The assessments identify the type and extent of mental health disorders and make recommendations for treatment interventions. Assessments routinely include individualized data collection, often including psychological testing, clinical interviewing, and reviewing of past records. Typically, the expertise of a licensed mental health professional is required to conduct the assessment and develop a comprehensive report. The purpose of a diagnostic assessment is to define the child or adolescent's concerns and use the information to develop a comprehensive treatment plan (**Table 7-11**).

How to Get a Child or Adolescent to Agree to a Mental Health Screening

Some children and adolescents resist mental health screenings because they don't want to be blamed for the family's problems; others are fearful that people (e.g., the person doing the screening, peers, teachers) will think they are crazy.

TABLE 7-10 Mental Health Diagnostic Assessment Concern Areas				
	Child	Caregiver or Parent 1	Caregiver or Parent 2	Describe others:
History of neglect		NA	NA	
Physically abused		NA	NA	
Sexually abused		NA	NA	
Sexually acting out		NA	NA	
Emotionally abused		NA	NA	
Suicide ideation/attempt				
Intentional self-harm				
Violent or chronic aggression or hostility				
Delusions or hallucinations				
Substance/alcohol abuse				
Prenatal drug exposure				
Intentional delinquent acts				
Psychiatric illness				
History of boarding school				
Felony convictions				

And of course, many resist just because their parents or caregiver wants the screening. Here's how you can enlist their cooperation.

❖ Be clear that the screening is confidential and private. Only those with a legitimate need to know will be told the results (parents, and with consent, others in school who are in a position to help and support the child). The results are not shared with school staff or the child's peers. The purpose of the screening is to make decisions.

❖ Tell them that the parents and caregivers will meet with the psychiatrist (or psychologist, social worker, or other mental health professional) to review the family situation. They will hear the parents' side of the story, but it is really important to hear the child's side. Many young people find this invitation enticing because they want the professional to know how difficult their parents are.

TABLE 7-11 Mental Health Assessment and Plan				
Name			Date of Birth	
Address				
			Gender	
Cell Phone		Home		Work	
Staff Name				
Date of Assessment	/ /			

Description of Presenting Complaint/Problem

Mental Health History/Previous Treatment	Family History of Mental Illness

Social History Including School, Alcohol or Other Substance Use, Current Relationships, etc.

Current Medications	Relevant Medical Conditions/Investigations/ Allergies

Mental Status Examination (Please indicate relevant details)	
Appearance and behavior:	Mood:
Thinking:	Affect:
Perception:	Sleep:
Anhedonia:	Appetite:
Attention/concentration:	Motivation/energy:
Memory:	Judgement/insight:
Orientation:	Speech:

Risk Assessment					
Suicidal thoughts	Yes ☐	No ☐	Suicidal intent	Yes ☐	No ☐
Current plan	Yes ☐	No ☐	Risk to others	Yes ☐	No ☐

ICD-10 Provisional Diagnosis

F1   Alcohol and drug use disorder   ☐   F2   Psychotic disorder   ☐
F3   Depression   ☐   F4   Anxiety disorder   ☐
F5   Unexplained somatic disorder   ☐   Other / Unknown:

Mental Health Plan

Date of Mental Health Plan *(if different from date of assessment)*		/ /
Problem (e.g., **Sleep disturbance, panic attacks, etc.**)	**Goal** (e.g., **Improve sleep, reduce panic attacks, etc.**)	**Action/Task** (e.g., **Refer to allied health, medication, engagement of family/other supports, etc.**)
1.		
2.		
3.		

Emergency Care *(e.g., family contact/others to be contacted by patient or staff in emergency)*

1.
2.
3. Mental Health Service Provider Hospital (24-hour service)   Phone:

(Continues)

TABLE 7-11 Mental Health Assessment and Plan *(Continued)*			
Child, Parent, and Staff to sign sections below:			
I understand the above Mental Health Plan and agree to the outlined goals/actions.			
Child Signature:		**Staff Signature:**	
Parent/Caregiver Signature:			
Parent/Caregiver Signature:			
Has a copy of the Plan been given to the family?		Yes ☐ No ☐	
Proposed date for review of Plan (1–6 months after Plan completed)		/ /	
Review of Mental Health Plan *(Complete this section at the review consultation)*			
Problem	**Goal**	**Outcome**	**New Action/Task (if necessary)**
1. As above	As above		
2. As above	As above		
3. As above	As above		
Complete the following sections to help the patient look out for signs of relapse and how to manage it.			
Early Warning Signs *(Be specific: e.g., sleep disturbance, irritability, etc.)*			
1.		2.	
3.		4.	
Relapse Prevention Plan *(Reassess at review consultation)*			
1.		2.	
3.		4.	

❖ Acknowledge that the parents and caregivers are probably unhappy with the family situation, and tell them you assume that they feel the same way. Then ask if they are willing to do their part by helping themselves and their family. Make it clear that the parents and caregivers are ready and willing to be a part of the process.

❖ Express your concern about them, calling attention to their recent moods and behavior (for example, being angry, sad, defiant). Then suggest there are experts who can help them to feel better and thus make their life easier.

❖ Ask them to meet with a psychologist once, and leave it up to the therapist to enlist their cooperation. Most therapists are well prepared for the initial resistance that children and teenagers present.

❖ If it becomes necessary, insist on a screening as a condition for driving the family car, getting an allowance, or receiving other privileges.

❖ Use all of the available leverage of the school as well as other important sources of support. For example, the school can require an evaluation as a condition for remaining enrolled in school, participating in team sports practice and games, and participating in community and school activities, although care needs to be exercised not to antagonize the youth and defeat the purpose of your action.

Summary

Mental health program decisions are structural decisions related to school district policies for programs and services that do not require parent permission for students to access and participate in mental health programs and services. Families make formal decisions about their child's participation in mental health programs and services to address an identified mental health concern or problem. The decisions are made with the support of the student support team and reflect a process that has determined the child is not in crisis (i.e., sexual abuse, neglect, suicidal, violence) and initial information has been collected. The information gathered and needs identified shape the child and family program and service decisions. Likewise, the information clarifies needs and goals, serving as the foundation for a plan and recommendations. As part of the process, screening can occur. Screening is a relatively brief process designed to identify children and adolescents who are at risk of having disorders that warrant immediate attention, intervention, or more comprehensive review. Identifying the need for further assessment is the primary purpose of screening. The child must make the decision and agree to the screening.

For Practice and Discussion

1. There are lots of tools available to help educators evaluate curriculum. **Table 7-12** shows a sample page of a form used by the Connecticut State Board of Education to evaluate curricula in school districts throughout the state.

TABLE 7-12   Connecticut Curriculum Evaluation Form

I. Curriculum Development and Support

This section of the guide addresses district-level planning that is essential to curriculum development. Evidence may be presented from related documents, such as a curriculum development plan or a professional development plan.

The following are important aspects of curriculum development and should be evidenced:	Yes, there is evidence.	No, there is not evidence.	Comments/ Next Steps
A. A philosophy and/or mission statement about the teaching and learning of all students (including special education and ELL students) across all curricula guides the curriculum development (general philosophy sample, content-specific philosophy).			
B. An overall plan for curriculum development exists, involves and indicates where each curriculum area is in the development, implementation, or evaluation cycle with timelines. Plans for data-driven evaluation of the curriculum at the district/program level and for the content areas are also included (plan sample 1, plan sample 2).			
C. A defined model (e.g., Understanding by Design, Making Standards Work, Balanced Curriculum, The High/Scope Approach) governs the curriculum.			
D. A system to orient teachers and administrators in the use of the curriculum includes professional development and training of new staff as needed.			
E. A list of current references/research guided the curriculum development (references sample 1).			
F. A plan showing alignment with a standards-based report card/child profiles.			

(Continues)

II. Curriculum Components

This section of the guide proposes elements likely to be part of planning high-quality curriculum for all learners. These elements represent current professional understanding of what it means to plan so all learners have opportunities to achieve. Many of the elements are supported in education literature. Indicators are categorized as Goal or Advanced. Check those indicators that are evident in the curriculum. To meet either category, all indicators in the category must be checked.

Curriculum Document Addresses	Indicators Reflecting Goal and Advanced Performance	Comments/ Next Steps
A. Alignment to Standards — the matching of district grade-level/course-level/ learner expectations to standards	**GOAL** ☐ The curriculum aligns with the current state/national standards. ☐ The curriculum aligns with current state grade-level expectations. ☐ The curriculum aligns with current state/ national assessments. ☐ The curriculum aligns with other state-level resources.	
B. Learner Expectations (locally designed or CSDE GLEs) — statements about what students should know and be able to do	**GOAL** ☐ Learner expectations state what students should know and be able to do by the end of each grade level/course/program. ☐ Learner expectations are prioritized to reflect district/program goals. ☐ Learner expectations are included and organized into units/themes/chapters (based on the district's curriculum model, as appropriate) for a set period of time. ☐ Learner expectations address all six levels of cognitive domain (Bloom's taxonomy) **ADVANCED** ☐ Learner expectations are organized in three stated levels of priority from the most important to the least important based on the big ideas.	

CSDE = Connecticut State Department of Education; GLE = Grade Level Expectations; ELL = English Language Learner

Source: Reprinted by permission from Connecticut State Department of Education. (2009). Connecticut Curriculum Development Guide. Retrieved from http://www.sde.ct.gov/sde/lib/sde /pdf/Curriculum/Curriculum_Development_Guide_2009.pdf

Use this form to do a sample evaluation of the school curriculum in a local school district.

2. Your local school district curriculum committee, which you are a member of, has recently been exploring the adoption of a new school-wide violence prevention program. The committee has studied several evidence-based choices and some that are not. The committee has reduced the list to three programs. You have to help present the three programs to the faculty for their vote on which one to implement next year. Prepare the list of questions you would ask or qualities you would look for in the program of your choice to guide your presentation. Use the answers as the basis of your presentation.

3. Student support teams work in schools with a variety of student needs. List five mental health issues that complicate academic success. Explore the major warning signs you might see the student manifest at school. How does documentation from the multiple sources at school and home provide you with a more complete picture of the student's needs? What is the danger in using subjective or cursory information?

4. In your own words, outline five key actions that effective student support teams must complete in order to provide students and families with needed mental health services. How do the actions complement and build upon each other? Where do you anticipate struggles? What solutions might you recommend?

5. Explain the difference between a mental health screening and a formal mental health assessment. How would you work with a student resisting the mental health screening?

Key Terms

Evidence-based mental health programs   146

Formal decisions   140

Goal setting   155

Health Education Curriculum Analysis Tool (HECAT)   144

Individualized healthcare plans   149

Mental health diagnostic assessment   164

Mental health screening   161

National Registry of Evidence-Based Programs and Practices (NREPP)   146

Research-Tested Intervention Programs (RTIPs)   148

SMART goals   159

Structural decisions   140

References

Bogden, J.F. (2003). *How Schools Work and How to Work with Schools.* Alexandria, VA: National Association of State Boards of Education.

Centers for Disease Control and Prevention. (2011). Health education curriculum analysis tool. Division of Adolescent and School Health. Retrieved from http://www.cdc.gov /HealthyYouth/HECAT/

Connecticut State Department of Education. (2009). Curriculum development guide. Hartford CN. Retrieved from http://www.sde.ct.gov/sde/lib/sde/pdf/Curriculum/Curriculum _Development_Guide_2009.pdf

Corey, G. (2012). *Theory and Practice of Counseling and Psychotherapy.* Belmont, CA: Brooks/Cole Publisher.

National Health Education Standards, Joint Committee on. (2007). *National Health Education Standards: Achieving Excellence* (2nd ed.). Atlanta, GA: American Cancer Society.

National School Boards Association. (2013). [NSBA website]. Retrieved from http://www.nsba.org

Silkworth, C., Arnold, M., Harrigan, J., & Zaiger, D. (2005). *Individualized Healthcare Plans for the School Nurse: Concepts, Framework, Issues, and Applications for School Nursing Practice.* North Branch, MN: Sunrise River Press.

Telljohann, S.K., Symons, C.W., Pateman, B., & Seabert, D.M. (2012). *Health Education: Elementary and Middle School Applications* (7th ed.). New York: McGraw-Hill.

Weist, M.D., Rubin, M., Moore, E., Adelsheim, S., & Wrobel, G. (2007). Mental health screening in schools. *Journal of School Health*, 77(2): 53–58.

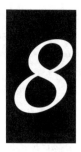

Sustaining Programs and Services

In this chapter, we will:

✦ Explore how to sustain mental health programs and services

✦ Discuss building school community social support and recovery support

✦ Describe case and resource management

✦ Discuss advocacy by youth, parents, caregivers, families, and staff

Scenarios

It is not enough for the student support teams to make the plans and get the children to participate in the mental health programs and services. We need to think detail and big picture. We need to be thinking about all of the details of offering programs and services (e.g., logistics such as scheduling, materials, staff). We need to think about how to nurture our student support teams. Without support, the team members burn out. Without support, our partnerships and collaborations just do not work. And all the while, the kids and families need ongoing attention; otherwise, pretty quickly they can get lost. It is hectic keeping track of everything and everybody. However, we can't just be thinking details. We need to think big about the school community and how we keep everything up and running. How we learn what works. How we deal with change.

Source: Marcia Andrews, assistant superintendent of safety, culture, and learning environment for a large Florida school district

I've been smoking cigarettes since I was about 10. They helped me calm down. I'm not addicted. I can stop anytime. My parents smoke cigarettes and it was no big deal my smoking at home. I started using weed when I was in sixth grade. Yeah, I was about 12 then. Some of the older kids on the bus would talk about how high weed made you feel and I knew I wanted to try it. My friend offered me a hit when we were hanging out and I liked the way it made me feel. I mean it made me feel like I could do or be anything. Eventually I started smoking weed every day. A couple of times my parents caught me when I was high. They told me it was bad for you and to stop. Yeah, right. Marijuana costs money and they stopped giving me money. I stole money from their wallets and alcohol from stores as well as other stuff that I could sell to younger kids. Then to pay for my habit, I started selling it in school. Eventually I was caught in school with a bag of marijuana. Following school policy, I was suspended from school for 5 days and was referred to the local drug and alcohol agency for an evaluation. The agency sent the school a letter stating that they recommended me for intensive outpatient treatment. So I went and did okay and hung out with lots of kids into more stuff than me. My parents wanted me clean and were talking to the school counselor so I could get some help staying clean there. I was attending my individual and group counseling sessions. I saw the drug and alcohol counselor at school and participated in a group at school, too. My old friends made fun of me. I felt kind of alone because not too many kids were trying to stay clean. Dad said to join the wrestling team. I don't know, I didn't have the energy. Kids kept bothering me. My grades began to slip and I got into a fight at school because some of the potheads started calling me names. I don't know why I punched out one of them, but yeah, I got suspended. The drug and alcohol counselor got to me pretty quickly after the fight. We talked and he asked me if he could call my parents in and have the four of us talk about what was going on. I don't like this recovery crap. The marijuana made me feel so good. I don't know how I'm going to stay clean or if I even want to. School is a waste right now. The counselor told me that it's normal to feel this way when you stop smoking weed.

Source: John, a middle school student recently suspended for marijuana possession

Sustaining Programs, Services, Teams, Partnerships, and Collaborations

Sustaining high quality programs, services, teams, partnerships, and collaborations requires that teams, partnerships, and collaborations take a number of actions (**Figure 8-1**). The actions include a focus on quality programs, ongoing training to prevent staff burnout, building **social support** as a buffer to stress, and a clear message of recovery and hope for youth and families struggling with mental health concerns and problems. Youth and family case and resource management is required: a systematic procedure of continual feedback and

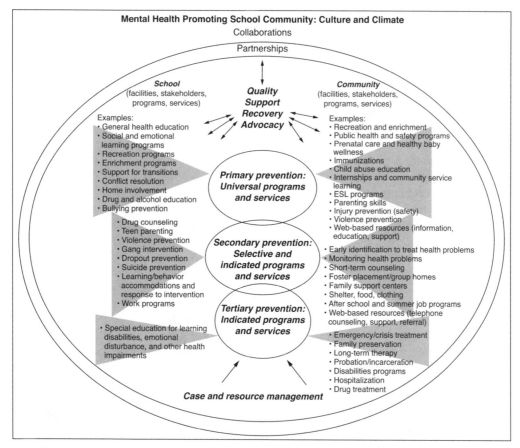

FIGURE 8-1 Sustainability for a mental health promoting school community.
Source: Adapted from Center for Mental Health in Schools at UCLA. (n.d.a.) School-community partnerships: A guide. UCLA Department of Psychology School Mental Health Project. Retrieved from http://www.smhp.psych.ucla.edu

monitoring of individual children and adolescents' participation in planned activities and progress toward stated goals (Center for Mental Health in Schools at UCLA, n.d.a.). Finally, advocacy takes place at a number of levels including working with children, adolescents, parents, caregivers, and families to be their own advocates; working on changes within existing systems; and working on public policy.

Fidelity and Adaptation

Fidelity and adaptation are indicators of quality programs and services. They focus on program and service implementation and how well the program or service addresses the needs of the children and adolescents. It takes a lot of effort to sustain a program or service. When programs and services are implemented in the field, practitioners rightly wonder whether they will realize the same outcomes as those reported from the original implementations. To increase that likelihood, program developers recommend that others implement the program consistent with prescribed protocols. In this way, developers seek maximum program fidelity. Realistically, though, field replications often must adapt to local needs and conditions.

Fidelity defines the extent to which the delivery of a program or service conforms to the curriculum, protocol, or guidelines for implementing that program or service. A program or service delivered exactly as intended by its originator has high fidelity. A program or service delivered quite differently than intended by its originator has low fidelity. Because programs and services delivered with high fidelity are more likely than those with low fidelity to achieve their original intended results—results that identified them as effective—fidelity is important for mental health programs and services. We want to know that our programs and services are effective. Resources are limited, and competition for people's time is high. High fidelity programs and services send the message that kids matter. They contribute to sustaining an environment that is safe in which to address concerns and problems.

Adaptation defines the degree to which a program or service undergoes change in its implementation to fit the needs of a particular delivery situation. The apparent antithesis of fidelity, adaptation could alter program integrity if a program is adapted so drastically that it is not delivered as originally intended. Paradoxically, however, the adaptation process may render a program more responsive to a particular group of children and adolescents. Adaptation could increase a program's cultural sensitivity and its fit within the new implementation setting. The quality of adaptation may represent the *sine qua non* of a program or service's acceptance by the intended end-users. Indeed, cultural adaptation has been found necessary to engage the interest of children and adolescents. It contributes to children and adolescents' feelings of being cared for and listened to. It adds to the psychological safety of the school community. Absent such interest and feelings, the program or service is less likely to result in positive outcomes for the youth and families.

Ongoing Skill Development to Prevent Staff Burnout

Sustaining teams, partnerships, and collaborations is accomplished by **ongoing skill development** and **problem solving**, but in particular by preventing **staff burnout**. Staff attends to the details and logistics that surface during the implementation and ongoing operation. One serious consequence of the work is staff burnout. They can experience physical and emotional exhaustion involving the development of negative job attitudes, a poor professional self-concept, and a loss of empathic concern for the youth and families they are trying to help. People in helping professions consistently put themselves at risk because they care so much and because they are expected by everyone else to take care of everyone other than themselves. Approaches to prevent burnout among staff are system- and person-centered. System-centered approaches are part of the coordinated school health staff promotion component. Eliminating or modifying worksite stressors (e.g., limiting workloads); enhancing the job experience (e.g., giving employees voice in policy decisions and job functions); offering training (e.g., self-care, conflict resolution, time management); creating an open, supportive, well-communicating work environment; and offering regular recognition of staff achievement are all examples of a system-centered approach to preventing burnout. Person-centered approaches focus on changing work patterns (e.g., decreasing hours, avoiding unnecessary meetings, setting priorities daily), professional development (e.g., developing new skills and interests, increasing skills for utilizing and managing technology), and creating your own growth-promoting workplace (e.g., seeking out leaders or mentors who promote balance, seeking professional social support).

As with all fields, school mental health issues, laws, and best practices are evolving and changing. It is essential that team members have opportunities to network with professionals from other schools and agencies on a regular basis. Partnerships and collaborations frequently convene quarterly or monthly gatherings of student support teams to problem solve challenges, share knowledge of and contacts with community organizations and human services, seek funding, share resources, and support each other in the work. Although funding continues to shrink, it is essential that teams have opportunities to evaluate their work and create improvement plans. Student support team meetings need to include team maintenance. Maintenance can be a regular meeting held monthly, or it can be held during an in-service training and externally or internally facilitated. School staff also need regular in-servicing on current trends in substance abuse, mental health concerns, appropriate crisis response and drills, and new programs and services.

Social Support as a Stress Buffer

Social support is an important protective factor and buffer to stress. The school community is the primary social structure for children and adolescents. Friendships and social relationships with peers are a central part of young people's lives. A positive and supportive school community environment encourages communication and interaction and does not tolerate harassment, bullying, or violence of any kind. No factor is more important for positive school outcomes than the children's and adolescents' perception of the school community staff's (e.g., teachers, counselors, social workers, principals, nurse, etc.) attitude toward them. When students believe that the school community staff care about them, see them as competent, respect their views, and desire their success, they tend to work toward fulfilling those high expectations. Examples of opportunities for youth peer-to-peer and youth–staff interaction are:

❖ Small learning communities, because lower student–staff ratios promote interaction

❖ Block scheduling, with longer classes that foster greater interaction

❖ Looping, in which a teacher is with the same class for more than 1 year

❖ Class meetings, where students share their thoughts daily or weekly

❖ Cooperative learning projects, which studies show eliminate cliques and widen friendship networks, especially across racial divides

❖ Staff members who are assigned as mentors or advisors to individual students or groups

Clear Message of Recovery and Hope

To sustain a supportive health promoting school community, teams, partnerships, and collaborations have to give a clear message of **recovery** and **hope** for youth and families struggling with mental health concerns and problems. Recovery from mental disorders and substance use disorders is a process of change through which individuals improve their health and wellness, live a self-directed life, and strive to reach their full potential. The 10 guiding principles of recovery (**Table 8-1**) provide a vision of how to approach a discussion with youth and families about mental concerns and problems. They set a culture and climate of acceptance and empathy at a time when people (youth and families) are most vulnerable.

TABLE 8-1   Guiding Principles of Recovery

1. *Recovery emerges from hope:* The belief that recovery is real provides the essential and motivating message of a better future—that people can and do overcome the internal and external challenges, barriers, and obstacles that confront them. Hope is internalized and can be fostered by peers, families, providers, allies, and others.

2. *Recovery is person-driven:* Self-determination and self-direction are the foundations for recovery as individuals define their own life goals and design their unique path(s) towards those goals. Individuals optimize their autonomy and independence to the greatest extent possible by leading, controlling, and exercising choice over the services and supports that assist their recovery and resilience.

3. *Recovery occurs via many pathways:* Individuals are unique with distinct needs, strengths, preferences, goals, culture, and backgrounds—including traumatic experiences—that affect and determine their pathway(s) to recovery. Recovery is built on the multiple capacities, strengths, talents, coping abilities, resources, and inherent value of each individual. Recovery pathways are highly personalized. They may include professional clinical treatment, use of medications, support from families and in schools, faith-based approaches, peer support, and other approaches. Recovery is nonlinear, characterized by continual growth and improved functioning that may involve setbacks. Because setbacks are a natural, though not inevitable, part of the recovery process, it is essential to foster resilience for all individuals and families.

4. *Recovery is holistic:* Recovery encompasses an individual's whole life, including mind, body, spirit, and community. This includes addressing self-care practices, family, housing, employment, education, clinical treatment for mental disorders and substance use disorders, services and supports, primary health care, dental care, complementary and alternative services, faith, spirituality, creativity, social networks, transportation, and community participation. The array of services and supports available should be integrated and coordinated.

5. *Recovery is supported by peers and allies:* Mutual support and mutual aid groups, including the sharing of experiential knowledge and skills, as well as social learning, play an invaluable role in recovery. Peers encourage and engage other peers and provide each other with a vital sense of belonging, supportive relationships, valued roles, and community. Through helping others and giving back to the community, one helps one's self. Peer-operated supports and services provide important resources to assist people along their journeys of recovery and wellness. Professionals can also play an important role in the recovery process by providing clinical treatment and other services that support individuals in their chosen recovery paths. Although peers and allies play an important role for many in recovery, their role for children and youth may be slightly different. Peer supports for families are very important for children with behavioral health problems and can also play a supportive role for youth in recovery.

6. *Recovery is supported through relationships and social networks:* An important factor in the recovery process is the presence and involvement of people who believe in the person's ability to recover; who offer hope, support, and encouragement; and who also suggest strategies and resources for change. Family members, peers, providers, faith groups, community members, and other allies form vital support networks.

7. *Recovery is culturally based and influenced:* Culture and cultural background in all of its diverse representations—including values, traditions, and beliefs—are keys in determining a person's journey and unique pathway to recovery. Services should be culturally grounded, attuned, sensitive, congruent, and competent, as well as personalized to meet each individual's unique needs.

8. *Recovery is supported by addressing trauma:* The experience of trauma (such as physical or sexual abuse, domestic violence, war, disaster, and others) is often a precursor to or associated with alcohol and drug use, mental health problems, and related issues. Services and supports should be trauma-informed to foster safety (physical and emotional) and trust, as well as promote choice, empowerment, and collaboration.

9. *Recovery involves individual, family, and community strengths and responsibility:* Individuals, families, and communities have strengths and resources that serve as a foundation for recovery. In addition, individuals have a personal responsibility for their own self-care and journeys of recovery. Individuals should be supported in speaking for themselves. Families and significant others have responsibilities to support their loved ones, especially for children and youth in recovery. Communities have responsibilities to provide opportunities and resources to address discrimination and to foster social inclusion and recovery.

10. *Recovery is based on respect:* Community, systems, and societal acceptance and appreciation for people affected by mental health and substance use problems, including protecting their rights and eliminating discrimination, are crucial in achieving recovery. There is a need to acknowledge that taking steps towards recovery may require great courage. Self-acceptance, developing a positive and meaningful sense of identity, and regaining belief in one's self are particularly important.

Source: Substance Abuse and Mental Health Services Administration. (2011). Guiding principles of recovery. Retrieved from http://www.samhsa.gov/samhsanewsletter/Volume_17_Number_5 /GuidingPrinciples.aspx

Case and Resource Management

Critical for the youth and family who are struggling with a mental health concern or problem is **case and resource management**, a systematic procedure of continual feedback and monitoring of participation in planned activities and progress toward stated goals (**Table 8-2**). Case management is how to attend to the children, adolescents, and their families who are participating in secondary and tertiary prevention programs. These are children who the team has worked with to move through the individual mental health concerns and problems intervention process. They are participating in agreed-upon programs and services, and progressing on personal goals. We want them to know that, as individuals, they are important and deserve attention as they address their concerns and problems. Resource management is about looking at the system and identifying the gaps and places where the process breaks down and fixing it. It is about making sure that the system wraps around the child and family and meets their needs instead of requiring them to fit into an existing box. It is also about identifying new or more intensive resources and avoiding duplication of services by different entities.

TABLE 8-2 Student Support Team Case Management and Resource Management	
Focus on the Child and Adolescent: Case Management	**Focus on the School Community: Resource Management**
❖ Identification and referral ❖ Crisis intervention ❖ Information gathering ❖ Goals and plans developed ❖ Case monitoring ❖ Case progress review ❖ Case reassessment ❖ Advocacy	❖ Map school resources as well as community-based resources. Look strategically at schools within a district and around a district. ❖ Identify the most pressing issues and program development needs at the school level. ❖ Coordinate and integrate school resources and connect with community resources. ❖ Establish priorities for strengthening programs and developing new ones. ❖ Plan and facilitate ways to strengthen and develop new programs and services. ❖ Recommend how resources should be deployed and redeployed. ❖ Identify where additional resources exist and develop strategies for accessing them. ❖ Provide advocacy. ❖ Plan and deliver social marketing to constituents.
Source: Adapted from Center for Mental Health in Schools at UCLA. (n.d.b.) School-community partnerships: A guide. UCLA Department of Psychology School Mental Health Project. Retrieved from http://www.smhp.psych.ucla.edu	

At the core of this work is monitoring that is focused on the appropriateness of the programs and services to address the needs of youth. It is about the details of helping people change their behavior. John, the young person introduced at the beginning of the chapter, highlights the need for case and resource management.

One important note about the term *case management* is that it is widely used by medical personnel to describe the medical management of the care concerning an individual patient's particular disease or symptoms. In human services, case management is not purely oriented to medical treatment; rather, management of care takes into account all aspects of the person's life and environment, not only the biological problems. Likewise, we have added the word *resource* to the term *case management* to highlight the importance of navigating and utilizing the available school community (including classroom) programs and services.

Effective case management is critical to the overall success of any type of action plan with students at any level. Case management is defined as a variety of activities designed to engage the student, the school staff, and the family in the process in a way that serves their interests effectively (Ballew & Mink, 1986; Rothman, 1992). At the core of this work is consistent monitoring that is focused on the appropriateness of the interventions. Is the student involved? Are the child and family's goals being met? Does the plan need to be improved or changed? What are the outcomes, and do they show that we are being effective?

In case management, we want to ensure that youth and families connect with at least one member of the student support team. Furthermore, it is important that children, adolescents, parents, and caregivers are using the plan developed in the team process to guide what is happening. The plan is regularly checked for progress and revised to attain goals.

Resource management is about the big picture that Marcia Andrews, associate superintendent of safety, culture, and learning environment, talked about at the beginning of the chapter. Andrews, as part of the student support team, looks for gaps in the infrastructure and evaluates the outcomes of students to determine if the system is meeting their needs. The student support team continually seeks and maps new resources, and looks for opportunities to share resources between schools and between districts. Resource management facilitates building the infrastructure that supports the team's work with individual children and adolescents while also expanding the school community capacity to meet the unique needs of all youth. The case and resource management provides quick feedback to all levels of the socio-ecological model.

Case and resource management is an ongoing process, not a single event. Through the process, the youth and family participate in the planned programs and services to achieve the agreed-upon goals. Furthermore, members of the team (or the partnership or collaboration) work to make the best match between needs and available programs and services. Team members focus on getting a high quality of care, access to appropriate services, and services in the most cost-effective way possible (Kane, 1990; Weil & Karls, 1985). Case and resource management can be very intense in the beginning of the relationship with the children, adolescents, and families seeking help or if they are in a crisis. Contact can be less frequent when things are going well. Case and resource management is confidential. Student support teams may have families and youth re-sign (renew) consents signed during the initial connections.

Elements of Case and Resource Management

Case and resource management as part of a student support team flows from goals and plans developed by the young person, parents, caregivers, and family. Although mainly focused on the individual child or teenager, case and resource management has its roots in advocacy. Partnerships and collaborations are not directly involved in the case and resource management with individual students, but are critical to making sure programs and services that are serving youth are supported and sustained. Case and resource management as part of a student support team has six elements:

1. *Monitoring:* Monitoring refers to periodically checking with the youth, parents, caregivers, and family to determine whether the plan is working, the care is of high quality, and all of the planned connections were made. The case and resource manager follows up on the appropriateness of programs and services, monitoring service delivery. The case and resource manager, as part of monitoring, wants to build a one-to-one connection with the young person and family and be viewed as a trusted source of support, guidance, and resources. It can be anticipated that there will be struggles and problems implementing the plan. In the monitoring process, the team member working with the youth and family problem solves what is best for the youth. It is not the role of the team member to have the answers or to reprimand the youth and family for not following the plan. Rather, through the development of the relationship and over the course of implementing the plan, the hope is to positively impact the child or adolescent's behavior and mental health. As part of monitoring, feedback from teachers, programs, and services are collected. It is common to collect information on specific skill development (**Figure 8-2**) and behaviors (**Figure 8-3**).

2. *Crisis intervention:* Children and adolescents as well as family members are vulnerable to crisis. They may feel traumatized and off balance. One of the consequences of being involved with the student support team is that youth and family are more visible to others and their feelings are more exposed. The result is their stress level may be higher. The student support team needs to be prepared to take action in the event of a crisis. Crisis has its own set of procedures/protocols to be implemented when the crisis occurs, which ensures that immediate needs are met. Case and resource management may be instrumental in aligning resources for intervention, recovery, and follow-up (Center for Mental Health in Schools at UCLA, n.d.b.).

3. *Reassessment:* Be proactive; try to anticipate what crises or challenges could arise, and plan for them. The lives of children and adolescents are not static;

Student's Name _____ Age _____ Grade Level _____ RtI Status _____ PBIS Status _____ 4 = Making good progress; move on to another skill 3 = Making progress; continue working on this skill 2 = Understanding beginning to develop; continue working on this skill 1 = No progress; need to review and respond with new strategies						
Skill Development or Other Strategy Goal	**Date**	**Date**	**Date**	**Date**	**Date**	**Comments**
Stress Management – deep breathing						
Plot for Goal #_____			4. _____ 3. _____ 2. _____ 1. _____			
Plot for Goal #_____			4. _____ 3. _____ 2. _____ 1. _____			

Key: RtI = Response to Intervention; PBIS = Positive Behavioral Interventions and Supports

FIGURE 8-2   Student support team skill monitoring chart.

Please return this progress monitoring checklist to _____ by _____.

Your Name_____ Date _____

Student's Name _____ Age _____ Grade Level ____

RtI Status_____ PBIS Status_____

Please check the items in which you have seen progress for this student during the past
_____ weeks.

Behaviors: Check all that apply

___ Disorganized   ___ Forgetful

___ Defiant of rules

___ Fails to accept responsibility

___ Fails to follow behavior expectations

___ Blames others

___ Uses attention-getting behaviors

___ Hyperactive or nervous

___ Appears agitated   ___Demonstrates anger

___ Regular day dreaming

___ Isolated or withdrawn   ___ Mood swings

___ Sexually preoccupied

___ Cheats on assignments   ___ Dishonest

___ Inappropriate language

___ Inappropriate crying

___ Bullies others

___ Demonstrates aggressive behavior

___ Steals others' belongings

___ Lies to teacher and others

___ Vandalizes others' property

___ Overly concerned about achievement

___ Overly sensitive to criticism

___ Talks about personal substance use

___ Talks about family issues that cause concern

___ Other: _____

Physical Concerns: Check all that apply

___ Frequent absences due to illness

___ Frequently fatigued

___ Sleeping in class

___ Hygiene problems

___ Frequent physical complaints

___ Slurred speech

___ Overly concerned about body image

___ Evidence of multiple cuts or skin abrasions

___ Requests passes to see school nurse

___ Talks about physical issues that raise concern

___ Other: _____

Key: RtI = Response to Intervention

FIGURE 8-3   Student support team progress monitoring checklist for grades 1–6.

expect change. Make sure that on a regular basis you conduct a brief reassessment to determine whether program and service needs have changed. It is best to talk with the child, adolescent, parent, caregiver, and family about how to check in. Telephone calls, texts, emails, and face-to-face conversations are all possible.

4. *Resource management:* We learn a lot working with individual children and adolescents through case management of monitoring, crisis intervention, and reassessment. Resource management is where we use and apply what we learn working individually to build capacity and hopefully promote the mental health of all young people. Table 8-2 lists a number of elements involved with resource management. They are all related to an ongoing assessment process to determine what is working, what needs to be modified, and how we might go about making the changes. For teams, partnerships, and collaborations, resource management encourages creative problem solving to best utilize resources that are effective and economical.

5. *Feedback:* The experience of working with children, adolescents, parents, caregivers, and families provides continuous information, data, and experience about the school community mental health promoting culture and climate. You know what programs and services are working well with whom and which are not working. This information both informs decisions at the level of the children and adolescents and provides feedback to all levels of the socio-ecological model.

6. *Advocacy:* Youth, parents, caregivers, and family members need to advocate for themselves. Team members need to advocate within the school community for programs and services. Members of the partnerships and collaborations need to be public policy advocates. We will talk more about advocacy later in this chapter.

Role of Documentation in Case and Resource Management

The management of a case and resources involves keeping **documentation**, an accurate written record of the child or adolescent's involvement with the team. Most student support teams will have minimum standards for maintaining a case record, such as having a consent form signed by the parents for services, filing a progress note for each personal or telephone contact, updating the file when a child's situation changes, and having a consistent system for the order in which forms are filed. **Figure 8-4** is an example of a form to track communications and information flow. Secure electronic and Web-based records are common and offer the advantage of automated reminders and easy access. Documentation is important because of the following reasons:

❖ *Consistency in communication and service provision:* Others on staff can pick up the case record and understand the plan, and thus be able to assist the child, adolescent, and family member when he or she calls or drops by.

Date: _____	Grade/Team/Section: _____
Student Name: _____	Date of Birth: _____
Parent Name: _____	Home #: _____
Address: _____	Work #: _____
City/State/Zip: _____	Case Mgr.: _____

Date Sent	Date Received	Data Sources
		Classroom teacher
		PE
		Speech pathologist
		Music
		Art
		RtI coordinator
		Other _____
		Staff follow-up
		Follow-up reminder
		Student evaluation sheet
		Nurse data form
		Counselor data form
		Parent letter and questionnaire
		Release of information
		Report cards (last 1 year)
		Attendance report
		Discipline chronology

Date	Action Taken
	Summarized staff data responses
	Reviewed referral with counselor
	Reviewed referral with team
	Reviewed alternatives and options

Summary of Action (use reverse side of paper):

Key: RtI = Response to Intervention

FIGURE 8-4 Student support team case and resource management documentation, grades 1–6.

❖ *Data for evaluation reports and funding requests:* School and community organization administrators must satisfy contract and grant requirements by providing accurate data on services and must have accurate information to develop grant proposals. They must also keep data to file fiscal reports and justify funding.

❖ *Monitoring quality of care:* Teams, partnerships, and collaborations can use case records as one tool for determining whether programs and services are responding to children, adolescents, parents, caregivers, and family most appropriately, and whether the available resources are adequate. In this way, gaps and errors can be caught, and unmet needs can be discovered.

❖ *Tracking progress and changes:* Reading a case record can give team members a good sense of how a child or adolescent has been doing over time and whether the goals of the plan have been met.

❖ *A "tickler system":* By keeping a schedule of when visits or calls should occur in the future, team members are reminded to maintain regular contact. These systems of reminders, often called *tickler files,* can be kept electronically. Computer-generated e-mails and text messages are commonly used for these purposes.

It is important to balance paperwork with service provision. Team members' time and energy are limited. There is always competition for people's time. Good case and resource management records are accurate, thorough, and succinct, so that the work is documented but the time with the individual or family does not suffer.

Barriers in the Provision of Case and Resource Management

Case and resource management can have several **barriers** if team members are not careful. The following are a few things to watch for (Poindexter, Valentine, & Conway, 1999):

❖ *Biased program and service plans:* One pitfall is the tendency to connect children and adolescents only with those programs and services with which you are familiar and enjoy a good relationship with the staff. It is important to offer all possible programs, services, and benefits, and to allow the children, adolescents, and families to choose for themselves. When there are problems and changes in the plan, team members need to be diligent not to pressure for particular decisions based on their own feelings and experiences with a program and service.

❖ *Favoritism:* It is common to spend more time or effort on young people whom you like or feel close to and slight others whom you experience as more difficult or demanding. It is vital that decisions about frequency of contact are based on the real needs of the child and family, not on whom you like the best! Good case and resource management treats everyone equally, taking into account the needs of the individual rather than the convenience or preference of the team member.

❖ *Turfism:* Conflicts happen between programs and services. With limited resources, staffing, and funding it is almost expected. Territorial battles among disciplines or agencies interfere with the coordination of services (Kane, 1985). Sometimes competition develops between programs, and staff in other organizations may be hesitant to coordinate services or make referrals to an organization. Effective staff strive to work through these problems in order to meet the needs of the children and adolescents.

❖ *Neglecting to involve the child or adolescent requesting help:* It is easy to make decisions about what needs to happen; however, without the agreement of the child, adolescent, parent, caregiver, and family, probably nothing will happen. In a crisis situation, time is critical, and decisions need to be made quickly to address the crisis. However, in situations that are not a crisis, you will be wasting time if you make decisions without talking directly with the child, adolescent, and family to get their approval (even on what you think are small decisions with positive outcomes and consequences).

Advocacy for Mental Health Programs and Services

Mental health programs and services exist with the tension that on any given day, changes may happen: funding may be cut for political reasons, regardless of program performance; legislation may divert funding to new, higher-priority initiatives; changes in program participants' eligibility criteria may affect the priority population's access to a program; economic factors such as recession might make money tight; or a new national (or state, local, school, business, hospital, or community) health priority might usurp a program's place in funders' and people's consciousness, leaving the program and its staff, stakeholders, and participants vulnerable to program closure. And if that is not enough, within the school community, change can happen at any moment. Expect staff comings and goings, new programs, curricula mandates, and policies. And all the while, children and adolescents and their families will move through their lives in the school community.

Advocacy is an important part of case and resource management. The role of advocacy in sustaining the mental health promoting school community goes beyond case and resource management. Advocacy is action in support of a cause or proposal. It can be political, as in lobbying for specific legislation, or social, as in speaking out on behalf of those without a voice. Broadly, advocacy is part of being a professional. At the same time, from the narrow perspective of a member of a team, partnership, or collaboration, advocacy is championing the mental health promoting school community, fighting for funding, and engaging others in order to sustain the programs and services required to address the needs of children and adolescents. You will work with parents and students to be their own advocates. You will work within your own school community system. And you will work across the broader system to promote public policy change. In all cases, as an advocate, you perform several functions: support, help, assist and aid, speak and plead on behalf of others, and defend and argue for people, programs, and services.

Promoting Self-Advocacy Skills

Significantly involving consumers (i.e., children, adolescents, parents, caregivers, and family members) who use mental health programs and services in system planning and evaluation is essential to the development of effective and responsive programs and services. Strong input from consumers is required to determine which services families and students find useful and appropriate, what type of alternatives or modifications are needed, and which processes need to be improved. After gathering information from all stakeholders, team, partnership and collaboration members need to determine which services might be run by professionals and which are better run by consumers, family members, or others. Finally, there is a need for consumers to become more empowered in their own recovery by advocating for programs and services.

A major challenge is that most children, adolescents, parents, caregivers, and family members do not have the skills to identify their needs and express their opinions in a clear, positive, and assertive manner. Most do not have the experience or training to allow them to effectively influence political systems. Working with consumers to be their own advocates means preparing them. To make an impact on their environments, they need assistance to feel empowered to make changes. Training youth, parents, caregivers, and family members to be advocates focuses on seven advocacy tasks (**Table 8-3**). Consumers as advocates not only impact the programs and services they or their child receives, but potentially, consumers as advocates impact the broader range of primary, secondary, and tertiary programs and services.

Advocating for Services and Change in Your Own System

Advocacy for change within one's own school community can bring with it some ethical dilemmas. The loyalty of an advocate is to the persons or groups who are being neglected by society or the service system; your complete loyalty cannot go to the school community organization that employs you. This conflict of values requires a strong sense of purpose and mission, as well as a strong identity as a professional with professional responsibility to be an advocate. Dilemmas faced by many professionals include questions such as: Will I jeopardize my job if I am too outspoken for the rights of those I serve? Is it safe to make waves in my organization? Workers in large organizations (such as hospitals, schools, and government agencies) often find themselves faced with rigid legal rules and restrictions that hamper their ability to be advocates, but they know changes are needed to provide empowering, appropriate services. These individuals often must decide how to best serve those who need help within their own service provision system.

TABLE 8-3   Youth, Parents, Caregivers, and Family Members' Advocacy Tasks

1. *Learn the rules of the game:* Advocates educate themselves about their local school community. They know how decisions are made and by whom. Advocates know about legal rights. They also know the procedures parents must follow to protect their rights and their child's rights.
2. *Gather information:* Advocates gather facts and information. As they gather information and organize documents, they learn about the child's educational and mental health history. Advocates use facts and independent documentation to resolve disagreements and disputes with the school.
3. *Plan and prepare:* Advocates know that planning prevents problems. Advocates do not expect school community staff to tell them about rights and responsibilities. Advocates read school laws, regulations, and cases to get answers to their questions. They learn how to use information to monitor a child's progress in programs and services as well as in school. They prepare for meetings, create agendas, write objectives, and use meeting worksheets and follow-up letters to clarify problems and nail down agreements.
4. *Keep written records:* Because documents are often the keys to success, advocates keep written records. They know that if a statement is not written down, it was not said. They make requests in writing and write polite follow-up letters to document events, discussions, and meetings.
5. *Ask questions, listen to answers:* Advocates are not afraid to ask questions. When they ask questions, they listen carefully to answers. Advocates know how to use "Who, what, why, where, when, how, and explain questions" (5 Ws + H + E) to discover the true reasons for positions.
6. *Identify problems:* Advocates learn to define and describe problems from all angles. They use their knowledge of interests, fears, and positions to develop strategies. Advocates are problem solvers. They do not waste valuable time and energy looking for people to blame.
7. *Propose solutions:* Advocates know that consumers can negotiate with school community teams, partnerships, and collaborations as well as the school and community organization staff for programs and services. As negotiators, advocates discuss issues and make offers or proposals. They seek win–win solutions that will satisfy the interests of consumers and school community programs and services.

One of your most important tasks as an advocate within your own system is to determine what can be changed. For example, if you are restricted by federal guidelines, then you may have to exist within those parameters. However, if the decision about a certain policy has been made locally, you may be more successful in changing the way things are currently done. That is not to say that you cannot advocate for change of the guidelines at the state or federal level in the long term.

You probably will (or already) have a good idea about why your issue is important. You probably also know something about its history, and what brought the situation about. That is great, but before you face the world in a big-time arena (or even small-time), you will need to be armed with quite a lot of extra knowledge about the background of your issue, as well as the way it affects your school community. The bottom line is that before you proceed with the specific plans, recommendations, and suggestions, you will need a nice, solid, comforting layer of knowledge on which to base your actions.

Why do you need a thorough understanding of your issue? For many reasons:

❖ You'll need to have arguments at your fingertips that can convince your members that the issue is important and keep them fired up.

❖ You'll need to persuade allies to join your cause by presenting them with facts that they won't be able to ignore or refute.

❖ You'll need to know why your opponents are taking the side they take, and what financial or other interests they may have in continuing to take that side.

❖ With research, you'll know better what needs to be done to correct a situation. Furthermore, you'll know which of the necessary steps are fairly easy to take, and which may be a major stretch for your organization.

❖ You'll know what strategic style is likely to work best, whether you're going to run an "in your face" type of initiative, or act behind the scenes, or something in between.

❖ When and if the dispute becomes public—as you may want it to do—you will have the answers. If a reporter asks you for a reaction, or shoves a microphone in your face, you will be sure of your facts.

❖ You'll be ready with facts any time you are challenged by your opponent, by the establishment (such as city hall), or by the media.

The facts are important but you also need to know more:

❖ You'll need to know how people feel about the issue, and what they believe.

❖ You'll need to know how the issue links or divides different segments of the community.

❖ You'll need to understand who is pulling the strings to make your opponents take the line they do.

❖ You'll need to know what forces might be at work in the local political scene to make officials drag their feet—or even jump in to oppose you.

❖ You might need to know what it will take to make people give up the old way of doing things and try something else.

❖ You might need to know the belief systems of people who oppose you on ideological grounds.

As you start to advocate within your system, be strategic. Consider who is affected by the issue. Who is affected the most? Who loses, and what do they lose? Who gains, and what do they gain? What are the consequences of the issue for the individuals most affected? Their families? The school community?

You also need to ask about the economic impact of the issue. What are the economic costs of the issue, and who bears these costs? What are the economic benefits of the issue, and who benefits?

What is the social impact of the issue? What are the social costs of the issue, and who bears these costs? What are the social benefits of the issue, and who benefits?

What are the barriers to addressing this issue? How can they be overcome?

What resources will be needed to address this issue? Where and how can they be tapped?

As you work within your system to make changes, look outside your system and community. In many cases, other communities and national organizations are involved with similar issues. You may be able to learn from smaller advocacy groups who may be tackling issues similar to yours. However, you'll need to be careful about taking over facts and figures prepared by other organizations. In certain cases, these might not be accurate, or might give a slant that is not helpful to your needs.

One thing you can learn from other groups is their process—the way they went about their work. Look at how they approached the school district. What worked and what did not? Use the partnership and collaboration to develop relationships with key stakeholders who can influence decisions about programs and services at the school community level.

Advocating for Public Policy Change in Broader Systems

Public policy advocacy creates environments in which mental health promotion programs and services can be successful. Advocacy for funding, legislation, regulations, governmental infrastructure, or research ensures the continuation of programs and services. Partnerships and collaborations are involved with public policy.

In order to build skills in advocacy, it is necessary to learn the terminology of advocacy (Galer-Unti, Alley, & Pulliam, 2010). **Table 8-4** lists key advocacy terms. The terms reflect the interactions of organized political and government structures in the making and administering of public decisions for a society. Advocates and lobbyists have the task of getting the public involved in the decision-making and administration processes and influencing the decisions made within them.

Legislative advocacy is, essentially, advocating for or against bills, ordinances, and laws. A bill is a piece of legislation that has been introduced as a proposed law. At the federal level, when a bill has been approved by the Senate and the House, it is signed into law by the president. The federal government has developed Web sites to track bills' progress toward becoming law. States vary widely in their processes of passing a bill to create a law. You can use the state and local government legislative Web sites to track local and state legislation.

Municipalities typically pass ordinances, which are enforced within the confines of the city. So an ordinance that applies within the confines of one town may not exist in the next town over. This is often confusing to people.

TABLE 8-4 Key Advocacy Terms and Definitions	
Advocacy	The processes by which individuals or groups attempt to bring about social or organizational change on behalf of a particular health goal, program, interest, or population
Appropriations	Legislation that designates or appropriates specific funding to a program at or below the authorization limit
Authorizations	Legislation that sets policies or programs and an upper spending limit
Bill	A proposed law presented for approval to a legislative body
Direct lobbying	Communication with a legislator or a member of a legislator's staff that gives a viewpoint on a specific piece of legislation
Electioneering	Persuasion of voters in a political campaign
Grassroots lobbying	Any attempt to indirectly influence legislators by motivating members of the public to express specific views to legislators and legislative aides
Law	A local, state, or federal bill that has been passed by a legislative process (e.g., a federal law passed by the U.S. Senate and the House of Representatives and signed by the president)
Lobbyist	An individual hired to represent the legislative interests of an organization (or related group of organizations) to members of a legislature, or other governing body
Media advocacy	Strategic use of news media and, when appropriate, paid advertising to support community organizing to advance a public policy initiative
Ordinance	A statute or regulation, usually enacted by a city or other municipal government

Source: From Fertman, C.I., & Allensworth, D.D. (2010). *Health promotion programs: From theory to practice* (p. 188). San Francisco: Jossey-Bass. Copyright © 2010 by the Society for Public Health Education. All rights reserved.

One town may allow drivers to use cell phones, whereas an adjacent community requires a hands-free device. Driving across the city limit, then, while talking on a cell phone, might result in a fine.

Two types of legislative processes are of significant interest to us. An authorization is a law that authorizes a program. It sets in place a policy or program. Appropriations differ from authorizations in their emphasis. Whereas authorizations set policies or programs, appropriations designate money for

specific purposes. The federal government and state legislatures have clear dead-
lines for their budget approvals. Unlike bills, which can be debated throughout
the legislative calendar, appropriations occur at a set point in the legislative calendar and are generally tied to the budget process. It is a good idea to keep an eye
on these funding cycles in order to know when arguments for funding for health
promotion programs will be most effective.

Influencing the legislative process occurs in a variety of ways. Different
types of lobbying might be used to influence passage of a bill or approval of an
appropriation.

As a public policy advocate, you do a range of activities. The activities all
involve your passion for and interest in promoting the mental health of children
and adolescents. **Table 8-5** provides a sample of possible activities. You do not
need to do them all. Working in advocacy is truly a team effort. Some people
are good at researching facts, whereas others are comfortable speaking out at
public meetings. Many people find visiting elected officials, whether it is the
local mayor, state officials, or representatives in Washington, D.C., to be worthwhile, influential, and important to the quality of school community program
and services.

Being a public policy advocate for mental health promoting school communities, you are involved with many organizations. Two large national advocacy organizations are the National Federation of Families for Children's Mental
Health and the National Alliance on Mental Illness. Both have active advocacy
that works across the socio-ecological levels.

TABLE 8-5   Public Policy Advocacy Activities
1. Presenting testimony to a local funding source about the needs of the community and its residents
2. Presenting written or oral testimony to the state legislature about a proposed bill that would be detrimental to the residents of the community
3. Working with a lobbyist from a large state agency to craft or change a piece of legislation
4. Talking directly to members of Congress or their staff members about legislation and issues that directly affect the population whom you serve
5. Providing information and technical assistance to a legislator on your agency or its service recipients
6. Developing or participating in coalitions that are formed to affect social change
7. Helping with a voter registration drive, perhaps with your agency's service recipients and their families, so that your agency or interest group can have a greater voice in the political process
8. Helping a local agency or support group to launch a letter-writing campaign to legislators about a particular important issue
9. Organizing or participating in demonstrations to bring attention to a certain issue or to protest a particular policy

The **National Federation of Families for Children's Mental Health (FFCMH)** is run by consumers (families) and arose 20 years ago from a grassroots movement. The membership includes more than 120 chapters and state organizations representing the families of children and youth with mental health needs. It supports that families have a primary decision-making role in the care of their own children as well as in the development of policies and procedures governing care for all children in their community, state, tribe, territory, and nation. It provides advocacy at the national level for the rights of children and youth with emotional, behavioral, and mental health challenges and their families. It provides leadership and technical assistance to a nationwide network of family-run organizations. It collaborates with family-run and other child-serving organizations to transform mental health care.

The **National Alliance on Mental Illness (NAMI)** is the largest national grassroots mental health organization dedicated to building better lives for the millions of Americans affected by mental illness. NAMI advocates for access to services, treatment, support, and research, and is steadfast in its commitment to raising awareness and building a community of hope for all of those in need. From its inception in 1979, NAMI has been dedicated to improving the lives of individuals and families affected by mental illness (NAMI, 2012).

The message of the organizations is that mental health concerns and problems affect all children, adolescents, and families, and that programs and services work and need to be supported and funded. Cuts in funding and support are devastating to children, adolescents, families, and our communities. One consequence of cuts is that the cost of not getting needed programs and services produces even higher costs in the long run. Addressing mental health concerns and problems is everyone's problem, and the solution is everyone's responsibility. We must protect and strengthen our mental healthcare system—it's a real investment that returns real benefits.

Summary

Sustaining mental health programs and services requires that teams, partnerships, and collaborations take a number of actions. The actions include a focus on fidelity and adaptation related to program and service quality. Action is needed to sustain teams, partnerships, and collaborations through ongoing skill development and problem solving, and in particular preventing staff burnout. Approaches to prevent burnout among staff are system- and person-centered. Likewise, sustaining programs and services requires social support, which is created through youth peer-to-peer and youth–staff interactions. It is also important to give a clear message of recovery and hope to youth and families struggling with mental health concerns and problems. Recovery from mental disorders and substance use disorders is a process of change through which individuals improve their health and wellness, live a self-directed life, and strive to reach their full potential. Youth and family case and resource management is required: a systematic procedure of continual feedback and monitoring of individual children and adolescents' participation in planned activities and progress toward stated goals. Finally, advocacy takes place at a number of levels including working with children, adolescents, parents, caregivers, and families to be their own advocates, working on changes within existing systems, and working on public policy.

For Practice and Discussion

1. Why are fidelity and adaptation important? What makes educators quick to adapt a program to meet their needs? Discuss the pros and cons of fidelity and adaptation.
2. Your local school district superintendent has recruited you to develop the student support team, a yearlong skill development in-service program. Where do you start? Draft a sample plan, taking into account the needs of the team and the school. Compare your plan to a local district's plan. How did you do?
3. Use John's story from the beginning of the chapter to differentiate case management from resource management. Based on the story, what feedback might you provide to the local partnerships? What are potential program and service gaps?
4. Liza and her family have a multitude of issues that have presented themselves after her initial referral to the student support team for anger issues. They live in a rural area, her dad lost his job recently, and her mom is underemployed working at a low paying job and exhibits signs of depression. What services might Liza and her family need, and how can they get the most from them?
5. There is a growing need for recreational and after-school activities for teens in your town. A few friends thought of a plan to use an old storefront as an after school hangout that would focus on recreational and skill-building activities for adolescents, but you have no funds. You think you can get volunteer workers and mentors to help staff the place. Now what do you do? Prepare a plan detailing the steps to take and the people/organizations to involve.

Key Terms

Adaptation   178
Advocacy   190
Barriers   189
Case and resource management   182
Documentation   187
Fidelity   178
Hope   180
National Alliance on Mental Illness
  (NAMI)   197

National Federation of Families
  for Children's Mental Health
  (FFCMH)   197
Ongoing skill development   178
Problem solving   178
Public policy   194
Recovery   180
Social support   176
Staff burnout   178

References

Adelman, H., & Taylor, L. (2007). Best practices in the use of resource teams to enhance learning supports. In A. Thomas & J. Grimes (Eds.), *Best Practices in School Psychology V* (pp. 2–17). Bethesda, MD: National Association of School Psychologists.

Ballew, J., & Mink, G. (1986). *Case Management in the Human Services*. Springfield, IL: Thomas.

Center for Mental Health in Schools at UCLA. (n.d.a.). Case management in the school context. Retrieved from http://www.smhp.psych.ucla.edu/pdfdocs/quicktraining/casemanagement .pdf

Center for Mental Health in Schools at UCLA. (n.d.b.). Mental health assistance at schools: Overview of practices for problem identification, triage, referral, and management of care. Retrieved from http://smhp.psych.ucla.edu/pdfdocs/practicenotes/developingsystems.pdf

Galer-Unti, R.A., Alley, K.B., & Pulliam, R.M. (2010). Advocacy. In C. Fertman & D. Allensworth (Eds.), *Health Promotion Programs: From Theory to Practice* (pp. 181–199). San Francisco: Jossey-Bass.

Kane, R.A. (1985). Case management in health care settings. In M. Weil, J.M. Karls, & Associates (Eds.), *Case Management in Human Services Practice: A Systematic Approach to Mobilizing Resources for Clients* (pp. 170–203). San Francisco: Jossey-Bass.

Kane, R.A. (1990). Case management and assessment of the elderly. In R. Kane, J. Grimley Evans, & D. MacFadyen (Eds.), *Improving the Health of Older People: A World View* (pp. 398–416). New York: Oxford University Press.

National Alliance on Mental Illness (NAMI). (2012). About NAMI. Retrieved from http://www .nami.org/template.cfm?section=About_NAMI

Poindexter, C., Valentine, D., & Conway, P. (1999). *Essential Skills for Human Services*. Belmont, CA: Wadsworth.

Rothman, J. (1992). *Guidelines for Case Management: Putting Research to Professional Use*. Itasca, IL: Peacock.

Substance Abuse and Mental Health Services Administration. (2011). Guiding principles of recovery. Retrieved from http://www.samhsa.gov/samhsanewsletter/Volume_17 _Number_5/GuidingPrinciples.aspx

Weil, M., & Karls, J.M. (1985). *Case Management in Human Service Practice*. San Francisco: Jossey-Bass.

ENGAGING FAMILIES

In this chapter, we will:

✦ Discuss family engagement in mental health programs and services

✦ Explain family engagement capacity building

✦ Describe strategies to address challenges to family engagement

✦ Present family engagement and family-centered mental health policy and practice

Scenarios

I hurt when I hear about other parents' kids getting into trouble. I feel bad because part of me feels relief that it isn't my child. I've had plenty of tough times with my own kids. It isn't easy. I feel bad because sometimes I have wished that the kids would just run away. You can call me a bad mother if you want. Sometimes I was too tired and exhausted to care. But I have never stopped loving my children. At some point I realized that it can't be all about my kid. I am not quite sure when the switch happened. I realized that it (the problem) has to be larger. It's got to be about everyone's children. What I really needed was to feel connected with other parents and school people. To feel supported and to know we had a voice and that people saw us. We were not invisible, dismissed as uninterested, disconnected.

Source: Deja Diamond, mother

My son started showing problems at the age of 12. I started pushing for services and [it] wasn't until 14 that I actually got [him] services. I did learn a little bit, like I needed to ask for an IEP, but all they did was test him for academics. He didn't qualify because his academics were fine, but then tested for ADHD and he was put on medicine. (I initially refused medicine.) When I went to a therapist they were just explaining to me that I had this horrible kid and if I didn't do something quick, he was going to turn into a psychopath and I felt they were slamming me and I had poor parenting skills, so I took offense to that. When he got tested for ADHD [the] school wanted thousands of dollars per semester and saying that they could work out all his problems within the school, but I couldn't afford that. I took a parenting class when he was 15 for parents with an adolescent with behavioral problems and it was not until I took that class, that I was able to understand and modify how I treat my child. The reason why the class was so effective was everyone was having trouble with their kids and the normal parenting skills didn't work. I was in a classroom full of parents who had experienced what I experienced so I didn't think that I was a bad parent.

Source: Unknown (Cooper et al., 2001)

Family Engagement in Mental Health Programs and Services

Parents and caregivers are the decision makers in their children's lives. To help children means working with and supporting their parents and caregivers; however, simply working with parents and caregivers to address the needs and concerns of their child is insufficient. Parents and caregivers need to be full partners with school community staff and other members of the community in the work of creating and sustaining mental health programs and services. A symbol of this expanded view of the family's role is represented by the research-informed shift in terminology from **parental involvement**, representing supportive activities that occur primarily in the home between parent and child, to **family engagement**, broadening the role of families from at-home activities to full partnerships with school community staff and other parents and community members in the overall improvement of the school community. A similar shift is also seen in the mental health system. Researchers, advocates, and policy makers acknowledge family- and youth-driven programs and services are a core component in promoting the transition from a child-centered perspective to a family-centered perspective in mental health policy and practice.

This broader definition and view requires that family engagement be a **shared responsibility** among families, school community staff, and community members in which families are committed to actively supporting their children's learning and healthy development (including mental health), and school community personnel and community members are committed to engaging and partnering with families in meaningful and culturally respectful, culturally competent, and culturally proficient ways. This shared responsibility must be continuous across a child's lifespan, from cradle to career. And it must occur in multiple settings where children and adolescents learn, live, and play: at home, at school, and in community settings.

Family Engagement Capacity Building

Schools, school districts, and community organizations' capacity and approaches to parent engagement have evolved over the last 40 years. Mapp (2012) discusses five themes (**Table 9-1**) that shape and undergird parent engagement, all of which flow from the parent involvement provisions of the Title I Elementary and Secondary Education Act passed in 2002, known more familiarly as the No Child Left Behind Act, and which addresses family engagement in a number of sections. These themes provide us with a context for the current legislative environment for how schools operate. They provide a picture of and explanation for why family engagement initiatives may struggle as well as leverage points for family engagement. They point toward increasing **organizational capacity** to train school community staff and parents, caregivers, and family members on how to create and support family engagement.

Throughout the history of parental engagement in schools, parents and school staff have been asked to engage in ways for which neither side was prepared. The antipoverty programs of the 1960s provided technical assistance and capacity building to poor communities and communities of color, resulting in the cultivation of a cadre of parents who were ready and able to participate in district and school councils. Over the past few decades, however, the overall federal emphasis on capacity building has dissipated, and there has been a steady decrease in the focus on the capacity-building side of parental engagement. For example, recent national legislation places a heavy emphasis on the role of parents in the development of parent involvement policies at the district

---

TABLE 9-1   What Needs to Be Done to Support Parent Engagement

❖ Increase the focus on and commitment to building the capacity of families and school community personnel to create and sustain partnerships that support children's learning and healthy development
❖ Promote systemic initiatives of family engagement versus "random acts"
❖ Focus on an improvement mindset for family engagement versus compliance
❖ Shift the emphasis of family engagement from individual development to collective growth
❖ Increase commitment to monitoring and evaluation

Source: Mapp, K. L. (2012). Title I and parent involvement: Lessons from the past, recommendations for the future. Reprinted with permission of the Center for American Progress and American Enterprise Institute, Washington, DC.

and school levels and the development of school–parent compacts, but lacks an equal and corresponding emphasis on the type of capacity building required for parents to fulfill these **roles** (Elmore, 2002).

Similarly, state-, district-, and school-level staff receive little to no training on the skills and competencies required to partner with families. There has been and continues to be little leadership from any source demanding or providing pre- or in-service training of teachers in this area. Teachers are also unprepared to work with families in supporting these roles. Many new teachers identified working with families as their greatest challenge and the area where they feel least well prepared (Mapp, 2012). The limited capacity of both parents and states, school districts, and communities to partner with each other and share the responsibility of improving child and adolescent learning and health performance factors heavily as we think about how to build capacity.

The **Harvard Family Research Project (HFRP)** has provided leadership to address the family engagement capacity building void. The project has developed family engagement capacity-building principles (**Table 9-2**) that clearly emphasize ongoing shared responsibility across a school community. In a joint effort with United Way Worldwide, the Harvard Family Research Project developed **Family Engagement for High School Success** (discussed in the following section). The initiative's two-part focus is on the comprehensive planning and early implementation of a family engagement initiative. The Centers for Disease Control and Prevention (CDC), within the family component of the coordinated school health program, has developed materials for teachers and school district personnel to support parent engagement as part of school health, including promoting mental health. The CDC materials encourage school district capacity building in how school community staff can connect and engage with parents, and then sustain parent engagement (Centers for Disease Control and Prevention, 2012).

TABLE 9-2   Family Engagement Capacity-Building Principles

❖ Family engagement is a shared responsibility in which schools and other community agencies and organizations are committed to reaching out to engage families in meaningful ways and in which families are committed to actively supporting their children's learning and development.

❖ Family engagement is continuous across a child's life and entails enduring commitment, but parental roles change as children mature into young adulthood.

❖ Effective family engagement cuts across and reinforces learning in the multiple settings where children learn—at home, in prekindergarten programs, in school, in afterschool and summer programs, in faith-based institutions, and in the community.

Source: Weiss, H., & Lopez, M.E. (2009). Redefining family engagement in education. *FINE Newsletter*, I(2). © 2013 President and Fellows of Harvard College. Reprinted with permission from Harvard Family Research Project. Since 1983, HFRP has helped stakeholders develop and evaluate strategies to promote the wellbeing of children, youth, families, and their communities. To learn more about how HFRP can support your work with children and families, visit hfrp.org.

Family Engagement for High School Success Initiative

This family engagement capacity-building initiative models how to bring families, school leaders, community partners, and students together to build a network of support to keep students on the path to high school graduation, college or advanced training, and successful lives beyond. Developed as a part of the initiative is the Family Engagement for High School Success Toolkit, which details how to plan and implement parent engagement capacity building in local school communities. The outcome-focused approach aims to design family engagement strategies to remove obstacles to engagement, and, ultimately, build stronger connections between families and schools. Local United Ways are the initiative brokers convening the parents of the school communities along with the local organizations including the school districts. The Family Engagement for High School Success Toolkit helps local United Way chapters, nonprofits, schools, and other community organizations to achieve three goals:

1. Identify how to spot ninth graders who are at risk of dropping out, considering factors such as attendance, behavior, and academic performance.

2. Enlist and enroll the right partners and work creatively to reach parents of at-risk kids.

3. Work with parents, schools, and partners to apply research-based strategies and promising practices to get at-risk students back on track to graduate from high school.

It is important to note that this toolkit is based on an initiative that deliberately focused on improving academic outcomes for students at high risk of not graduating from high school, yet the principles contained in the toolkit are applicable to a wide array of K–12 family engagement initiatives. Although the toolkit was created for larger community organizations such as United Way chapters, schools and smaller nonprofits will find the planning and implementation guidance useful as they look to connect with other organizations that can contribute to the development of a comprehensive family engagement initiative.

The toolkit reflects two important family engagement principles. First, family engagement is shared and co-constructed, necessitating the participation of students and families in designing family engagement strategies. Second, school communities can work to address the obstacles to family engagement—including those related to social disadvantage and cultural differences—and provide meaningful opportunities for families to take action.

Emerging Family Engagement Strategies

Emerging family engagement strategies reflect the challenges of family engagement. The challenges are many, and vary by the individual and community, ranging from poverty, single parenting, co-parenting, and housing to health status and religious beliefs. The challenges reflect the lives of parents, caregivers, and family members. Many of the challenges come from the environments in which we live and work. Increasingly, these environments are full of turbulence and anxiety produced by ever-changing economic conditions and developments, governmental programs and policies, social relations, communities, families, and cultural tensions. Over time, new strategies evolve as social, economic, and political societal forces impact families and produce new challenges to family engagement. Emerging family engagement strategies operate in synchrony and across mental health programs and services and are carried out with high intensity over a sustained period of time. They are produced when a school community has taken the time and expense to build the capacity of both institutions (schools, agencies, government) and individuals (parents, caregivers, family members), as discussed in the previous section. Four emerging strategies are discussed in this section: **parent- and caregiver-friendly school communities**, **family network organizations**, **parent and family education**, and **out-of-school-time programs**.

Parent- and Caregiver-Friendly School Communities

Creating a school community environment that is parent- and caregiver-friendly eases tension and creates the opportunity for schools and families to partner and collaborate to meet the mental health needs of children and adolescents. Parents, agency staff, teachers, counselors, social workers, and principals in discussions have suggested strategies that lend support to efforts to build good school community and family relationships (Bickham et al., 1998; Jordon, Orozco, & Averett, 2002; Prior & Gerard, 2007):

❖ *Be flexible and creative:* It takes time to build a relationship with parents and to engage them in meaningful activities and conversations. Providing flexibility regarding the time to meet with parents, talking on the telephone, using social media, and having impromptu feedback sessions when parents and family members are available all help to build trust and rapport.

❖ *Assess and respect the needs of families:* Assess the ongoing needs of families. Regularly talk with families individually and in small groups about their needs and goals. This is useful when working with families of a different culture than your own.

❖ *Provide resources for families:* Make space for families and parents in the school and community organization buildings. If we want parents to come, we have to take time to make them feel welcomed. Simple procedures such as offering a beverage and a snack are helpful. Try to provide access to telephones and transportation, if necessary.

❖ *Establish a family feedback loop:* We constantly want to be checking to ensure that the activities and services of the school community are addressing the needs of the child or adolescent. Ask the parents, family members, and youth directly about the programs and services. Ask the community providers to assess the family's satisfaction with the services. Talk with the local family support organization about conducting a feedback and brain-storming session on how to improve services and service gaps.

❖ *Give clear and consistent messages about mental health:* Let students, parents, and families know that (1) every child's mental health is important, (2) many children have mental health problems, (3) these problems are real and painful and can be severe, (4) mental health problems can be recognized and treated, and (5) caring families and communities working together can help.

❖ *Look for activities to involve families:* School community activities are places where teachers and families spend time together in a nonthreatening environment. Sporting events, religious gatherings, and holiday celebrations are all potentially common grounds. Invite families to class activities, send birthday and holiday greeting cards, and e-mail and telephone when their child is doing well. These activities provide a means to have a shared experience and to be a part of the school community that is not necessarily focused on the student. They can serve as a basis for more personal sharing of interests and emotions.

❖ *Create a welcoming, culturally competent school:* Be clear about the school's procedures and rules for parent visitation so that an unsuspecting parent doesn't meet with disapproval rather than welcome when coming to the school. Be aware of the cultures represented in your school and how their home country's education systems compare to ours so that you are somewhat familiar with parents' expectations and actions. The disproportionate and inappropriate identification of culturally and linguistically diverse students as being in need of mental health programs and services raises concerns of miscommunications and stereotyping.

Family Network Organizations

The major family mental health promoting network organization is the National Federation of Families for Children's Mental Health (FFCMH), which was formed in 1989. Its purpose is to bolster family members' individual voices across states, to gather and disseminate information, and to collectively address the needs of families dealing with emotional, behavioral, and mental health issues across child- and family-serving systems. Families wanted their own access to information, and they wanted to affect national-level policy and the development of those policies within states.

Family participation and support in a system of care is fundamental to the FFCMH. Therefore, it works to develop and implement policies, legislation, funding mechanisms, and service delivery systems that utilize the strengths of families in the following ways:

❖ Ensuring that they are equal partners in planning, implementation, and evaluation of services

❖ Viewing the child as a whole person and family as a whole unit rather than emphasizing the disability

❖ Educating and empowering families and children to make decisions about their own lives

❖ Encouraging innovative programming that increases options and promotes the integration of services

A visit to the FFCMH Web site (www.ffcmh.org) links families to the federation's state and local affiliates, newsletter, and technical assistance. The FFCMH has created a national network of family network organizations. The state and local affiliates focus on establishing and strengthening family networks to provide family-to-family support and resources. The Federation's newsletter, *ReClaiming Children*, provides parents and families practical actions and tips for working with schools, community providers, and mental health professionals. Likewise, it gives parents information on advocacy and program evaluation. Technical assistance from the organization supports the system of care that communities have funded to operate the Comprehensive Community Mental Health Services for Children and Their Families Program. Support is also provided to families to develop leadership and advocacy skills.

A number of other national and local organizations also provide families mental health information, resources, support, access, and linkages to programs and services for their child or adolescent. **Mental Health America** (MHA; www.mentalhealthamerica.net) is a consumer-based advocacy group heavily committed to helping people affected by mental illnesses to achieve mental and physical wellness and to performing outreach efforts to help all Americans manage day-to-day stress. MHA is very active in lobbying for mental health legislation and reform on issues such as healthcare reform, mental health parity, comparative effectiveness research, federal prevention initiatives, mental health funding and appropriation, health information technology, and Medicare and Medicaid.

The National Alliance for the Mentally Ill (NAMI) is a nonprofit, grassroots, self-help, support, and advocacy organization of consumers, families, and friends of people with a severe emotional disturbance, such as schizophrenia, major depression, bipolar disorder, obsessive-compulsive disorder, and anxiety disorders. Working on the national, state, and local levels, NAMI provides education about severe brain disorders, supports increased funding for research, and advocates for adequate health insurance, housing, rehabilitation, and jobs for people with serious psychiatric illnesses. Consumers, family members, and friends are encouraged to contact NAMI on the Web at www.nami.org or to call the toll-free NAMI HelpLine at 1-800-950-NAMI (6264) for information and referral to the NAMI affiliate group in their area. The Substance Abuse and Mental Health Services Administration (SAMHSA) Center for Mental Health Services supports the **Statewide Family Network Program**. The purpose of this program is to enhance state capacity and infrastructure to be more oriented to the needs of children and adolescents with serious emotional disturbances and their families by providing information, referrals, and support to families who have a child with a serious emotional disturbance, and to create a mechanism for families to participate in state and local mental health services planning and policy development. Nearly every state has active family organizations dedicated to promoting systems of care that are responsive to the needs of children and adolescents with serious emotional disturbances and their families. Although significant progress has been made, further support will ensure self-sufficient, empowered networks that will effectively participate in state and local mental health services planning and healthcare reform activities related to improving community-based services for children and adolescents with serious emotional disturbances and their families.

Local family network organizations with their roots in the school community needs, economics, cultural diversity, and families exist in most communities. Common are organizations that provide support and information to families who are concerned about a family member or friend's mental health. An example of such an organization in Pennsylvania is the Bridge to Hope sponsored by the Passavant Hospital Foundation as part of their outreach programs. It runs support groups for those impacted by the addiction of a loved one. The Bridge to Hope has worked with over 800 parents since its inception. The group is composed of parents with adult children in recovery, those who continue to abuse drugs, and also those who have lost their children to overdoses. The Bridge to Hope's mission and vision (**Table 9-3**) are to educate and support families confronted with substance abuse and addiction, so they will know they do not walk alone. As a refuge for families, they provide hope, encouragement, support, and education through sharing of experiences with the process of treatment and recovery of a loved one. Through mutual sharing of experiences, the members learn the value

---

TABLE 9-3   Local Family Network Organization Mission and Vision Statements

Bridge to Hope Mission Statement

As a focused support group, our mission is to provide a refuge for the families of those affected by substance abuse and addiction. We will provide encouragement, support, reinforcement, empathy, and education, and share the experiences we have endured while navigating through this arduous process. Our members will be shown a pathway to hope en route to a full recovery of family members and their affected loved ones. We will share our experiences with our communities and educate the public on the epidemic of substance abuse that is occurring locally, regionally, and nationally while respecting the privacy of every individual.

Bridge to Hope Vision Statement

The Bridge to Hope will be an indispensable resource for families and a dynamic, influential force throughout our region and beyond as families and communities confront the difficult task of managing their issues surrounding addiction. Our program, hallmarked by experience, education, dedication, tenacity, value, success, and growth, will be recognized as a model for groups in other locales as the need for support becomes more widespread and its benefits more apparent.

We will be a beacon of enlightenment in a society which today is largely lost in the darkness of misconceptions, stereotypes, and apathy. We will, in fact, create HOPE in what would otherwise be a hopeless epidemic.

Source: Courtesy of Bridge to Hope.

of taking care of themselves. The support groups are generally oriented toward wellness by providing family members with information, coping, and problem-solving skills. In addition, they have a strong advocacy and outreach to local, state, and federal government agencies as well as managed care organizations providing feedback to shape legislation and needed community services.

Parent and Family Education

Over the last 20 years, family education programs have been created to address families' concerns and to lend support. They are by far the easiest to implement, low budget, and manageable for most schools and community agencies. They are practical, accessible, frequently designed for specific groups, and widely available. School professionals that have worked to build strong relationships with parents and have made their schools culturally and family-friendly find these programs a logical extension of their efforts. Clearly, not every community can or will implement a family, school, and provider collaboration. However, parent and family education is a step that most schools and agencies can take.

Education programs to enhance family functioning, prevent behavior problems, and promote mental health have been developed with support from the U.S. Department of Health and Human Services, Center for Substance Abuse Prevention (CSAP) (www.samhsa.gov/about/csap.aspx). Largely, the programs identified through these initiatives have an "academic" orientation with an emphasis on curricula, activities, and psycho-educational processes for specific populations. They are developed in universities through demonstration grants and research studies. The programs are frequently implemented by community agencies in collaboration with a school. The following paragraphs describe a number of programs that focus on parents and might be considered as an offering by a school community in collaboration with parents and community organizations.

The Strengthening Families Program (SFP) is a family skills training program designed to increase resilience and reduce risk factors for behavioral, emotional, academic, and social problems in children 3–16 years old. SFP comprises three life-skills courses delivered in 14 weekly, 2-hour sessions. The Parenting Skills sessions are designed to help parents learn to increase desired behaviors in children by using attention and rewards, clear communication, effective discipline, substance use education, problem solving, and limit setting. The Children's Life Skills sessions are designed to help children learn effective communication, understand their feelings, improve social and problem-solving skills, resist peer pressure, understand the consequences of substance use, and comply with parental rules. In the Family Life Skills sessions, families engage in structured family activities, practice therapeutic child play, conduct family meetings, learn communication skills, practice effective discipline, reinforce positive behaviors in each other, and plan family activities together. Participation in ongoing family support groups and booster sessions is encouraged to increase generalization and the use of skills learned.

Familias Unidas is an intensive family-based intervention for Hispanic families with children ages 12–17. The program is designed to prevent conduct disorders; use of illicit drugs, alcohol, and cigarettes; and risky sexual behaviors by improving family functioning. Familias Unidas is guided by ecodevelopmental theory, which proposes that adolescent behavior is affected by a multiplicity of risk and protective processes operating at different levels (i.e., within family, within peer network, and beyond), often with compounding effects. The program is also influenced by culturally specific models developed for Hispanic populations in the United States. The intervention is delivered primarily through multiparent groups, which aim to develop effective parenting skills, and family visits, during which parents are encouraged to apply those skills while interacting with their adolescent. The multiparent groups, led by a trained facilitator, meet in weekly 2-hour sessions for the duration of the intervention. Familias Unidas also involves meetings of parents with school personnel, including the school counselor and teachers, to connect parents to their adolescent's school world. Family activities involving the parents, the adolescent, and his or her peers and their parents allow parents to connect to their adolescent's peer network and practice monitoring skills.

WATCH D.O.G.S. (Dads of Great Students) is a program of the National Center for Fathering focusing on prevention of violence in schools by using the positive influence of fathers and father figures to provide an unobtrusive presence in the schools, and to be a positive role model for students. Through WATCH D.O.G.S. participation, schools get an enhanced sense of security at their buildings, students gain positive male role models, and fathers learn about the complex challenges facing today's youth and gain awareness of the positive impact they can have on a student's academic performance, self-esteem, and social behavior. WATCH D.O.G.S. is for fathers and father figures who volunteer at least 1 day each year at an official WATCH D.O.G.S. school. During the day, WATCH D.O.G.S may read with students, eat lunch with them, watch school entrances and hallways, mentor students, and any other assigned activities.

Out-of-School-Time Programs

Out-of-school-time programs encompass a broad array of opportunities that support children and youth, including before- and afterschool programs and summer learning programs. One constant across these multiple settings where children learn is families. Families are essential partners in successful out-of-school-time (OST) programs and play many important roles: consumers, advocates, allies, and volunteers.

One initiative to strengthen programs' capacity for engaging families to improve youth outcomes was the Engaging Families Initiative (EFI), a 4-year program of the Boston Build the Out-of-School Time Network (BOSTnet) that resulted in the preparation and dissemination of an Engaging Families Toolkit.

The EFI was designed to work with after school service providers focused on black and Latino children's academic and informal learning by increasing parental engagement. BOSTnet continues to provide technical assistance, operational support, and connection to community resources from local organizations. A number of tools were developed to increase staff capacity in the area of parent engagement. The tools are for self-assessment of program practices and feasible and practical strategies for enhancing parent engagement in after-school programs.

Family Engagement and Family-Centered Mental Health Policy and Practice

Family-centered mental health policy and practice is the emerging model to deliver programs and services to youth and their families. It reflects an evolution in thinking about how best to serve young people and their families. Although the concept of family-centered policy and practice is new and evolving, there are emerging definitions in the field (**Table 9-4**). The family-centered mental health policy and practice is designed to create positive outcomes for children and families through:

- ❖ Policy that advocates for resources and system change and ensures the quality of family engagement
- ❖ School community mental health programs and services that are collaborative, built on the strengths of families, based on core principles, driven by quality standards, and evaluated based on best practices
- ❖ Parent, caregiver, and family member leaders that serve as advocates, policy makers, and champions of quality
- ❖ School community partnerships where all segments come together and begin the process of identifying and achieving mutual goals and objectives

Family-centered mental health policy and practice links family, community support, and school community organizations to establish continuity of care. The programs and services are family-centered and are designed and delivered according to the particular needs and preferences of the family members. Plans are designed to build on strengths and resources, rather than weaknesses and deficits. Consensus is gathered from the group to determine the needs that

---

TABLE 9-4   Definition of Family-Centered Mental Health Policy and Practice

Family-driven means families have a primary decision-making role in the care of their own children as well as the policies and procedures governing care for all children in their community, state, tribe, territory, and nation. This includes:

- ❖ Choosing culturally and linguistically competent supports, services, and providers
- ❖ Setting goals
- ❖ Designing, implementing, and evaluating programs
- ❖ Monitoring outcomes
- ❖ Partnering in funding decisions

Source: Working Definition of Family-Driven Care, January 2008. Rockville, MD: National Federation of Families for Children's Mental Health. Reprinted by permission of National Federation of Families.

are in the best interests of the child. Parents, caregivers, and family members serve as leaders for advocacy. Professionals and families are seen as equal partners. Educational and behavioral goals are agreed upon. Programs and services are comprehensive, and efforts are made to ensure that they are accessible to the family and youth. The concepts of *equality*, *mutuality*, and *teamwork* are terms used to describe the collaborations (Osher & Osher, 2002; Worthington, Hernandez, Friedman, & Uzzell, 2001).

The concept of family-centered mental health policy and practice has roots in both the education and mental health systems. For many years now, school special education programs utilized Individualized Education Programs (IEPs), and Positive Behavioral Interventions and Supports (PBIS) have promoted person-centered planning and have engaged families in the treatment of children. In the mental health field, the system of care model and wraparound services have promoted a planning process for treatment that is family focused. Today, both education and mental health systems use family-driven language. For transformation to be effective requires attitudinal change, new skills, redeployment of resources, and time for all of this to occur. Transformation to family-centered mental health policy and practice is complex, multidimensional, and, in some cases, revolutionary. Osher and colleagues (2006) list 10 principles (**Table 9-5**)

TABLE 9-5   Principles of Family-Centered Mental Health Policy and Practice

❖ Families and youth, providers, and administrators embrace the concept of sharing decision making and responsibility for outcomes.

❖ Families and youth are given accurate, understandable, and complete information necessary to set goals and to make informed decisions and choices about the right services and supports for individual children and their families.

❖ All children, youth, and families have a biological, adoptive, foster, or surrogate family voice advocating on their behalf and may appoint them as substitute decision makers at any time.

❖ Families and family-run organizations engage in peer support activities to reduce isolation, gather and disseminate accurate information, and strengthen the family voice.

❖ Families and family-run organizations provide direction for decisions that impact funding for services, treatments, and supports and advocate for families and youth to have choices.

❖ Providers take the initiative to change policy and practice from provider-driven to family-driven.

❖ Administrators allocate staff, training, support and resources to make family-driven practice work at the point where services and supports are delivered to children, youth, and families and where family and youth-run organizations are funded and sustained.

❖ Community attitude change efforts focus on removing barriers and discrimination created by stigma.

❖ Communities and private agencies embrace, value, and celebrate the diverse cultures of their children, youth, and families and work to eliminate mental health disparities.

❖ Everyone who connects with children, youth, and families continually advances their own cultural and linguistic responsiveness as the population served changes so that the needs of the diverse populations are appropriately addressed.

Source: Working Definition of Family-Driven Care. January 2008. Rockville, MD: National Federation of Families for Children's Mental Health. Reprinted by permission of National Federation of Families.

that guide the development of family-centered mental health policy and practice, and these principles illustrate the multi-faceted nature of the task. For many practitioners, the adoption of these principles is visionary and definitely revolutionary, but for parents and their children, it is viewed as obligatory.

Family-centered mental health policy and practice present an opportunity for family engagement in the mental health promoting school community. It can reinforce the underlying principle (Table 9-2) of family engagement being a shared responsibility of the school community and families. As part of this opportunity all members of student support teams, partnerships, and collaborations are required to (1) share the vision of how to engage families for decision making and action; (2) use common language—communication is informative, efficient, effective, and relevant to all the members of the team, especially families; and (3) share a common experience—the actions, procedures, and operations are experienced by all the members of the teams, partnerships, and collaborations (Kutash & Duchnowski, 2007) .

As in most reform movements, both small and large steps can be taken to achieve the desired change. Family-centered mental health policy and practice provides opportunities for families' voices to be included in how school communities promote the mental health of youth and families. Increasing family voice means ensuring that family and youth voices are heard and valued; that families and youth have access to useful, usable, and understandable information and data; that school communities provide sound professional expertise to help families make decisions; and that schools share power, authority, resources, and responsibility for plans and choices (Osher, Osher, & Blau, 2006).

Challenges in Engaging Those with Serious Mental Health Concerns and Problems

Engaging families of children and adolescents with serious mental health concerns and problems (e.g., youth with substance disorder, depression, emotional disturbance, in recovery) is a priority within family-centered mental health policy and practice. Families, students, mental health professionals, school teachers, principals, social workers, and counselors may have differing ideas about how and what it means to involve families in programs and services. Family members who interact with their child's school frequently report feeling marginalized and feeling as if they are perceived as uncaring or too overwhelmed in their own lives to be an effective parent. Families often feel exhausted, ashamed, isolated, and lacking support. The opening chapter vignette from Deja Diamond reflects this perspective.

The families may struggle with multiple stressors, including poverty, single parenting, joblessness, racism, violence, drug abuse, alcoholism, and their own mental health issues. Parents' own mental health and life concerns can impair their parenting abilities. Misconceptions about the roles of school systems and mental health services can cause additional confusion (Federation of Families for

Children's Mental Health, 2001). Some parents themselves have had problems in school, and may avoid working with school personnel due to painful memories of these problems (Harry, 1992).

Families often have concerns about maintaining a sense of control over parenting their children. Professional jargon used by both educators and mental health professionals can be perceived as condescending and cause parents to feel ineffective in addressing their concerns about their own children. Family members may fear that they will be blamed for a teenager's problems. In addition, many, if not most, families view school and mental health issues and services with suspicion and stigma and have concerns about the confidentiality of information shared with school and mental health professionals. Such negative perceptions perpetuate negative school and family relationships.

Students, particularly adolescents, are adept at keeping parents and teachers at odds. They are establishing independence and autonomy and may not want family members involved in their school and mental health treatment. A variety of factors may influence students' willingness to involve their families with their school. Family members may not approve of the child's behavior in school. Students want to conceal the problems (e.g., disruptive behavior, sexuality, substance abuse) that are apparent to school personnel. This is especially true when there is potential for volatile family reaction, family conflict, or abuse (Bickham et al., 1998).

Additional challenges to family involvement may be created by administrative structures and problems associated with service systems and schools. The social service community, including schools, has often used the challenging nature of the symptoms and many of the issues that these families face to place blame onto parents and other family members for their children's behavior (Osher, Penn, & Spencer, 2008; Perry, Kaufmann, Hoover, & Zundel, 2008). Just the sheer number of professional adults involved with their child can seem overwhelming and intimidating to parents. Although mental health treatment is available, it is often difficult for families to access. It can be expensive and time consuming. Community mental health programs may lack the resources (e.g., funding, staffing) to provide families with evening and weekend appointments, child care, and transportation. Programs also may lack resources to provide the training and support needed by clinicians to facilitate family involvement. Students often require services from several sources. Parents are challenged to coordinate services and activities. They may encounter conflicting requirements, different atmospheres and expectations, and contradictory messages. Furthermore, as schools strive to meet the needs of these children, many teachers and support staff are cast in unfamiliar roles and acquire new responsibilities with little preparation and support. Low teacher expectations for students with an emotional disturbance reinforce their generally poor performance in schools, and such students have been pushed out of their local schools by transfer, suspension, and hostility (Lehr, Johnson, Bremer, Cosio, & Thompson, 2004).

Helping Relationships

Engaging families of children and adolescents with serious mental health concerns and problems requires a relationship between the families and school community organizations. Without underlying trust and honesty between school community professionals and family members, there can be no expectations for positive outcomes for anyone: student, family, or school. Of all the places where children and adolescents with a mental health concern spend time, schools are where many families feel their children and adolescents are the most vulnerable. Family members say their relationships with school community professionals make or break their willingness to be involved in school community organizations (i.e., schools, agencies). And although families and organizations recognize the value of collaborating and working together, the reality of the relationships can be frustrating for everyone involved. In **Box 9-1**, John, a parent, reflects on his experience, reinforcing the struggles and importance of family engagement when a child has a serious mental health concern and problem.

Box 9-1
John, a Parent, Reflects on Family Engagement

Family denial is as natural a reaction as any other defense mechanism, and it is pervasive. With substance abuse at epidemic levels, it is affecting just as many "good" homes as "troubled" homes. Parents who have instilled a traditional value system into their family life just can't believe that the problem has come to their home to roost. Usually, the denial ends only when the abuse reaches "crisis" level, and the child's health, performance, or social interaction is severely damaged. It also tends to end when the addict gets expelled from school or arrested. Once the family really gets the enormity of the situation, denial can be the only thing that stands between them and the bridge.

The school and community organizations, likewise, are in conflict between their perceived roles and their moral obligation to recognize and confront symptoms of drug use. There is generally no reward for teachers, agency counselors, or school districts that become active in ferreting out drug users and informing the parents of their suspicions; on the contrary, parental reaction is often angry, hostile, and litigious. With school community violence on the rise (often due to drug use), the "zero tolerance" policy that now prevails throughout the country also interferes with good communications.

How do we deal with these impediments? I think some of the answers are: keeping the epidemic in the forefront of media coverage; giving our schools and communities more confidence in the outcome if they try to help identify kids in trouble; actively supporting all organizations and groups; and most importantly, helping families understand that this affliction can and does affect any family, regardless of the social, economic, or religious environment in which the children are raised.

Forming **helping relationships** with family members as individuals allows staff to establish connections with family members separate from their child. The first step in forming the relationship is to recognize and validate the level at which families are already involved with their children. In most cases they live with the child or teenager whose behavior may be out of control and troubled. The daily living can be exhausting. Without the school community professionals' acceptance and knowledge of the current level of the child or adolescent's involvement in their own family, getting family members to be involved with the student support team is not realistic. Be aware that as the student moves through the school system, parents must adjust to new faces, attitudes, and the culture of a new school. They will bring with them their history with the school district and maybe their own negative past experiences. These changes should be recognized and validated.

School community professionals (e.g., teachers, school nurses, counselors, social workers, administrators) and family members each bring different perspectives and experiences to their relations (**Figure 9-1**). Both professionals and family members bring attitudes, values, feelings, communication skills, experiences, culture, roles, sense of efficacy, and personality, which may be similar or may be very different from those of each other and the family. In addition, the family members bring knowledge of their child, needs, problems, and expectations about what will happen, whereas the school people come with professional training and skills and knowledge of all students, ideally to assist and support the family. In building helping relationships, the focus must be on equality, listening, flexibility, sensitivity, and being available. Doing a self-check to examine personal biases and beliefs prior to meeting with family members will help to avoid conflict and facilitate establishing trust and helping relationships.

Relationship building takes time for families of children with a serious mental health concern and problem. Over a period of weeks and months, relationships between family members and school community professionals grow and develop. The relationships are best viewed as long term, spanning years. Difficult periods with troubled youth behavior are weathered, the disappointments of families, schools, and community organizations acknowledged. Better behavior and outcomes are designed and agreed upon. However, rewarding and satisfying communications may or may not balance out the difficult periods. Meeting expectations and demands may sometimes be beyond the reach of both families and professionals. Throughout these periods, persistent and consistent communication between school community professionals and parents is needed to build and maintain the relationships.

In an ideal world, relationships between professionals and families would be conflict-free and without failure; however, inevitably there are conflicts and failures in communication, hurt feelings, and unsatisfactory outcomes. Looking for opportunities to resolve conflict, the use of problem solving and anger management strategies should be viewed as part of the relationship-building process. Simply anticipating the conflicts, failures, hurts, and poor outcomes is unsatisfactory without taking preventive action.

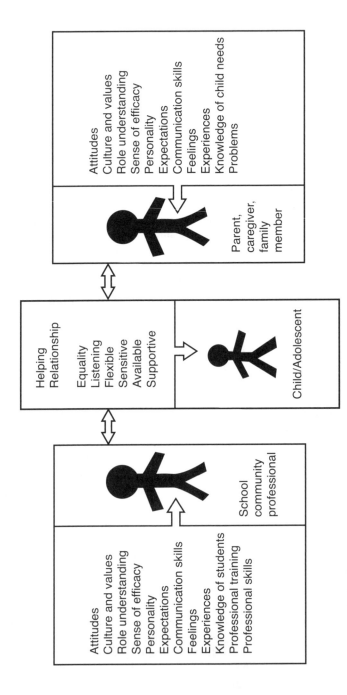

FIGURE 9-1 Helping relationship with family member focused on the child/adolescent.
Source: Adapted from Fertman, C. (2004). Schools and families of students with an emotional disturbance:Allies and partners. In D. Hiatt-Michael, (Ed.), *Promising Practices to Connect Schools and Families of Children with Special Needs.* Greenwich, CT: Information Age Publishers.

Matching families and school community professionals is often random, but there is considerable evidence that compatibility between the two is important for effective relationships and working together. The following questions (Rogers, 1958; Woodside & McClam, 2002) may help increase self-awareness in relationship-building skills with family members:

❖ Can I be perceived as trustworthy, dependable, and consistent?

❖ Can I express myself well enough that the family members understand what I am saying?

❖ Can I experience attitudes of warmth, caring, liking, interest, and respect for the family members?

❖ Can I separate my needs from those of the family members?

❖ Am I secure enough in myself to allow the family members to be separate and independent of me?

❖ Am I able to see the world as the family members do?

❖ Can I accept the family members as they are?

In the process of building relationships with families, consider what families bring and what the school community professionals bring to the relationship. Families are a rich source of information. They can provide an intimate knowledge and understanding of their child: their likes, hobbies, behaviors at home and in the community, beliefs, and the strengths of the family system. School community professionals bring a body of knowledge and expertise about learning and mental health. Parents must be aware that school community professionals abide by a code of ethics that sets standards of acceptable personal and professional behavior such as confidentiality. To engage parents and families in the school community requires thinking in new ways about relationships with them. Forming relationships goes a long way to engage families to support the success of youth with serious mental health concerns and problems.

Summary

Family engagement in mental health programs and services is a shared responsibility among families, school community staff, and community members in which families are committed to actively supporting their children's learning and healthy development (including mental health), and school community personnel and community members are committed to engaging and partnering with families in meaningful and culturally respectful, culturally competent, and culturally proficient ways. Schools, school districts, and community organizations' capacity and approaches to parent engagement have evolved over the last 40 years. They point toward increasing organizational capacity to train school community staff and parents, caregivers, and family members on how to create and support family engagement. Family engagement capacity-building initiatives model how to bring families, school leaders, community partners, and students together to build a network of support to keep students on the path to high school graduation, college or advanced training, and successful lives beyond. Emerging family engagement strategies operate in synchrony and across mental health programs and services and are carried out with high intensity over a sustained period of time. They are produced when a school community has taken the time and expense to build the capacity of both institutions (schools, agencies, government) and individuals (parents, caregivers, family members). Four emerging strategies are: parent- and caregiver-friendly schools, family network organizations, family education, and out-of-school-time programs. Family-centered mental health policy and practice is the emerging model for delivering programs and services to youth and their families. A priority for family-centered mental health policy and practice is to engage families of children and adolescents with serious mental health concerns and problems (e.g., youth with substance disorder, depression, emotional disturbance, in recovery) and to establish helping relationships with them.

For Practice and Discussion

1. Discuss the reasons for the change from parent involvement to family engagement.
2. In order to work effectively with parents, schools must build and maintain their capacity to create and sustain family engagement in their schools. You have just joined a team at the middle school tasked with improving parent engagement. The middle school is located in a distressed, multiethnic, multiracial neighborhood with recent immigrants. How would you go about creating family engagement?
3. During a wave of immigration, a large urban resettlement site was established in a formerly closed down public housing complex. The schools in the area receiving these new families had worked hard to create and sustain viable parent engagement in their schools. The assignment of the new immigrants posed enormous challenges in many areas, but none more than parent engagement. Everyone saw many challenges ahead. List them. Discuss the principles in Table 9-2 and explain how they would apply.
4. You are a parent with an adopted child from another country and culture who suffered deprivation and trauma. You would like the school to involve you in decisions they make about programs and services for your child. Cite examples of how the school could utilize your willingness to participate in your child's education.
5. List practices or activities that develop trust between parents/families and schools. Discuss barriers to achieving trust.
6. Why is parent engagement a shared responsibility? List partners and why they are important.
7. Describe a family-friendly school. Visit a school and compare it to your description. Were you welcomed? How did you feel? How would a new parent feel?
8. Conduct a search on the Web for three or four examples of family-centered mental health policies and programs. Identify those that apply to families in schools.

Key Terms

Family-centered mental health policy
and practice   212
Family engagement   202
Family Engagement for High School
Success   204
Family network organizations   206
Harvard Family Research Project
(HFRP)   204
Helping relationships   217
Mental Health America   208

Organizational capacity   203
Out-of-school-time programs   206
Parent- and caregiver-friendly school
communities   206
Parent and family education   206
Parental involvement   202
Roles   204
Shared responsibility   202
Statewide Family Network
Program   208

References

Bickham, N., Pizarro, J., Warner, B., Rosenthal, B., & Weist, M. (1998). Family involvement in expanded school mental health. *Journal of School Health*, 68(10): 425–428.

BOSTnet. Engaging Families in Out-of-School Time Programs Toolkit. Retrieved from http://www.bostnet.org/uploads/3/0/3/9/3039436/engagingfamiliestoolkit.pdf

Centers for Disease Control and Prevention. (2012). *Parent Engagement: Strategies for Involving Parents in School Health*. Atlanta, GA: U.S. Department of Health and Human Services. Retrieved from http://www.cdc.gov/HealthyYouth/

Cooper, J., Aratani, Y., Masi, R., Banghart, P., Dababnah, S., Douglas-Hall, A., Tavares, A., & Stagman, S. (2001). *Unclaimed Children Revisited: California Case Study*. New York: National Center for Children in Poverty. Mailman School of Public Health, Columbia University (65). Reprinted by permission of National Center for Children in Poverty.

Elmore, R. (2002). *Bridging the Gap Between Standards and Achievement: The Imperative for Professional Development in Education*. Washington, DC: The Albert Shanker Institute.

Fertman, C. (2004). Schools and families of students with an emotional disturbance: Allies and partners. In D. Hiatt-Michael (Ed.), *Promising Practices to Connect Schools and Families of Children with Special Needs* (pp. 79–99). Greenwich, CT: Information Age.

Harry, B. (1992). *Cultural Diversity, Families and the Special Education System: Communication and Empowerment*. New York: Teachers College Press.

Jordon, C., Orozco, E., & Averett, A. (2002). *Emerging Issues in School, Family, and Community Connections: Annual Synthesis, 2001*. Austin, TX: National Center for Family and Community Connections with Schools, Southwest Educational Development Laboratory.

Kutash, K., & Duchnowski, A. (2007). *The Role of Mental Health Services in Promoting Safe and Secure Schools: Effective Strategies for Creating Safer Schools and Communities*. Washington, D.C.: Hamilton Fish Institute on School and Community Violence and Northwest Regional Educational Laboratory.

Lehr, C., Johnson, D., Bremer, C., Cosio, A., & Thompson, M. (2004). Essential tools: Increasing rates of school completion: Moving from policy and research to practice – A manual for policymakers, administrators, and educators. University of Minnesota, National Center on Secondary Education and Transition. Retrieved from http://www.ncset.org/publications/essentialtools/dropout/dropout.pdf

Mapp, K.L. (2012). Title I and parent involvement: Lessons from the past, recommendations for the future. American Enterprise Institute for Public Policy Research. Retrieved from http://www.aei.org/paper/education/k-12/school-spending/title-i-and-parental-involvement/

National Federation of Families for Children's Mental Health. (2001). *Blamed and Ashamed*. Alexandria, VA: Author.

Osher, T.W., Osher, D., & Blau, G. (2006). *Shifting Gears to Family-Driven Care: Ambassador's Tool Kit*. Rockville, MD: National Federation of Families for Children's Mental Health.

Osher, T.W., & Osher, D.M. (2002). The paradigm shift to true collaboration with families. *Journal of Child and Family Studies*, 11(1): 47–60.

Osher, T., Penn, M., & Spencer, S. (2008). Partnerships with families for family-driven systems of care. In B. Stroule & G. Blau (Eds.), *The System of Care Handbook: Transforming Mental Health Services for Children, Youth, and Families* (pp. 249–274). Baltimore, MD: Brooks.

Perry, D., Kaufmann, R., Hoover, S. & Zundel, C., (2008). Services for young children and their families in systems of care. In B. Stroule & G. Blau (Eds.), *The System of Care Handbook: Transforming Mental Health Services for Children, Youth, and Families* (p. 491–516). Baltimore, MD: Brooks.

Prior, J., & Gerard, M. (2007). *Family Involvement in Early Childhood Education: Research into Practice*. Clifton Park, NY: Thomson Delmar Learning.

Rogers, C. (1958). The characteristics of a helping relationship. *Personnel and Guidance Journal*, 37(1): 6–16.

Weiss, H., Lopez, M.E., & Rosenberg, H. (2010). *Beyond Random Acts: Family, School, and Community Engagement as an Integral Part of Education Reform*. Cambridge, MA: Harvard Family Research Project.

Woodside, M., & McClam, T. (2002). *An Introduction to Human Services* (4th ed.). Pacific Grove, CA: Brooks/Cole.

Worthington, J., Hernandez, M., Friedman, B., & Uzzell, D. (2001). *Learning from Families: Identifying Service Strategies for Success. Systems of Care: Promising Practices in Children's Mental Health, 2001 Series, Volume II*. Washington, DC: Center for Effective Collaboration and Practice, American Institute for Research.

ADDRESSING SOCIAL DETERMINANTS

In this chapter, we will:

✦   Define social determinants of health and mental health
✦   Discuss the complexity of addressing social determinants
✦   Explain strategies to address poverty
✦   Define cultural competence
✦   Describe culturally competent programs and services

Scenarios

My stepfather was laid off and couldn't find a job because he hurt his back. He got involved with some guys and pretty soon he was working as a migrant crew leader because he could speak English and Spanish. Mom worked cleaning the house of a rich lady. That was good for a while because she sent us candy and chocolates and strawberries. The farmer where my stepfather worked sent us fresh vegetables. It isn't enough money. I have to get up and send my sister and brother to school. Then I have to walk for miles to get to school and then back home on time because I have to cook dinner. I help my brothers and sisters with their homework and clean up after dinner. When my mother gets home, she's too tired to do much except eat and sleep. I don't get a chance to spend time with friends. My stepfather decided that we would rent rooms to people, so we had boarders and no privacy. I wish I could get away. I like school, but my grades are not too good.

Source: Olivia is in the ninth grade at a rural high school

I have one older sister and two young brothers and one of these younger brothers was born in the States. My family left Vietnam by boat through Indonesia. We stay in a refugee camp for two years. It was very crowded and dirty. I don't know why we were there; something to do with my father's job. We were sent to a city in the U.S. where other refugees were sent from the camp. In beginning, we were help by the Catholic Charities and members of the local parish that have church volunteers who helped refugees. They set us up in an apartment, but my parents had to start working quickly. The apartment was better than the refugee camp, but my parents felt so closed off. They did not know what to expect. My dad got a job ironing clothes in laundry, and my mom in bakery where other refugees worked. Sometimes my belly hurt, and when mom gets home from work, she give us bread and rolls and I feel better. Some of the people in the town were not nice to us. When we walk outside, we hear names like, "asshole" and "jing." They did not like us, they make fun of us. Dad say to just ignore them. I could not. We be with our church volunteer group and each other. We were most lonely for our country, but there we were not free. I missed my grandparents, relatives, and friends from the refugee camp. When I started school, I was so scared everyday that I cried and cried. I was afraid of everyone and everything. I did not like the rules. I had to wear shoes to school. My mother was the only one I felt safe with. I did not let go of her no matter how hard she tried to get me on the school bus in the morning. I missed first two weeks of school because I was so scared that I cried and cling to my mom's legs and not let go. Mom hit me, cried with me, but I can't make myself go. I can't leave her. School officer came to our apartment and tell mom that if I don't go to school, she will have to pay a big fine. My dad punished me, but I cried harder. Nobody knew what to do to help me.

Source: Huy grew up in Vietnam until he was 4 years old.

Addressing Social Determinants of Mental Health

Although genes, behavior, and medical care play a role in how well we feel and how long we live, such factors as **economics**, **social conditions**, and the culture in which we are born, live, learn, work, and play have the most significant impact on our mental and physical health. These are called **social determinants of health** (physical and mental), and include gender, economics, education, disability, geographic location, culture, ethnicity, social conditions, and sexual orientation.

Among children and adolescents, differences (disparities) in health status often result from social determinants (U.S. Department of Health and Human Services, 2010). Disparities occur in physical health (e.g., higher rates of obesity, asthma, tooth decay, sexually transmitted infections), mental health (e.g., higher rates of depression, anxiety, stress, substance use), and built environments (e.g., higher rates of violence, crime, inadequate housing, and recreation facilities).

It is fundamental to know, identify, and address the social determinants of mental health among children and adolescents. Each child and adolescent is a **mosaic of identity** (**Figure 10-1**) with multiple identities. The life experiences (identities) of many children and adolescents may be full of instability, uncertainty, and stress that are the result of social determinants. These experiences (identities) contribute to their vulnerability and the disparities in their health status. Addressing social determinants is complicated. The social determinants cause significant barriers and circumstances that make children and adolescents

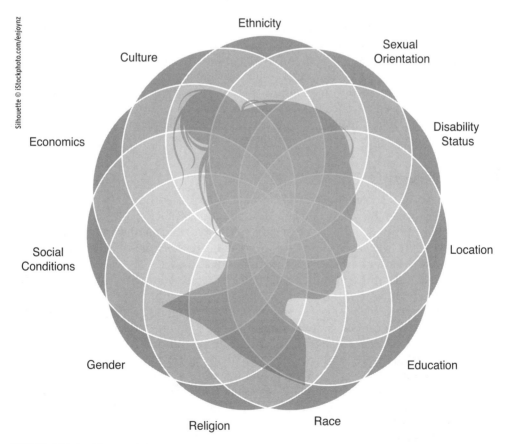

FIGURE 10-1 Mosaic of identity.
Source: Adapted from Adams, M., Bell, L. A., & Griffin, P. (2007). *Teaching for Diversity and Social Justice.* New York: Routledge.

vulnerable to poor health (physical and mental). Three critical points when addressing the mental health of vulnerable populations of children and adolescents are:

1. Long before a child becomes part of a school community, his or her health (physical and mental) has an established history.

2. Neighborhoods and homes shouldn't be hazardous to a child's health.

3. Youth, families, and caregivers should have the opportunity to make the choices that allow children and adolescents to live a long, healthy life, regardless of their income, education, or ethnic background (Robert Wood Johnson Foundation, 2010).

According to Adams, Bell, and Griffin (2007), to address the disparities that result from the social determinants, we need to focus our work in a number of areas. First is to appreciate social differences without an emphasis on power dynamics or differential access to resources and institutional support needed to live safe, satisfying, productive lives. Second is to understand the social power dynamics that result in some groups having privilege, status, and access, whereas other groups are disadvantaged, oppressed, and denied access (i.e., vulnerable children, adolescents, and families). Third, we need to focus on actions (teams, partnerships, collaborations) to address the vulnerabilities of groups and individuals (children and adolescents) that are produced by the social differences and social dynamics (social determinants).

Strategies to Address Poverty

Poverty is a social determinant of mental health with negative mental health consequences for youth and families and for the school community. It is not the responsibility or purpose of mental health programs and services to eradicate poverty. However, they can do a lot to mobilize the broader school community, families, and staff to lessen the negative consequences.

Schools and community agencies that are educating and serving high numbers of poor children and adolescents can employ innovative strategies to promote health (physical and mental) and academic achievement. Many of these strategies have a direct impact on the academic success of children and adolescents, such as offering incentives to recruit and retain highly effective teachers and staff, implementing a challenging yet accessible curriculum, and providing additional learning, program, and service opportunities beyond the traditional school day. Yet it is just as important to directly address the negative impacts of poverty on children's mental health (Soto Mas, Allensworth, & Jones, 2010).

Support for young children's mental health and family well-being is one of the key strategies to combat the negative consequences of poverty of children and adolescents (Smith, Stagman, Blank, Ong, & McDow, 2011; Zorn & Noga, 2004). **Table 10-1** lists examples of strategies that can be employed as part of

TABLE 10-1	Strategies for Team, Partnership, and Collaboration Focus on Support for Young Children's Mental Health and Family Well-Being

❖ Promoting early childhood mental health in home visiting and parenting programs
❖ Enhancing supports for early childhood mental health in early care and education programs
❖ Screening parents for depression
❖ Screening children for social-emotional problems
❖ Supporting the well-being of exceptionally vulnerable children
❖ Increasing awareness of the effects of family poverty
❖ Increasing the economic health of families to self-sufficiency

Sources: Data from Zorn, D., & Noga, J. (2004). *Family Poverty and Its Implication for School Success.* Cincinnati, OH: University of Cincinnati Evaluation Service Center; and Smith, S., Stagman, S., Blank, S., Ong, C., & McDow, K. (2011). *Building Strong Systems of Support for Young Children's Mental Health.* New York: Mailman School of Public Health, Columbia University, National Center for Children in Poverty.

a school community plan to combat the negative consequences of poverty on children's mental health. The strategies are proactive, moving to address root causes of mental health concerns and problems by intervening early in the life of a child and family.

Home Visiting and Parenting Programs

Home visiting and parenting programs offer unique opportunities to address young children's mental health needs. Through outreach and targeting of services, these programs can reach infants, toddlers, and preschoolers at high risk of mental health problems due to family economic hardship and other risk factors. Although varied in their scope and content, these programs typically aim to promote nurturing parent–child relationships and healthy child development beginning very early in life. For example, the Nurse–Family Partnership (NFP) home-visiting program is an evidence-based program that serves first-time mothers living below 200% of the federal poverty level (www .nursefamilypartnership .org). The visiting nurses address a wide range of mental health problems that can affect the mother's ability to provide safe and nurturing care to her infant. The problems include major mental illnesses such as depression, anxiety, and, less frequently, psychotic disorders. Parenting problems related to the mother's own history of abuse and neglect as well as current family discord, violence, and instability can also be addressed.

The nurses are matched with a mental health consultant who is available during case conferences to offer guidance to the nurses. Topics that a consultant might discuss with the nurses include indicators of depression, how to respond to aspects of parent–infant interactions that cause concern, and strategies for working with clients who resist additional mental health support that they may need. The mental health consultants spend about half to two-thirds of their time providing direct, home-based services to NFP mothers whom the nurses think would benefit from this intervention. If a mother agrees, the nurse introduces the consultant to the woman, and the consultant can then schedule a separate time to provide further assessment and services such as guidance on caregiver–infant interaction or psychotherapy. The number and length of visits as well as the type of interventions provided are tailored to the needs of the mother and child. The consultants also help the NFP nurses access appropriate psychiatric or other supportive services for the women they visit when it is determined these services are needed and available. The consultants work closely with the nurses and supervisors to ensure that the services to which the women are referred are accessible and coordinated.

Faith-based programs and services are also active in this arena. They employ a holistic approach to care, integrating spiritual, emotional, and physical health in the safe, familiar, and comfortable environment of a person's faith community. An example of such a program is the Aurora Parish Nurse Program, which expands the traditional model of the hospital as the primary place of health care and healing by creating access points within faith communities to help empower congregations to provide education, programs, and services that address the spiritual, mental, and physical health of its members. A local hospital partners with local faith communities to encourage and support ministries of health and healing across the lifespan. They will work with young mothers and their young children much the same as Nurse–Family Partnership but will be introduced to it through their faith community with services provided as part of faith-based activities and gatherings. (www.aurorahealthcare.org/services/parish/index.asp)

Enhanced Supports for Early Childhood Mental Health

More than 11 million infants, toddlers, and preschoolers are in early care and education settings, including home-based and center-based child care, Head Start, and prekindergarten programs (National Association of Child Care Resource and Referral Agencies, 2011). Promising approaches include early childhood mental health consultation, training of teachers and child-care providers that focuses on strategies for supporting young children's social-emotional growth, and curricula that provide explicit supports for social-emotional learning (Gillman, 2005). Early childhood mental health consultants typically help teachers learn strategies for promoting children's social-emotional growth and reducing challenging behaviors. Consultants may focus their work with teachers on building supports for all children in the early childhood setting, on addressing the needs of individual children, or on both. They may also work directly with children and parents (Perry, 2005). Training for teachers and providers in the area of social-emotional growth is highly varied in format and scope. This training may range from one-time workshops to more intensive on-site assistance to help a teacher or provider practice new skills in promoting children's social-emotional development. Sometimes group training is linked to on-site coaching.

There is growing evidence that teachers and practitioners need more than brief workshop-style training to acquire complex new skills and to apply them in early care and education settings (Zaslow, Tout, Halle, Whittaker, & Lavelle, 2010). Another strategy, implementing a social-emotional curriculum, can help teachers provide intentional supports for social-emotional learning through read-alouds, small-group activities, and explicit instruction. Examples of social-emotional curricula that have been found to promote young children's social-emotional competence and positive behavior include Dinosaur School (Webster-Stratton, Reid, & Stoolmiller, 2008) and PATHS (Domitrovich, Cortes, & Greenberg, 2007).

Screen Parents for Depression

Low-income mothers with young children have shown rates of depression ranging as high as 40–60% across several studies. One important reason for concern about the high prevalence of maternal depression is that depressive symptoms in a child's primary caregiver are associated with increased risks of problems in early development and learning (Earls, 2010). Mothers who experience depression during pregnancy and after giving birth often lack the energy and enthusiasm needed to provide their children with responsive caregiving. These mothers may be unable to provide consistent comforting or engage in playful interactions that help children acquire a sense of security along with social-emotional and language skills. The negative effects of maternal depression on young children include lower cognitive functioning, weaker language skills, and behavior problems. Several states have taken action to increase identification and treatment of mothers with depression. One example is Ohio's Help Me Grow home-visiting program (www.ohiohelpmegrow.org/About%20Us/abouthelpmegrow.aspx), which identifies and helps to secure treatment for women who may be experiencing depression during pregnancy or after giving birth. Help Me Grow, which operates in all 88 of Ohio's counties, provides home visitation to first-time parents with family incomes up to 200% of the federal poverty level. Most families enter the program during pregnancy or the first 6 months of the infant's life.

Screen Children for Social-Emotional Problems

Social-emotional and behavior problems are fairly common among young children, with the prevalence of these problems ranging from about 20–30% in samples of children from low-income families (Qi & Kaiser, 2003). Without intervention, behavioral difficulties tend to persist (Blandon et al., 2010). Identifying and addressing the social-emotional problems of young children as early as possible can limit the negative effects of these difficulties on learning, school performance, and relationships with peers and teachers. There is evidence that reliable identification requires the use of a standardized developmental screening tool, and that tools focused on social-emotional screening are more reliable than global screening tools (Jee et al., 2010). Developing effective social-emotional screening practices at the state level is a complex task requiring the development of resources and training for the professionals who will administer the screenings and help connect families to needed evaluation and intervention services. An example of one such effort is the California Statewide Screening Collaborative (CSSC), which was first convened in 2007 as part of the Early Childhood Comprehensive Systems to bring together state agencies, organizations, and special initiatives that focus on young children's mental health and wellness. The collaborative aims to increase coordination across state agencies and organizations involved in early identification of developmental challenges. The group also seeks to promote the use of standardized screening tools, particularly by healthcare professionals, and to identify funding opportunities to do this work. CSSC has developed a Web site with information about child screening. This Web site provides a review of validated screening tools, including social-emotional measures, and a guide to help providers determine when a referral is necessary and what developmental services and resources are available (California Department of Public Health, 2007).

Support the Well-Being of Exceptionally Vulnerable Children

A critical element of a comprehensive system of supports for young children's mental health is intentional outreach to exceptionally vulnerable children whose life circumstances place them at very high risk for the development of mental health problems in early childhood and beyond. These children include infants, toddlers, and preschoolers involved in the child welfare system; young children who are homeless; and young children whose families are experiencing multiple risks, such as extreme poverty, parental psychiatric or physical illness, substance abuse, or domestic violence. All states participate in early intervention programs, which provide assessment and intervention services to address a range of developmental delays. New Mexico is among several states whose programs incorporate strong supports for addressing the mental health needs of infants and toddlers. The assessments include many child, parent, and family risks known to increase the chances that infants and toddlers will experience developmental or mental health problems. Examples of these risks are low birth weight; feeding difficulties; the child's experience of trauma, such as a significant loss; homelessness; parent substance abuse; parent psychiatric illness; domestic violence; and evidence of parenting difficulties.

Increase Awareness of the Effects of Family Poverty

Community awareness of the effects of family poverty is an essential first step to developing community solutions. Getting the data you need to make your case is often difficult. Programs and services typically have anecdotal reports of services provided and demographic data used for annual reporting to funders. Furthermore, it is not unusual for programs and services within the same school community to use data from different sources and years or to not separate out the data by income, making comparisons and conclusions difficult. Given high rates of poverty for families and children and low rates of academic proficiency, efforts to develop data sharing or a centralized source of information on local poverty can play an important role in better understanding the face of family and child poverty (Kulick & Dalton, 2011). Increasing the economic health of the family in ways that lead to income stability is an important step in improving developmental outcomes for children in poverty.

Increase Economic Health of Families to Self-Sufficiency

Employment provides benefits for low-income adults that extend beyond the provision of income. However, employment that does not bring income stability for families may actually result in negative outcomes for the children of the family. Long-term, stable employment that is not under-employment or earning poverty-level wages is essential for families to build a cushion of benefits and savings that can sustain them during emergencies. Employment programs must integrate basic job training with educational, social, and emotional supports that are targeted to improving low-income parents' prospects for long-term, stable employment. Moving families from poverty to self-sufficiency must become the focus of a broad-based community effort that extends beyond traditional human service agencies alone. These agencies cannot be expected to work in a vacuum. Broad-based community support is essential to facilitate the creation and maintenance of services to families living in poverty. A first step must be involvement of community residents and employers in conversation around these issues. However, it is the critical second step that must then occur—translation of the conversation on family poverty into action that ultimately improves the lives of children and families.

Cultural Competence and Culturally Competent Programs and Services

Culture and ethnicity are social determinants of mental health. Culture contributes to beliefs about gender, health, work, school, religion, death, and sexual orientation. Differences are found between white and racial/ethnic (e.g., black, Hispanic, Native American) groups in the manner in which mental health concerns and problems are perceived and expressed. This has a direct effect on how youth and families present themselves, and consequently on how mental health professionals interact with them.

Culture is often described as the combination of a body of knowledge, a body of belief, and a body of behavior. It involves a number of elements, including personal identification, language, thoughts, communications, actions, customs, beliefs, values, and institutions that are often specific to ethnic, racial, religious, geographic, or social groups. These influence beliefs and belief systems surrounding health, healing, wellness, illness, disease, and delivery of mental health programs and services. The concept of

cultural competence has a positive effect on how we deliver programs and services by enabling them to be respectful of and responsive to the health beliefs, practices, and cultural and linguistic needs of the diverse youth and families we serve.

Cultural competence is critical to reducing mental health disparities and improving access to high-quality mental health care. When developed and implemented as a framework, cultural competence enables schools, agencies, and groups of professionals to function effectively to understand the needs of groups accessing health information, programs, and services.

Cultural Competence Continuum

Acquiring the skill of cultural competence is critical for effective helping. Most people do not intend to be disrespectful to members of other cultures, but they still make mistakes because they have not learned about other world views. Cross, Bazron, Dennis, and Isaacs (1989) wrote about a variety of stages or phases toward becoming competent to work with persons of other cultures. They call this five-step journey a **cultural competence continuum**, meaning a line from one end to the other. Not only can individual helpers travel along this continuum, but so can agencies and organizations. The first three stages relate to being unaware, and the final two involve being more appropriate and responsive.

1. *Cultural destructiveness:* When a person, organization, or culture completely and purposefully disregards another culture, it sets out to destroy that culture. Examples include genocide, or the purposeful mass killing of an entire culture. Cultural destruction can start as simply as denying children the right to speak their native language.

   Sometimes cultural destructiveness is evident to a lesser extent when a person or a system operates out of hate and prejudice, labeling anyone different as "those people." Ethnocentrism, meaning the view that one's culture of origin is the best possible culture, can lead to many destructive practices and attitudes.

2. *Cultural incapacity:* In this stage, the incompetence may be unintentional, but the individual or organization lacks the capacity to help others of different cultural membership. Use of practitioners with language skills or interpreters with limited experience in a cultural group while treating, screening, or assessing students and families can lead to incorrect diagnosis and treatment. Sometimes people are simply unaware of differences and appear to be rude because of that (for example, a mother that doesn't shake hands with you, a child that doesn't look you in the eye). A person therefore may be measured or judged based on culturally biased standards about age, gender, or behavior.

   Another effect of this accidental incompetence is to give the message or signal to people seeking help that they are not really welcome in our school community. We may behave as if these visitors are actually inconveniences, rather than the reason the organizations are open for business. An example of this is a community agency where persons are immediately treated rudely by a receptionist and made to wait an unreasonable amount of time before they are seen.

3. *Cultural blindness:* At this phase, staff may think that they are culturally competent when they are not. This is a dangerous pitfall because staff and agencies are then not taking steps to correct cultural biases. For example, perhaps agency policies are not really person-driven and person-centered, but we think that they are. The result is that policies and practices that may be ageist, sexist, classist, racist, or homophobic are never questioned. Actions are justified with statements like, "We've always done it this way."

4. *Cultural precompetence*: Moving along the continuum toward being culturally competent, attempts to improve are made during the precompetence stage. There is a definite movement toward being more aware, sensitive, and competent, although the staff or organization may have not yet fully arrived. In this phase, the agency has realized its pitfalls, and staff are talking about what can be done to be more culturally appropriate. At this point, the agency staff may make an attempt to be more welcoming by adding reading material or posters in the waiting room that relate to a variety of cultures. Another example is at a shelter for women who are abused, the staff realized that the program was not welcoming to lesbians experiencing relationship violence and began to correct that situation through aggressive outreach and training of staff. A third example is schools that offer all school forms in languages spoken by community members. When an organization is in the precompetence stage, staff might be discouraged by false starts, failures, and difficulties, or so pleased with initial efforts that they do not go far enough. It is therefore important always to be on your guard and monitor school community programs and services with cultural competence in mind.

5. *Cultural competence:* At this point, the school community staff accepts and respects differences, continues to monitor behavior and attitudes, pays attention to dynamics, and strives to adapt to the demands of a diverse clientele. Organizations that are culturally competent actually welcome and celebrate diversity, holding all cultures in high esteem. Organizations that are culturally appropriate try to achieve a goodness of fit between programs and services and the youth and families being served. They are perceived as part of and reflective of their youth and families. Staff understands that some universal human experiences transcend culture (such as joy or grief), and that the commonalities between cultural groups are just as important as differences. A culturally competent staff and organization validate similarities as well as celebrating differences.

Culturally Competent Programs and Services

Schools and communities facilitate students' access to and engagement in mental health programs when they design mental health programs and services with the goal of eliminating health disparities and promoting equity. They promote rapport and cooperation and increase youth and family engagement. They honor the families' autonomy, including their right to retain their own cultural orientation in regard to their health. At the same time, each organization has its values and ways of doing things, its own culture. These assumptions of organizations and staff sometimes can create challenges to being a culturally competent organization. Examples of organizational culture ideas that may get in the way include the following:

❖ People who ask for help must be on time.
❖ Eye contact from the person seeking help is desirable.
❖ Technology is useful and not to be feared.
❖ Paperwork is essential.
❖ The individual is more important than the family, neighborhood, or community.
❖ Staff should be distant and uninvolved with service recipients or applicants.
❖ All programs and services are suitable for all persons.
❖ Everyone should be treated exactly the same.
❖ Persons seeking help should follow our rules.
❖ The causes of problems are logical and rational.
❖ Experts know what is best for persons who ask for help.
❖ Drop-in care is impossible.
❖ Formal settings such as schools, program offices, hospitals, and clinics are the best places in which to provide care.
❖ Visiting hours in institutions should be limited.
❖ Medication is good.
❖ Mental health problems can be dealt with by strangers.
❖ People should be responsible for paying for their health care.

Culturally competent programs and services are not designed with the notion that "one size fits all"; rather, such programs and services offer a variety of alternatives and options to fit a variety of people. Youth and families have access to as much choice as possible in a culturally competent organization. In addition, culturally competent programs and services realize and acknowledge that society has not always been fair to everyone and that oppression and **discrimination** are real. Culturally competent programs

TABLE 10-2	**Questions Programs and Services Ask to Assess and Reflect Upon Their Attempts to Be Culturally Competent**

❖ How do staff, volunteers, and leadership represent the diverse population served by the organization?

❖ Do youth and families genuinely have a voice in program and service planning and implementation?

❖ Is there outreach to populations that may be underserved or may not feel welcome or safe in approaching the organization?

❖ Are programs and services offered in neighborhoods and communities that are underserved or most greatly affected? If not possible, are connections made and networks built with local religious communities or businesses?

❖ Is the organization linguistically and culturally competent?

❖ Does the organization aggressively advocate for the rights of all youth and families who are affected by the social problems (i.e., social determinants) of concern within the school community?

and services have as an underlying philosophy that each and every person deserves dignity and has value. **Table 10-2** lists a number of strategies that programs and services use to assess and reflect upon their practices to be culturally competent.

Culturally Competent Mental Health Programs and Services

Culturally competent programs and services promote mental health among youth and families from diverse cultures that reflect the mosaic of identity (Figure 10-1). To be effective, they employ varied and multiple strategies that span the socio-ecological model, working from national and state policy and programs to the individual level.

Racial and Ethnic Approaches to Community Health (REACH) Program

The **Racial and Ethnic Approaches to Community Health (REACH)** program began in 1999 as the cornerstone of the Center for Disease Control and Prevention's (CDC's) efforts to eliminate racial and ethnic health disparities in the United States. REACH partners use community-based, participatory approaches to identify, develop, and disseminate effective strategies for addressing health disparities across a wide range of health priority areas. Because the causes of racial and ethnic health disparities are complex and include individual, community, societal, cultural, and environmental factors, REACH communities engage a variety of strategies in their work, from counseling and education to systems and policy change.

REACH identified the following key principles and supporting activities for effective community-level work to reduce physical and mental health disparities in racial and ethnic minority communities across the United States:

❖ *Trust:* Build a culture of collaboration with communities based on trust.

❖ *Empowerment:* Give individuals and communities the knowledge and tools needed to create change by seeking and demanding better health and building on local resources.

❖ *Culture and history:* Design health initiatives that are grounded in the unique historical and cultural context of racial and ethnic minority communities in the United States.

❖ *Focus on causes:* Assess and focus on the underlying causes of poor community health, and implement solutions that will stay embedded in the community infrastructure.

❖ *Community investment and expertise:* Recognize and invest in local community expertise and motivate communities to mobilize and organize existing resources.

❖ *Trusted organizations:* Enlist organizations within the community that are valued by community members, including groups with a primary mission unrelated to health.

❖ *Community leaders:* Help community leaders and key organizations forge unique partnerships and act as catalysts for change in the community.

❖ *Ownership:* Develop a collective outlook to promote shared interest in a healthy future through widespread community engagement and leadership.

❖ *Sustainability:* Make changes to organizations, community environments, and policies to help ensure that health improvements are long-lasting and community activities and programs are self-sustaining.

❖ *Hope:* Foster optimism, pride, and a promising vision for a healthier future.

National Alliance for Hispanic Health (NAHH)

The **National Alliance for Hispanic Health (NAHH)** has been an advocate at the national level for health issues in the Latino community since 1973. Its members are health and human service providers working at the community level, seeking community-based solutions to health and mental health problems. NAHH is a nonprofit and does not accept funds from alcohol or tobacco companies; it is funded by private donations. It is widely recognized as the leading agency representing Latino health issues at the national level. NAHH operates several programs, among them Hispanic Health Link, ¡Vive tu Vida! (Live Your Life!)—Understanding and Taking Action to Treat and Manage Depression, Proyecto Informar Training and Technical Assistance Network (PITTAN), and Nuestras Voces: National Hispanic Leadership Network for Tobacco Control. It develops resource materials and provides training in a number of areas, including culturally proficient services; *Buena Salud: Guide to Overcoming Depression and Enjoying Life* is an example. You can read about the organization's vision and mission at www.hispanichealth.org.

National Latino Behavioral Health Association (NLBHA)

The **National Latino Behavioral Health Association (NLBHA)** was formed as a nonprofit in 2002 to address the mental health and substance use issues of the Latino community. It is an outgrowth of the Substance Abuse and Mental Health Services Administration (SAMHSA)-sponsored National Congress on Hispanic Mental Health. It works to influence policy, improve treatment outcomes and the quality of services, eliminate disparities in access to services and funding, and highlight the underutilization of services and the lack of appropriately trained personnel and practical research. The Community Defined Evidence Project seeks to gather examples of community-based practices that work, thus building a database to inform policy makers, researchers, and others. The Tenemos Voz National Latino Consumer Network gives voice to consumer desires for advocacy, education, prevention, intervention, and support. Further information about the association's initiatives is available at www.nlbha.org.

California Strategic Plan on Reducing Mental Health Stigma and Discrimination

Discrimination against people with special needs, such as individuals with mental health disabilities, is still a problem, even though there are laws protecting people with disabilities. Discrimination includes stereotypes about people with special needs and prejudices toward them. A model for school community actions to eliminate discrimination toward individuals with mental disabilities is the **California Strategic Plan on Reducing Mental Health Stigma and Discrimination** (California Department of Mental Health, 2009). The plan has four strategic directions.

Strategic direction 1: Creating a supportive environment for all consumers and those at risk for mental health challenges, family members, and the community at large by establishing social norms that recognize that mental health is integral to everyone's well-being. Create widespread understanding and recognition within the public and across all systems that people at different points in their lives experience different degrees of mental health from wellness to crisis, and persons living with mental health challenges have resilience and the capacity for recovery.

Strategic direction 2: Promoting awareness, accountability, and changes in values, practices, policies, and procedures across and within systems and organizations that encourage the respect and rights of people identified with mental health challenges. Initiate systematic reviews to identify and address stigmatizing and discriminatory language, behaviors, practices, and policies.

Strategic direction 3: Upholding and advancing federal and state laws to identify and eliminate discriminatory policies and practices. Increase awareness and understanding of existing laws and regulations that protect individuals living with mental health challenges and their family members against discrimination. Promote the compliance with and enforcement of current antidiscrimination laws and regulations. Work to enhance and/or amend current statutes and regulations to further protect individuals and their family members from discrimination.

Strategic direction 4: Increasing knowledge of effective and promising programs and practices that reduce stigma and discrimination using methods that include community-led approaches. Develop and implement a plan to address the information gaps on how to reduce stigma and discrimination to build effective and promising antistigma and antidiscrimination programs. Increase the skills and abilities of community participants to evaluate programs. Disseminate the lessons learned, promising practices, and other outcome findings.

Immigrant and International Advisory Council

Immigrants often find themselves facing different laws, lifestyles, language, and most significantly, a new culture. An **Immigrant and International Advisory Council** was formed in 2008 to help make Allegheny County Department of Human Services (DHS) accessible to all residents of the city of Pittsburgh and surrounding Allegheny County, Pennsylvania, regardless of their country of origin (Allegheny County Department of Human Services, 2013).

As a way to help DHS staff members increase their understanding of different cultures, the council provides occasional cultural competency trainings. Information is presented on providing services that are accessible and culturally sensitive, and includes communications and assessment tips and resources to help with specific service needs. These presentations feature individuals from various cultures who provide a brief overview of the language, religion, customs, and beliefs of their own cultural group. Past presentations have included Latino, Muslim, West African, Bhutanese, and Iraqi cultures. The council is able to provide trainings focusing on other cultural groups as well, such as Russian, Burmese, and Chinese.

Communication is one of the biggest barriers for cultural understanding and has been a main focus of the council's efforts. Language Line, a call center with the ability to provide immediate interpreting services for more than 170 languages, is one tool that DHS staff use to communicate with English-language learners. To date, more than 100 DHS staff members have been trained to use Language Line. Additionally, the council is developing more in-person interpretation services through a local language bank that will serve the broader community, including providers and consumers of human services, health care, education, and legal services.

These are just two of the activities of the Immigrant and International Advisory Council focused on specific human service needs. Others include the Refugee Career Mentoring Committee to pair highly educated and skilled refugees with peer mentors; the COMPASS AmeriCorps Project Committee (in conjunction with the Greater Pittsburgh Literacy Council) to deploy AmeriCorps volunteers to work with immigrant-serving agencies and provide ongoing support for the social service needs of immigrants and refugees; the Children and Youth Committee to expand access to mentoring and career development opportunities; and the Immigrant Family Childcare Project, which hopes to increase the quality of child care through home-based child-care programs.

Cultural Brokers

The goal of **cultural brokers** is to increase the capacity of school communities to design, implement, and evaluate culturally competent mental health promoting programs and services. A cultural broker focuses on how he or she can bridge the gap of communication between youth and families and the school community programs and services through knowledge and understanding of cultures by serving as a mediator or agent of change. **Box 10-1** illustrates how one cultural broker (Miss Chau), who worked with school community mental health programs and services that served the Vietnamese refugee boy, Huy, and his family (who shared his story at the beginning of this chapter), was a bridge between the school community and the family.

Cultural brokers are particularly important for refugee children. In 2008, 24% of all refugees resettled in the United States were school-aged children

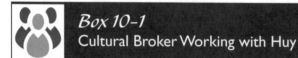

Box 10-1
Cultural Broker Working with Huy

Miss Chau (cultural broker) talks about Huy with a smile. "Huy could have been diagnosed with a mental health disorder because of the frequency, intensity, and duration of his behavior in the first few months of school. For me, he was a little lost boy who had left his home, lived in a refugee camp, and heaven knows what he endured there, and is living in chronic poverty where no one really understands him. We expected him to wear shoes, get on a yellow school bus, and come to a scary new school and just fit in.

"We mobilized our student support team. They wanted to invite mom and dad to help us plan, but they didn't speak English. I asked for a few days to put some strategies in place. I had worked before with the owner of the bakery where Huy's mother was working. Eight years ago, she had been a refugee. I stopped at the bakery and we had an informal conversation. She knew about Huy's challenges. She helped me understand the shame he was feeling and how embarrassed his parents were. I asked if she could share with Huy's mom and dad that she had worked with us before and that we had an understanding of their culture and community. Mom was washing pots in the bakery kitchen. The bakery owner told me she would talk with her and that I should come by tomorrow to sit awhile with them.

between the ages of 5 and 18 years. The need to provide services to this population is tremendous because many face significant challenges adapting to U.S. schools, whether academically, culturally, or psychosocially. Refugee students may arrive with minimal previous formal education, interrupted schooling, and no/or limited English. In addition, refugee students need time to adjust to U.S. culture, make friends, and develop a sense of belonging in their new school, community, and country. Refugee parents support their children to the best of their ability, but cultural, linguistic, and other barriers may prevent them from being involved in their children's education in the way that teachers expect them to be (Bridging Refugee Youth and Children's Services, 2012).

The characteristics, roles, and skills of cultural brokers are highly variable. Currently, the term *cultural broker* is used to denote a range of individuals from immigrant children who negotiate two or more cultures daily (Phillips & Crowell, 1994) to leaders in organizations who serve as catalysts for change (Heifetz & Laurie, 1997). The range and complexity of roles are equally varied. Cultural brokers in the mental health promoting school community vary (**Table 10-3**). They may serve as intermediaries at the most basic level—bridging the cultural gap by communicating differences and similarities between cultures. They may also serve in more sophisticated roles such as mediating and negotiating complex processes within organizations, government, or communities, and between interest groups or countries.

Cultural brokers are knowledgeable in two realms: (1) the mental health values, beliefs, and practices within their cultural group or community; and (2) the mental healthcare system that they have learned to navigate effectively for themselves and

---

TABLE 10-3   Cultural Broker Tasks in a Mental Health Promoting School Community
❖ Recognize the values that guide and mold attitudes and behaviors.
❖ Understand a community's traditional mental health beliefs, values, and practices and changes that occur through acculturation.
❖ Develop materials to help inform youth and families on mental health programs and services.
❖ Serve as guides for mental health programs and services that are in the process of incorporating culturally and linguistically competent principles, values, and practices.
❖ Understand and practice the tenets of effective cross-cultural communication, including the cultural nuances of both verbal and nonverbal communication.
❖ Advocate for the youth and families to ensure the delivery of effective mental health programs and services.
Source: National Center for Cultural Competence. (2004). *Bridging the Cultural Divide in Health Care Settings: The Essential Role of Cultural Broker Programs.* Washington, DC: Author. Adapted and included with permission of the National Center for Cultural Competence, Georgetown University Center for Child and Human Development, Georgetown University Medical Center.

their families. They serve as communicators and liaisons between the youth and families and the school community programs and services. Cultural brokers can play a critical and beneficial role—on a personal level, in the community in which they live, and on a professional level, in their respective agencies or practices.

Cultural brokers can help to ease the historical and inherent distrust that many racially, ethnically, and culturally diverse communities have toward many mental health programs and services. Two elements are essential to the delivery of effective services: (1) the ability to establish and maintain trust, and (2) the capacity to devote sufficient time to build a meaningful relationship between the staff and youth and families. Cultural brokers employ these skills and promote increased use of mental health programs and services within their respective communities.

In many ways, cultural brokers are change agents because they can initiate the transformation of a school community by creating an inclusive and collaborative environment for youth, families, schools, and community organizations. They model and mentor behavioral change, which can break down bias, prejudice, and other institutional barriers that exist in the school community. They work toward changing intergroup and interpersonal relationships so that the organization can build capacity from within to adapt to the changing needs (Heifetz & Laurie, 1997) of the communities they serve.

Summary

Among children and adolescents, differences (disparities) in health status often result from social determinants. Disparities are in physical health (e.g., higher rates of obesity, asthma, tooth decay, sexually transmitted infections), mental health (e.g., higher rates of depression, anxiety, stress, substance use), and built environments (e.g., higher rates of violence, crime, inadequate housing and recreation facilities). Three action areas to address the vulnerabilities that are produced by the social differences and social dynamics (social determinants) focus on buffering the negative consequences of poverty on children, building cultural competence, and providing culturally competent programs and services.

For Practice and Discussion

1. You have read about Huy in this chapter. List the social determinants you think affected his mental health, and explain why you think they posed a problem for his school attendance and success. How did the cultural broker help?
2. Social determinants affect all our lives. What are some that you think affect you? Olivia and her family were going through tough economic times. What effects do you feel this might have on Olivia and her siblings? Discuss what you, working as a member of a school community support team, would do to help Olivia's academic performance.
3. Think of your favorite school. Why is it your favorite? Where would you say it is on the cultural competency continuum, and why? Are there social determinants that you think are responsible? What are they, and why?

4. You are the newly hired director of a social service agency tasked with providing case management and mental health services to immigrant and refugee families in the region. Looking through the organization's literature, you find it is all in English. No one on staff speaks another language, but they say they tell clients to bring someone who speaks English with them to the appointments. They don't see the need to change anything. What do you do to provide culturally competent services to clients?

5. In your local school community, identify programs and services that focus on support for young children's mental health and family well-being. What are the local programs and services? What families and children do they serve? Select one strategy from Table 10-1 that you believe needs to be added to current program and services offerings in your school community. Prepare a statement advocating for the strategy. Include how it will impact the social determinates of mental health for school community members.

6. Culturally competent mental health promotion programs are not designed with the notion that one size fits all; rather, such programs offer a variety of alternatives and options to fit a variety of people. Culturally competent mental health promotion programs have as an underlying philosophy that each and every person deserves dignity and has value. What are ways that a mental health promotion program can be culturally sensitive and respectful?

7. Identify inclusion strategies currently being used in your local school communities' programs and services. What are the local programs and services? What children, families, and community members do they serve? Select one strategy from this chapter that you believe needs to be added to current inclusion strategies used by local program and services. Prepare a statement advocating for the strategy. Include how it will impact the social determinants of mental health for school community members.

8. Identity in your life where you have served as a cultural broker bridging two cultures to help address a friend's or family member's health need. What are personal challenges for you to be a cultural broker?

Key Terms

California Strategic Plan on Reducing Mental Health Stigma and Discrimination 237

Cultural brokers 239

Cultural competence 232

Cultural competence continuum 232

Discrimination 234

Economics 224

Immigrant and International Advisory Council 238

Mosaic of identity 225

National Alliance for Hispanic Health (NAHH) 236

National Latino Behavioral Health Association (NLBHA) 237

Poverty 226

Racial and Ethnic Approaches to Community Health (REACH) 235

Social conditions 224

Social determinants of health 224

References

Adams, M., Bell, L.A., & Griffin, P. (2007). *Teaching for Diversity and Social Justice.* New York: Routledge.

Allegheny County Department of Human Services. (2013). Your Culture Is Valued Here: Lessons from DHS Immigrant and International Advisory Council. Pittsburgh: Author. Retrieved from http://www.alleghenycounty.us/dhs/research.aspx

Aurora Health Care. (2012). Parish Nurse Program. Milwaukee, WI. Retrieved from www.aurorahealthcare.org/services/parish/index.asp

Blandon, A.Y., Calkins, S.D., Grimm, K.J., Keane, S.P., & O'Brien, M. (2010). Testing a developmental cascade model of emotional and social competence and early peer acceptance. *Development and Psychopathology,* 22: 737–748.

Bridging Refugee Youth and Children's Services. (2012). *Refugee Children in U.S. Schools: A Toolkit for Teachers and School Personnel.* Washington, DC: Author.

California Department of Mental Health. (2009). *California Strategic Plan on Reducing Mental Health Stigma and Discrimination.* Sacramento, CA: California Department of Mental Health Mental Health Services Oversight and Accountability Commission. Retrieved from http://www.dmh.ca.gov/peistatewideprojects/docs/Reducing_Disparities/CDMH_MH_Stigma_Plan_09_V5.pdf

California Department of Public Health. (2007). California Statewide Screening Collaborative. Sacramento, CA. Retrieved from http://www.cdph.ca.gov/programs/ECCS/Documents/MO-ECCS-FactSheet.pdf

Cross, T., Bazron, B., Dennis, K., & Isaacs, M. (1989). *Towards a Culturally Competent System of Care* (Vol. I). Washington, DC: Georgetown University Child Development Center, CASSP Technical Assistance Center.

Domitrovich, C.E., Cortes, R., & Greenberg, M.T. (2007). Improving young children's social and emotional competence: A randomized trial of the Preschool PATHS Program. *Journal of Primary Prevention,* 28(2): 67–91. PMID: 17265130.

Earls, M.F. (2010). Incorporating recognition and management of perinatal and postpartum depression into pediatric practice. *Pediatrics,* 126: 1032–1039.

Gilliam, W. (2007). *Early Childhood Consultation Partnership: Results of a Random-Controlled Evaluation.* New Haven, CT: Yale University School of Medicine, Child Study Center.

Heifetz, R.A., & Laurie, D.L. (1997). The work of leadership. *Harvard Business Review,* 75(1): 124–134.

Jee, S.H., Szilagyi, M., Ovenshire, C., Norton, A., Conn, A.-M., Blumkin, A., et al. (2010). Improved detection of developmental delays among young children in foster care. *Pediatrics,* 25(2): 282–289.

Kulick, E., & Dalton, E. (2011). *Disparities in Achievement: Human Services Involvement of Children in Pittsburgh Public Schools.* Pittsburgh, PA: Allegheny County Department of Human Services & Pittsburgh Public Schools Data Sharing Partnership.

National Association of Child Care Resource and Referral Agencies. (2011). *Capitol Connection Guidebook, 112th Congress: A Congressional Resource Manual for CCR&Rs.* Arlington, VA: Author.

National Health Service Corps. (2004). *Bridging the Cultural Divide in Health Care Settings: The Essential Role of Cultural Broker Programs.* Washington, DC: Author.

Perry, D.F. (2005). *Evaluation Results for the Early Childhood Mental Health Consultation Pilot Sites.* Washington, DC: Center for Child and Human Development.

Phillips, D., & Crowell, N. (1994). *Cultural Diversity and Early Education: Report of a Workshop.* Washington, DC: National Academy Press. Retrieved from http://darwin.nap.edu/html/earlyed

Qi, C., & Kaiser, A.P. (2003). Behavior problems of preschool children from low-income families: Review of the literature. *Topics in Early Childhood Special Education,* 23(4): 188–216.

Robert Wood Johnson Foundation. (2010). A new way to talk about the social determinants of health. Retrieved from http://www.rwjf.org/vulnerablepopulations/product.jsp?id=66428

Smith, S., Stagman, S., Blank, S., Ong, C., & McDow, K. (2011). *Building Strong Systems of Support for Young Children's Mental Health*. New York: Mailman School of Public Health, Columbia University, National Center for Children in Poverty.

Soto Mas, F., Allensworth, D., & Jones, C.P. (2010). Health promotion programs designed to eliminate health disparities. In C. Fertman & D. Allensworth (Eds.), *Health Promotion Programs: From Theory to Practice* (pp.29–56). San Francisco: Jossey-Bass.

U.S. Department of Health and Human Services. (2010). Healthy People 2020. Retrieved from http://www.healthypeople.gov/2020/default.aspx

Webster-Stratton, C., Reid, M.J., & Stoolmiller, M. (2008). Preventing conduct problems and improving school readiness: Evaluation of the Incredible Years teacher and child training programs in high-risk schools. *Journal of Child Psychology and Psychiatry*, 49: 471–488.

Zaslow, M., Tout, K., Halle, T., Whittaker, J.V., & Lavelle, B. (2010). Toward the identification of features of effective professional development for early childhood educators. Literature review. Retrieved from http://www2.ed.gov/rschstat/eval/professional-development/literature-review.pdf

Zorn, D., & Noga, J. (2004). *Family Poverty and Its Implication for School Success*. Cincinnati, OH: University of Cincinnati Evaluation Service Center.

FACEBOOK, CELL PHONES, AND MENTAL HEALTH COMMUNICATIONS

In this chapter, we will:

◆ Discuss the importance of mental health communication and social media to engage young people, parents, caregivers, and families

◆ Discuss mental health communication and social media strategies to reduce cyberbullying

◆ Explain social marketing strategies to reduce mental health stigma

◆ Describe effective mental health communication and social media plans

Scenarios

How do we get kids and parents to even know what we (the team) do? Flyers at home are old, emails are perceived as dangerous, texting is problematic, using Twitter is unknown, and we can't be friends on Facebook. Our principal likes robocalls—the automated phone call to deliver her prerecorded message. The school district is working on a dashboard where parents can log in to check on attendance, behavior, test scores, and homework. It is cumbersome. I don't think anyone uses it. Maybe we can develop an app. Frankly, I don't think they would ever post on any social media, "Hey, there is a drug and alcohol support group tomorrow, third period [at 9:45], at the middle school in room 236." It does turn out that there is some word of mouth about our team. If you have a problem or had a problem, you know us. Otherwise we are pretty well hidden, under the radar. I wonder how we can get heard above all of the noise.

Source: Sarah Wu, teacher and student support team member at the Franklin K–8 Educational Center

Technology has changed so much for education. It's opened a lot of doors to new ways to teach and communicate, but it's also changed the way kids interact. Cyberbullying happens all the time. Last year, one of my kids was being harassed all the time on Facebook. She was getting nasty comments on her wall and messages all the time from a group of girls telling her that she was ugly and stupid and that she should kill herself. She deleted her account, but the same kids started texting her. She was miserable, crying a lot, scared to come to school even. We were shocked to find phone apps that take kids to self-injury and "how-to" suicide sites. The other teachers and I were terrified that she was going to hurt herself. I was nervous every day waiting to see if she was going to be in class. I felt powerless. We couldn't control these other girls and what they were doing outside of school.

Source: Mike Murphy, an eighth-grade science teacher

Importance of Mental Health Communication and Social Media

We live in a media-savvy world where information is shared instantly across the globe. With e-mail, instant and text messaging, smartphones, apps, tablets, **social media**, and other forms of communication, it is hard to go even a few minutes without being contacted or updated in some way. Having so much information available at our fingertips is great for being able to keep in touch with friends and relatives and for finding out information about current events, our health, or really any possible topic of interest. However, it also is a stressor that people have to deal with, it is out of control, and it is ever-present. At any one moment, information and anxiety can show up on our doorsteps. At the same time, all of the information and all of the technology that keeps us up to date and in contact with friends and family can be a source of help, support, and resources when we need it.

The development of the Internet and other digital technologies during the past 2 decades has altered how people, especially children and adolescents, use media. By early 2012, more than 4 in 10 American adults owned a smartphone, while one in five owned a tablet. New cars are manufactured with the Internet built in. With more Internet access comes deeper immersion into social networking for adults and youth (Pew Research Center, 2012). The child advocacy group Common Sense Media surveyed 1,000 teenagers ages 13 to 17 and found 9 out of 10 use social media sites, and the same ratio say they text. Among those who text, two-thirds text daily and half use social networking sites daily (Common Sense Media, 2012). In a separate study, it was found that digital media has become a regular part of the media diet of children. For example, 42% of children under 8 years old have a TV in their bedroom. Approximately half (52%) of all 0- to 8-year-olds have access to a new mobile device such as a smartphone, video iPod, or iPad tablet. In a typical day, 1 in 10 (11%) of 0- to 8-year-olds uses a smartphone, video iPod, iPad, or similar device to play games, watch videos, or use other apps. In addition to the traditional digital divide, a new "app gap" has developed, with only 14% of lower-income parents having downloaded new media apps for their kids to use, compared to 47% of upper-income parents. (Common Sense Media, 2011). The rapid changes and widespread use of these new technologies has fueled concerns about the role of social media on young people's overall well-being (Bélanger, Akre, Berchtold, & Michaud, 2011; Romer, Bagdasarov, & More, 2013). Clearly school communities need to be assertive and proactive in the use of social media to promote the health of children and adolescents.

Social media (media for social interaction, using highly accessible and scalable publishing techniques and Web-based platforms) is now viewed as a tool to promote health with the options to communicate health (including mental health) information in the school community changing with each new technological advance. Land lines, replaced by cell phones, replaced by instant messaging, replaced by texting, replaced by tweeting, Facebook, Instagram, Snapchat, and Tumblr, create opportunities and challenges. Health communication (including **mental health communication**) is defined by Healthy People 2010 as the art and technique of informing, influencing, and motivating individual, institutional, and public audiences about important health (and mental health) issues (U.S. Department of Health and Human Services, 2000). It has been described further as "a multifaceted and multidisciplinary approach to reach different audiences and share health-related information with the goal of influencing, engaging, and supporting individuals, communities, health professionals, special groups, policy makers, and the public to champion, introduce, adopt, or sustain a behavior, practice, or policy that will ultimately improve health outcomes" (Schiavo, 2007, p. 7).

Technology, especially social media, has made communication increasingly accessible and provides new media for teams, partnerships, collaborations, and mental health programs and services to use. The dissemination of mental health messages can create awareness of an issue, change attitudes toward a health behavior, and encourage and motivate individuals to follow recommended health behaviors. It is important to recognize that mental health communication alone cannot change behavior. It can increase awareness and knowledge, prompt action, and reinforce attitudes, but it cannot compensate for inadequate mental healthcare services or for behaviors that are complex in nature and require more than just communication (National Cancer Institute, 2001). Two factors key to using social media as a tool of health communication are mental health literacy and plain language.

Mental Health Literacy

Families are increasingly responsible for making healthy decisions about family members' health and treatment. Frequently, families are challenged with seeking and understanding mental health information, communicating with professionals, managing and monitoring their own mental health, maintaining good mental health, navigating the mental healthcare system, filling out insurance forms, signing informed consent forms, seeking out options of and access to care, acting as caregivers, comprehending medications and correct dosages, advocating for their health or the health of their children, and the list goes on. Many parents and caregivers (as well as the general public) cannot recognize specific mental health disorders or different types of psychological distress. They differ from mental health professionals in their beliefs about the causes of mental health concerns and problems and the most effective treatments. Attitudes that hinder recognition and appropriate help-seeking are common. Much of the mental health information most readily available to the public is misleading.

With these many challenges, **mental health literacy** skills become a major factor in determining a successful outcome. Although experts are still debating the single definition of mental health literacy, the most commonly accepted definition is the degree to which individuals have the capacity to obtain, process, and understand basic mental health information and services needed to make appropriate mental health decisions (Selden, Zorn, Ratzan, & Parker, 2000; U.S. Department of Health and Human Services, 2000).

Because the word *literacy* is included in the phrase, people often misinterpret mental health literacy to be an issue of concern only for those who cannot read or write. However, mental health literacy expands beyond reading and writing skills to include the ability to comprehend and assess mental health information in order to make informed decisions about mentally healthy behaviors, emotional and social functioning, and stress management (Institute of Medicine [IOM], 2004; U.S. Department of Health and Human Services, 2004).

A range of factors contribute to mental health literacy, including social and individual factors such as cultural and conceptual knowledge, and listening, speaking, arithmetic, writing, and reading skills (IOM, 2004). Studies have shown that individuals with inadequate health literacy (including mental health literacy) report less knowledge about their medical conditions and treatment, worse health status, less understanding and use of preventive services, and a higher rate of hospitalization than those with marginal or adequate health literacy (Berkman et al., 2004; IOM, 2004).

A few assessment tools are available to help us address mental health literacy. They are most often used to assess a person's literacy in the context of printed health information. They are the Rapid Estimate of Adult Literacy in Medicine (REALM; Davis et al., 1993) and the Test of Functional Health Literacy in Adults (TOFHLA; Parker, Baker, Williams, & Nurss, 1995) and shortened version, the S-TOFHLA (Baker et al., 1999). The TOFHLA is also validated to be used with adolescents (Chisolm & Buchanan, 2007). The REALM is a medical word recognition and pronunciation test that asks a person to read from a list of 66 common medical words. This test provides a grade-level score for an individual who reads below the ninth-grade reading level. The TOFHLA and S-TOFHLA measure a person's ability to read health-related information and understand numerical information. TOFHLA scores are reported as inadequate, marginal, or adequate health literacy. Both the REALM and TOFHLA help us to determine a person's ability to understand health information and whether they have the needed skills to follow medication or other mental health instructions.

Mental health literacy is often talked about in terms of the individual (youth, family members); however, mental health programs and services, public health programs, policy makers, healthcare professionals, and schools are also responsible for mental health literacy. Although individuals' mental health literacy skills and capacities can be linked to their own education level, culture, or language, it is also important to acknowledge the communication and assessment skills of those whom people interact with regarding mental health, as well as the ability of the media, the marketplace, and the government to provide mental health information in a manner appropriate to the audience (IOM, 2004). The Ontario Centre of Excellence for Child and Youth Mental Health (2012) launched a model mental health literacy initiative designed to build common language and understanding among diverse professionals, families, children, youth, and decision makers. It highlights a socio-ecological approach to address mental health literacy by promoting basic knowledge to foster youth and families' best possible mental health, recognize concerns and problems, and help youth and families get support when needed.

As part of being culturally competent organizations, mental health programs and services require **linguistic competence** (Goode & Jones, 2009). Linguistic competence is the capacity of an organization and its personnel to communicate effectively and convey information in a manner that is easily understood by diverse audiences, including persons of limited English proficiency/English language learners, those who have low literacy skills or are not literate, individuals with disabilities, and those who are deaf or hard of hearing. Linguistic competency requires organizational and provider capacity to respond effectively to the health and mental health literacy needs of populations served. The organization must have policy, structures, practices, procedures, and dedicated resources to support this capacity. This may include, but is not limited to, the use of:

❖ Bilingual/bicultural or multilingual/multicultural staff
❖ Cross-cultural communication approaches
❖ Cultural brokers
❖ Foreign language interpretation services including distance technologies
❖ Sign language interpretation services
❖ Multilingual telecommunication systems
❖ Videoconferencing and telehealth technologies
❖ TTY and other assistive technology devices
❖ Computer-assisted real-time translation (CART) or viable real-time transcriptions (VRT)

❖ Print materials in easy to read, low literacy, picture, and symbol formats

❖ Materials in alternative formats (e.g., audiotape, Braille, enlarged print)

❖ Varied approaches to share information with individuals who experience cognitive disabilities

❖ Materials developed and tested for specific cultural, ethnic, and linguistic groups

❖ Translation services, including those of

◆ Legally binding documents (e.g., consent forms, confidentiality and patient rights statements, release of information, applications)

◆ Signage

◆ Health education materials

◆ Public awareness materials and campaigns

◆ Ethnic media in languages other than English (e.g., television, radio, Internet, newspapers, periodicals)

Plain Language Strategies to Improve Mental Health Literacy

Presenting information in **plain language** (or plain English) is an integral component of improving mental health literacy. Plain language has many definitions, but is fundamentally defined as communication your audience can understand the first time they read or hear it (PlainLanguage.gov, n.d.). Written material is in plain language if your audience can:

❖ Find what they need

❖ Understand what they find

❖ Use what they find to meet their needs

Although definitions vary, the essence of plain language focuses on the audience, clarity, and comprehension. Using clear and concrete words in a straightforward manner is the best way to organize information, particularly with health content. Using graphs and charts is recommended to clearly convey data and statistics, as shown in **Figure 11-1**, a plain language fact sheet example of binge drinking.

Using plain language is especially important when communicating with people with low health literacy, but all people can benefit from information in plain language. Something to note, though, is that plain language refers not only to the specific words that are used, but also *how* information is presented. Here are a few suggestions for presenting information so that it can be visually appealing, logically organized, and more comprehensible:

❖ Have ample white space. Break up dense amounts of text. Keep sentences short.

❖ Use a design and layout that can increase comprehension. Pictures or graphics, such as those used in Figure 11-1, are visually appealing and can help illustrate examples or important points.

❖ Use clear headings and bullets. **Figure 11-2** shows how using bullets breaks up the text and makes it easier to read.

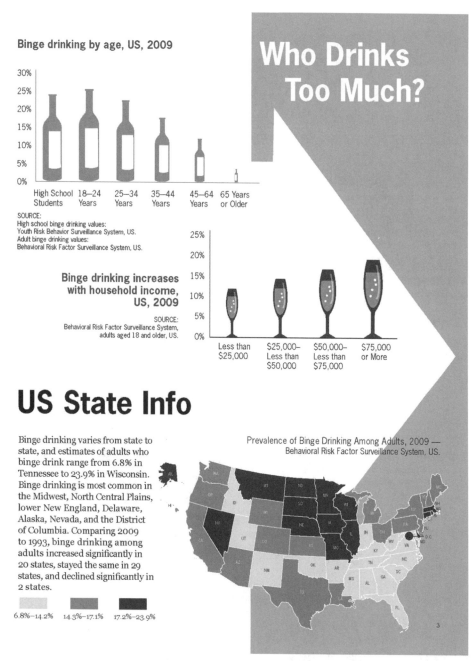

Binge drinking by age, US, 2009

SOURCE:
High school binge drinking values:
Youth Risk Behavior Surveillance System, US.
Adult binge drinking values:
Behavioral Risk Factor Surveillance System, US.

Who Drinks Too Much?

Binge drinking increases with household income, US, 2009

SOURCE:
Behavioral Risk Factor Surveillance System,
adults aged 18 and older, US.

US State Info

Binge drinking varies from state to state, and estimates of adults who binge drink range from 6.8% in Tennessee to 23.9% in Wisconsin. Binge drinking is most common in the Midwest, North Central Plains, lower New England, Delaware, Alaska, Nevada, and the District of Columbia. Comparing 2009 to 1993, binge drinking among adults increased significantly in 20 states, stayed the same in 29 states, and declined significantly in 2 states.

Prevalence of Binge Drinking Among Adults, 2009 —
Behavioral Risk Factor Surveillance System, US.

6.8%–14.2%   14.3%–17.1%   17.2%–23.9%

FIGURE 11-1   Binge drinking fact sheet with plain language techniques.
Source: Centers for Disease Control and Prevention. (2010). CDC Vital Signs. Retrieved from http://www.cdc.gov/VitalSigns/BingeDrinking/

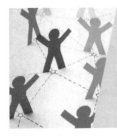

CHILDREN'S MENTAL HEALTH AWARENESS

Anxiety Disorders in Children and Adolescents Fact Sheet

Anxiety can be a normal reaction to stress. It can help us deal with a tense situation, study harder for an exam, or keep focused on an important speech. In general, it can help us cope. But when anxiety becomes an excessive, irrational dread of everyday situations, it has become a disabling condition. Examples of anxiety disorders are obsessive compulsive disorder, post-traumatic stress disorder, social phobia, specific phobia, and generalized anxiety disorder. Symptoms of many of these disorders begin in childhood or adolescence.

YESTERDAY

- The brain areas and circuitries underlying symptoms of anxiety disorders were unknown.

- No targeted psychotherapies for anxiety disorders existed.

- Clinicians did not have strong information to help them make treatment decisions between a specific psychotherapy, medication alone, or a combination of medication and psychotherapy.

TODAY

- A large, national survey of adolescent mental health reported that about 8 percent of teens ages 13–18 have an anxiety disorder, with symptoms commonly emerging around age 6. However, of these teens, only 18 percent received mental health care.

- Imaging studies show that children with anxiety disorders have atypical activity in specific brain areas, compared with other people. For example:

  — In one, very small study, anxious adolescents exposed to an anxiety-provoking situation showed heightened activity in brain structures associated with fear processing and emotion regulation, when compared with normal controls.

  — Another small study found that youth with generalized anxiety disorder had unchecked activity in the brain's fear center, when looking at angry faces so quickly that they are hardly aware of seeing them.

- Brain scans of teens sizing each other up reveal an emotion circuit activating more in girls as they grow older, but not in boys. This finding highlights how emotion circuitry diverges in the male and female brain during a developmental stage in which girls are at increased risk for developing mood and anxiety disorders.

- The Child/Adolescent Anxiety Multimodal Study (CAMS), in addition to other studies on treating childhood anxiety disorders, found that high-quality cognitive behavioral therapy (CBT), given with or without medication, can effectively treat anxiety disorders in children. One small study even found that a behavioral therapy designed to treat social phobia in children was more effective than an antidepressant medication.

NATIONAL INSTITUTE OF MENTAL HEALTH

FIGURE 11-2 Anxiety disorder fact sheet with plain language techniques.
Source: National Institute of Mental Health. (n.d.). Children's mental health awareness: Anxiety disorders in children and adolescents fact sheet. Retrieved from http://www.nimh.nih.gov/health /publications/anxiety-disorders-in-children-and-adolescents/index.shtml

❖ Try using question and answer formats with straightforward answers (**Tables 11-1** and **11-2**).

❖ Prepare materials in the language spoken in the home of the youth and family.

❖ Use active voice and strong verbs.

❖ Avoid medical jargon and use conversational language.

❖ Supplement written materials with audiovisuals or conversation.

TABLE 11-1 Parent Information Student Support Team Flyer	
Do You See Your Child Showing Any of These Behaviors? ❖ Withdrawing from family, friends, and/or school ❖ Changing friends; no longer spends time with old friends ❖ Unexplained physical injuries ❖ Talking about suicide ❖ Depressed ❖ Defying authority, both at home and at school ❖ Acting aggressively ❖ Lying ❖ Needing money without an explanation ❖ Sudden drop in grades ❖ Experimenting with drugs or alcohol **Are You Concerned About Your Child's Reaction to:** ❖ Recent death of a loved one ❖ Divorce of parents ❖ Family relocation ❖ A relationship problem ❖ Other traumatic event If your child is having trouble in or out of school, we can help you. There may be times when you just don't know how to help your child. That's okay; someone else may know how to help.	**What Is the Student Support Team?** Every school in our district has programs and services for students who experience barriers to learning. In each school building, we have a Student Support Team to assist parents and school personnel in removing these barriers. A Student Support Team, made up of school and agency staff, is available to help you access school and community programs and services for your child. Your school's Student Support Team will help you find programs and services within the school and, if needed, in the community. We do not diagnose, treat, or refer your child for treatment. Rather, we will provide you with information; you make the choices. Remember, you are part of our team. Our goal is to help your child succeed in school. **How Does My Child Become Involved in the Program?** Students come to the Student Support Team in different ways. Anyone can refer a student to the Student Support Team. Some students are referred by teachers and other school personnel. Any school staff member, a student's friend, or a family member can let the Student Support Team know that they are worried about someone. The student themselves can even go directly to the Student Support Team to ask for help. However, the Student Support Team will not become involved unless we receive your permission.

Source: Commonwealth of Pennsylvania, Pennsylvania Department of Education, Carl Fertman, Myrna M. Delgado, and Susan L. Tarasevich. Reprinted with permission.

TABLE 11-2   Folleto Informativo para Padres Sobre el Programa del Equipo de Apoyo Estudiantil

¿Ha visto a su hijo(a) con lo siguiente o comportandose de la siguiente manera?	¿Cual es el Equipo de Apoyo Estudiantil?
❖ Alejándose de la familia, sus amistades o la escuela ❖ Cambiando de amistades; ya no pasa tiempo con sus viejos amigos ❖ Lesiones físicas inexplicables ❖ Hablando de suicidio ❖ Parece estar deprimido ❖ Desafiando la autoridad, tanto en casa como en la escuela ❖ Actuando agresivamente ❖ Mentiendo ❖ Necesitando dinero sin explicación ❖ Caída repentina en las calificaciones (grados, notas) ❖ Experimentando con drogas ó alcohol	Cada escuela en nuestro distrito tiene programas y servicios para los estudiantes que enfrentan problemas/barreras o para quienes se le hace difícil aprender. En cada edificio contamos con un equipo de apoyo estudiantil para ayudar a los padres y el personal de la escuela superar estas barreras. Un equipo de apoyo estudiantil compuesto de personal de la escuela y agencias, está disponible para ayudarle con los programas y servicios escolares y comunitarios para su hijo(a).
¿Le preocupa la reacción de su hija(o) a las siguientes?	El equipo de apoyo estudiantil de la escuela le ayudará buscar programas y servicios dentro de la escuela y si es necesario, en la comunidad. El equipo no ofrece consultas ni diagnosis ni refiere su hija(a) a tratamiento. De lo contrario, le damos la información para que usted tome las decisiones. Recuerde que usted es parte de nuestro equipo. Nuestro objetivo es ayudar a su hijo(a) tener éxito en la escuela.
❖ Muerte reciente de un ser querido ❖ Divorcio de los padres ❖ Mudanza o reubicación de la familia ❖ Problemas con relaciones personales ❖ Otro evento traumático	
Si su hijo(a) tiene problemas en o fuera de la escuela, podemos ayudarle. Pueden haber ocasiones cuando usted no sabe cómo ayudarlo(a). Esté bien, no se preocupe o desanime. Otra persona puede saber cómo ayudar.	**¿Como se puede involucrar mi hijo(a) en el programa?** Estudiantes entran en el programa en diferentes maneras. Cualquiera puede referir un estudiante al equipo de apoyo estudiantil. Maestros y otro personal escolar puede referir algunos estudiantes. Cualquier miembro del personal escolar, una amistad del estudiante o miembro de la familia le puede informar al equipo que esta preocupado por algún estudiante. Hasta los mismos estudiantes pueden ir incluso directamente al equipo y pedir ayuda. Sin embargo, el equipo de apoyo estudiantil no se involucra a menos que no reciba su permiso.

Source: Commonwealth of Pennsylvania, Pennsylvania Department of Education, Carl Fertman, Myrna M. Delgado, and Susan L. Tarasevich. Reprinted with permission.

TABLE 11-3   Health Literacy Resources

❖ Centers for Disease Control and Prevention, Gateway to Health Communication and Social Marketing Practice
www.cdc.gov/healthcommunication/

❖ Health Literacy Month
www.healthliteracymonth.org

❖ Health Resources and Services Administration (HRSA) Effective Healthcare Communication 101: Addressing Health Literacy, Cultural Competency, and Limited English Proficiency (CEU/CE, CHES, CME, and CNE credits available)
http://www.hrsa.gov/healthliteracy/

❖ National Assessment of Adult Literacy (NAAL): Results from the 2003 National Assessment of Adult Literacy
http://nces.ed.gov/naal/

❖ National Center for Cultural Competence, Georgetown University Center for Child and Human Development
www11.georgetown.edu/research/gucchd/nccc/index.html

❖ National Cancer Institute, National Institutes of Health: Clear and Simple: Developing Effective Print Materials for Low-Literate Readers
www.cancer.gov/cancertopics/cancerlibrary/clear-and-simple

❖ Literacy Information and Communication System (LINCS)
http://lincs.ed.gov/

❖ PlainLanguage.gov
www.plainlanguage.gov

❖ U.S. Department of Health and Human Services, Office of Disease Prevention and Health Promotion: Health Literacy
www.health.gov/communication/literacy

Consideration of the mental health literacy of the youth and families served by programs and services is now an essential element of material design. For example, Tables 11-1 and 11-2 illustrate a flyer developed using plain English and plain Spanish for parents and caregivers with low mental health literacy. The two are excerpted from an introductory flyer of a student support team that is provided during the initial contact with the family and designed to improve mental health literacy of parents and caregivers about the student support team.

An increasing number of resources are available to help design effective health communications that consider health literacy, mental health literacy, and plain language use (**Table 11-3**). The growth in the resources and interest in the field of health literacy reflects the consensus and concerns about the need to tailor and fit what we say and how we say it with the people (youth and families) who are participating in programs and services in order for them to achieve their goals.

Health Communication and Social Media Strategies to Prevent Cyberbullying

Technology and electronic communications have brought with them unanticipated and unintentional consequences. Information is readily available online, but it is not always accurate. There are many reputable, verifiable sites with excellent mental health resources, but there are also Web sites that have inaccurate information, promote harmful behavior (i.e., promoting drug use and self-injury practices), or may not have reputable mental health professionals providing the content. Of particular concern is that instead of consulting with a professional for mental health advice, some youth and families may rely solely on what is available online to self-diagnose.

Technology also has brought advances in sexual exploitation, increasing access to pornography and making it available to anyone with Internet access, including children and adolescents. More than 28,000 people every second are looking at pornography, and in the United States, Internet pornography is a $3 billion industry. Seven of 10 youth have accidentally been exposed to online pornography, while one in three has intentionally viewed it (Enough is Enough, 2010).

Technology has changed not only how children and adolescents can be exploited sexually, but also how they present themselves to the world. In a study of how teens present themselves on a dating Web site, it was found that females ages 14–18 were more likely to include risky content on their profiles. Nearly 28% of all profiles had some form of risky content; 15.8% included sex-related content, 13.8% included references to alcohol use, 6.8% referenced smoking cigarettes, 1.6% referenced drug use, and less than 1% included content regarding violence. This study is just one example of why it is important to teach media literacy and help children and adolescents present themselves safely online (Pujazon-Zazik, Manasse, & Orrell-Valente, 2012).

One particularly troubling consequence of the technological communication advances for school communities is cyberbullying. **Cyberbullying** is an entirely new form of bullying that is hard to control and can have deadly consequences. Cyberbullying is defined as when a "child, preteen or teen is tormented, threatened, harassed, humiliated, embarrassed, or otherwise targeted by another child, preteen or teen using the Internet, interactive and digital technologies, or mobile phones" (WiredSafety, 2012). This can include mean or threatening e-mails, text messages, instant messages, or posts on social networking sites; embarrassing videos or photographs posted online; rumors spread through social networking; and fake Web sites or profiles on social networking sites. Six percent of students in grades 6–12 have reported experiencing cyberbullying (Devoe & Bauer, 2011). Children and adolescents who are victims of cyberbullying are more likely to be bullied in person, use drugs and alcohol, refuse to attend or skip school, earn poor grades, have health problems, and have low self-esteem (U.S. Department of Health and Human Services, n.d.).

Student support teams, partnerships, and collaborations and mental health programs and services have a significant role in dealing with the wide ramifications of cyberbullying once it occurs. The work is made difficult because cyberbullying tends to occur at times and in places where young people cannot be easily monitored. Many incidents do not occur on school grounds, and although young people and their parents may seek your help, the school doesn't have the authority to intervene in a punitive fashion when the events did not occur at school, on school property, or during the school day. There is limited case law to guide schools in taking appropriate actions to deal with these "gray zone" areas. Nancy Willard (2007) argues that school officials can formally intervene in incidents where the off-campus speech of students has, or reasonably could, cause a *substantial disruption* at school—violent altercations between students, significant interference with the delivery of instruction, significant interference with the ability of other students to receive an education, or significant interference in the ability of many students to feel safe at school. In other words, the school must be able to prove that a nexus or connection exists between the events occurring off-campus and disruptions to the school community. Some states are beginning to use this "substantial disruption" language in their statutes (New Hampshire's new bullying statute is an example), and districts are adding this language to their statutes and policies. This language is important because it provides better notice to students and their parents (Willard, 2012).

School teams, partnerships, and collaborations and mental health programs must find ways to support students through these searing experiences, regardless of whether disciplinary consequences occur or legal actions are taken. Connections with caring adults and linkage with school and community resources are significant strategies that can deal with the individual issues and needs as they emerge. Developing better social, communication, and conflict resolution skills are the core goals.

The **Children's Internet Protection Act (CIPA)** is a federal law enacted by Congress in 2000 to protect children using school, college, and library computers from offensive Internet content. It requires that school districts create an Internet safety plan that addresses the following elements:

- ❖ Access by minors to inappropriate matter on the Internet and the Web
- ❖ Safety and security of minors when using electronic mail, chat rooms, and other forms of direct electronic communications
- ❖ Unauthorized online access by minors, including "hacking" and other unlawful activities
- ❖ Unauthorized disclosure, use, and dissemination of personal information regarding minors
- ❖ Measures designed to restrict minors' access to materials harmful to minors

The CIPA Internet Safety Plan requirements provide an excellent framework for an analysis of the strategy developed by a school district to support the safe and responsible use of the Internet by students. Most school districts can easily comply with the CIPA requirements (Willard, 2007). Key Internet Safety Plan activities to prevent cyberbullying are (Shanahan & Kelly, 2012):

❖ *Review and update antibullying and social media policies:* Ensure the policies reflect the immediate harm that can be caused by online bullying and that policies are in place to prevent cyberbullying.

❖ *Communicate the school's rules and values to the students:* Be sure that students read and understand the school's student code of conduct. Teach students how to responsibly use social media, and explain how incidents of cyberbullying can be discovered and how they will be addressed.

❖ *Review how the school has handled cyberbullying in the past:* Ensure your school has clear procedures in place to deal with cyberbullying. Make necessary changes so that responses to cyberbullying are consistent and effective.

Because of their vision and synergy, teams, partnerships, and collaborations have a greater opportunity and responsibility to educate young people and change the social norms. Interesting work has been published demonstrating that when students were surveyed about their perceptions on the extent of bullying in a school, a high number of students said it was occurring. Yet, when students found out that their peers disapproved of bullying, rates of bullying were reduced (Perkins, Craig, & Perkins, 2011). The key to changing social norms is empowering students to make positive choices and enlisting their creativity, ideas, and credibility to promote the positive social norms.

Families are allies in preventing cyberbullying. Talking with family members, we encourage a number of strategies (Kevorkian, 2010). The following is a list of six family cyberbullying prevention recommendations:

1. Be aware of your kids' activities. Know the technology they are using, the sites they visit, and who they are interacting with.

2. Talk with your kids about Internet safety and cyberbullying. Have rules in place about how computers, cell phones, iPads, and other devices may be used.

3. Teach your children how to be smart about what they say online, what is permissible to be shared, and which sites are appropriate to visit. Remind them to never share passwords with friends or strangers.

4. Make sure your kids know that you will review their online communications if necessary. Ask for their passwords in case you need to check on things.

5. Friend or follow your kids on social networking sites.

6. Encourage them to confide in you if they are being cyberbullied or if they know someone who is.

Finally, look at what is happening nationally and internationally in the prevention of cyberbullying. For example, the National Crime Prevention Council's campaign to fight cyberbullying featured a public service announcement contest and has two PSAs available for download on its site, including one featuring

McGruff the Crime Dog. The program also includes banner ads available for anyone to post on their Web site, as well as resources for parents to help prevent and stop cyberbullying. The Family Online Safety Institute (www.fosi.org/) is an international, nonprofit membership organization that is focused on developing a safer Internet by identifying and promoting best practices, tools, and methods. The institute brings together Internet safety advocates from a variety of sectors, including global corporations, government, nonprofits, academia, and the media, to discuss the current pulse of online safety and develop new solutions to keep children safe in our Web 2.0 world.

Social Marketing Strategies to Reduce Mental Health Stigma

Social media as part of **social marketing** can serve as a tool to combat stigma against mental health concerns and problems. Social marketing is similar to traditional marketing, but instead of encouraging the purchase of goods or services, social marketing encourages behavioral change. Social marketing has been defined by many; however, it is typically defined as "the application of commercial marketing technologies to the analysis, planning, execution, and evaluation of programs designed to influence the voluntary behavior of target audiences in order to improve their personal welfare and that of their society" (Andreason, 1995). Social marketing is one strategy within health communications that we can use to create, communicate, and deliver health information and interventions using customer-centered and science-based strategies to protect and promote the health of diverse populations (Centers for Disease Control and Prevention, 2005).

A key principle of social marketing is really understanding your audience and learning what will motivate them to take action on the behavior you are trying to influence. Lessons learned from social marketing efforts stress the importance of strategically researching and identifying the intended audiences and the best strategies and methods to effectively reach and influence them. Social marketing can be an excellent health communications tool for reframing behavior, reducing barriers to change, motivating individuals to explore behavioral alternatives, reaching unserved or underserved populations, and nudging social norms toward positive change. Teams, partnerships, and collaborations using social media and social marketing strategies can be effective when addressing **mental health stigma**.

Stigma refers to attitudes and beliefs that lead people to reject, avoid, or fear those they perceive as being different. Three major categories of mental health-related stigma exist:

❖ *Public stigma* encompasses the attitudes and feelings expressed by many in the general public toward persons living with mental health challenges or their family members.

❖ *Institutional stigma* occurs when negative attitudes and behaviors about mental illness, including social, emotional, and behavioral problems, are incorporated into the policies, practices, and cultures of organizations and social systems, such as education, health care, and employment.

❖ *Self-stigma* occurs when individuals internalize the disrespectful images that society, a community, or a peer group perpetuate, which may lead many individuals to refrain from seeking treatment for their mental health conditions.

Stigma is often reflected in commonly used language. Some of the synonyms and slang terms used to describe individuals with mental health challenges are among the first words young children use to discount other children they do not like, indicating how deeply entrenched stigmatization is in today's culture. The use of clinical terms, such as a "schizophrenic" instead of the preferred phrase "an individual experiencing schizophrenia," also produces a stigmatizing effect for many mental health consumers who object to being defined by a diagnosis. In the school community, we want to be sensitive to use nonstigmatizing terms that mental health consumers prefer.

Stigma also affects the family members, companions, and co-workers of those living with mental health conditions. Family members and caregivers are frequently seen as responsible for a loved one's mental health challenge and are treated with suspicion or disapproval. Parents, in particular, are often blamed for causing a child's emotional difficulties, and they internalize that stigma, contributing to further isolation of the child and family members. This situation is known as *stigma by association*. As a result, families and caregivers may ignore the mental health symptoms, or may have fears that impede the pursuit of early intervention services and support for the child and family. Studies have shown that some family members who do seek treatment report experiencing social stigma and stigmatizing attitudes from mental health professionals. Family members affected may include parents, children, siblings, grandparents, and others close to individuals experiencing mental health challenges.

Over the years, anti-stigma campaigns have discovered that education alone is not enough. Education can produce a better informed public, but it does not significantly reduce the stigma. Social marketing has encouraged the use of multifaceted approaches that aim to influence attitudes and behaviors across the socio-ecological model: individual, family, community, system, local, regional, state, and national. In addition, social marketing has provided strategies for more thorough and reliable ways to benchmark and evaluate efforts.

The **What a Difference a Friend Makes** program provides a great example of how social marketing principles are used for a successful health education program to reduce stigma. Its priority population is youth ages 18–25 because mental health conditions are almost twice as prevalent in this age group as the general population, but with the lowest rate of help-seeking behavior.

One of the primary goals of the program is to provide information and resources for friends of those with mental health issues so they can learn to be supportive and accepting. The program employs strategies of education and making contact by providing information and encouraging support. Materials to spread the message include booklets, Web videos and PSAs, and Webcasts. There is a 21-page booklet, available in both English and Spanish (see **Figure 11-3**), full of easy to read explanations about mental health problems and how to be supportive and help a friend through a mental health issue.

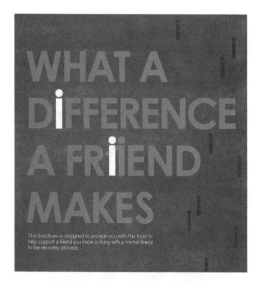 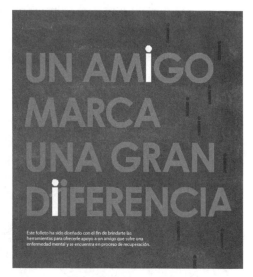

FIGURE 11-3   What a Difference a Friend Makes campaign booklet covers, in English and Spanish.
Source: Substance Abuse and Mental Health Services Administration. (2007). Mental illness: What a difference a friend makes. Retrieved from http://www.whatadifference.samhsa.gov/docs/NASC_English _web_508.pdf and http://www.whatadifference.samsha.gov/docs/NASC_Spanish_web.pdf

Another example of using social marketing to educate and combat stigma was Australia's 2006 national advertising campaign for the **beyondblue** organization. Using television commercials and print ads, as shown in **Figure 11-4**, the campaign had nine individual ads aimed at seven different audiences:

❖ People with depression and alcoholism

❖ People with bipolar disorder

❖ Women with postpartum depression

❖ People who experience depression in the workplace

❖ People with anxiety disorder

❖ Older individuals with depression

❖ Rural men with depression

The National Alliance on Mental Illness (NAMI) has developed a protest campaign to fight stigma called **StigmaBusters**. The program sends out e-mail alerts that list all instances of offensive portrayals and language about mental illness that have appeared in national media, films, television, magazines, advertisements, and major news outlets. The alerts include the name, e-mail address, and mailing address of the person responsible, and everyone who receives the e-mail alerts is asked to send a letter or e-mail to the responsible person to let them know that the portrayal or language used was hurtful or offensive. The StigmaBusters program will also send letters of commendation to television and film producers who accurately portray characters with a mental illness.

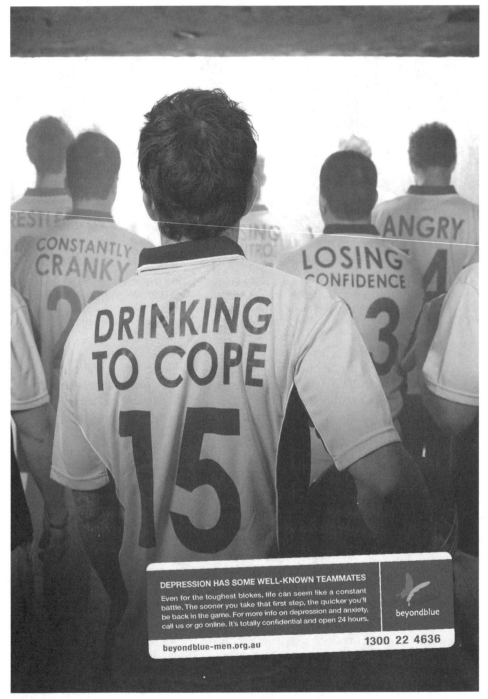

FIGURE 11-4 Print advertisement targeting rural men with depression.
Source: Courtesy of beyondblue.

New Zealand's national **Like Minds, Like Mine** program has drawn praise for its comprehensive, multilevel, long-term, social marketing-based approach to countering stigma and discrimination (www.likeminds.org.nz/page/5-home). It is widely regarded as one of the most successful mental health anti-stigma programs. In place since 1997, it is also the longest running national program.

The program has used a range of social marketing methods, including:

❖ Nationwide television and radio advertising campaigns

❖ Public speaking engagements by people with mental health challenges sharing their experiences

❖ Local programs and activities, such as photography and art exhibitions, public marches or protests, and Maori cultural events

❖ Media advocacy to disseminate positive personal stories, guidelines for journalists, training for journalism students, and other efforts to encourage nondiscriminatory reporting

The program is a collaborative effort involving a broad spectrum of agencies, such as mental health service providers, consumer-run organizations and networks, and nongovernmental organizations. It includes national public relations efforts and regional promotional and training activities. Over time, it has been adapted; it now incorporates an outcomes-based planning framework, and it is working to strengthen the role that people who have experienced mental challenges play in the program's leadership, management, and operation.

An emerging approach using social marketing strategies is the **Youth Mental Health First Aid (YMHFA)** course. Its roots are in an adult-oriented Mental Health First Aid course launched in 2001 in Wales (www.mhfa-wales.org.uk). The course is designed to teach members of the public how to support someone who might be developing a mental health problem or experiencing a mental health-related crisis, and to help them to receive professional help and other supports. YMHFA is an interactive public education program designed to increase mental health literacy. Just as CPR training helps a nonmedical professional assist an individual following a heart attack, YMHFA training helps an individual who doesn't have clinical training assist someone experiencing a mental health crisis. In both situations, the goal is to help support an individual until appropriate professional help arrives, with the added underlying intention to promote health literacy. The course's social marketing strategy encourages frank and honest discussion of mental health problems and concerns. **Figure 11-5** shows pages from the advertisement to recruit individuals to take the course.

The 14-hour YMHFA course, launched in 2007, teaches adults how to support adolescents who might be developing a mental health problem or in a mental health crisis, and to help them to receive professional help. The course content and manual are modified to provide information specific to adolescents. In addition to the mental health problems covered in the standard course, YMHFA covers eating disorders. Information is also provided about how to assist a young person who has been engaging in nonsuicidal self-injury. There is a strong theme throughout the whole program about the importance of early intervention to minimize

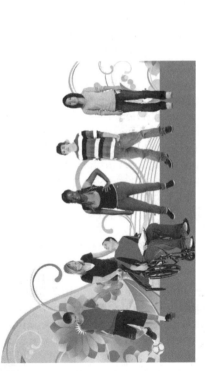

The course covers:

Mental Health First Aid
Common mental health problems
Depression
Anxiety disorders
Psychosis
Substance use disorders
Eating disorders
Non-fatal deliberate self-harming behaviour
All topics are regarding young people.

Participants will learn:

The signs and symptoms of these mental health problems
Where and how to get help
What sort of help has been shown by research to be effective.

Youth Mental Health First Aid (Wales) is for everybody

It is particularly relevant for those who work with adolescents and may come into contact with young people at risk of experiencing mental distress

Course aims

YMHFA (Wales) aims to help participants:

• Preserve life where a young person may be a danger to themselves or others
• Provide help to prevent mental distress developing into a more serious state
• Promote recovery of good mental health
• Provide comfort to a young person experiencing mental distress

Delivery

The 14-hour course can be delivered in either:

• **a 2-day training package**

or

• **4 separate modules**

Quotes from young people:

"Many young people feel isolated and the more people that are trained to listen the better".

"It would be great to get more teachers, school nurses and staff trained up in this."

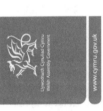

mind
Cymru

O blaid gwell
iechyd meddwl
For better
mental health

Youth mental health first aid

www.mhfa-wales.org.uk

Llywodraeth Cynulliad Cymru
Welsh Assembly Government

www.cymru.gov.uk

FIGURE 11-5 Youth Mental Health First Aid Course–social marketing.
Source: Courtesy of Mental Health First Aid (Wales), Mind Cymru.

the impact of mental health problems on adolescent development. Individuals trained in the course include adolescents, parents, school community professionals, adults involved in recreational activities with adolescents (e.g., sport coaches and scout leaders), and other adults who work with or care about adolescents.

Mental Health Communication and Social Media Plan

A **mental health communication and social media plan** guides and develops the information exchange between and among staff, youth, families, and school community members. Plans can be formal or informal, but the important element is that there is a consistent strategy for what information is communicated and how that communication will occur (**Table 11-4**). The most effective programs, services, teams, partnerships, and collaborations are in consensus on what messages are being communicated to the school community members. The communication plan is about details. It can provide guidelines for communications with families, staff, and community members. It can provide standardized formats for letters and e-mails. Even press releases and crisis management communications might be included in a communication plan. The most effective plans are a team effort. Members have spent time thinking about and discussing what they want to communicate. Likewise, they have considered the issues discussed earlier in the text: mental health literacy and use of plain language.

TABLE 11-4 Mental Health Communication and Social Media Plan

Intended audiences: Whom do you want to reach with your communications? Be specific.

Objectives: What do you want your intended audiences to do after they hear, watch, or experience this communication?

Obstacles: What beliefs, cultural practices, peer pressure, misinformation, etc. stand between your audience and the desired objective?

Key Promise: Select one single promise/benefit that the audience will experience upon hearing, seeing, or reading the objectives you've set?

Support Statements/Reasons Why: Include the reasons the key promise/benefit outweighs the obstacles and the reasons what you're promising or promoting is beneficial. These often become the messages.

Tone: What *feeling* or *personality* should your communication have? Should it be authoritative, light, emotional…? Choose a tone.

Media: What channels will the communication use, or what form will the communication take? Traditional (television, radio, newspaper, poster, brochures, flyer); New (e-mails, texts, Facebook, YouTube, blogs, apps, webinars); Devices (cell phones, tablets, videos, podcast, games)? All of the above?

Opportunities: What opportunities (times and places) exist for reaching your audience?

Creative Considerations: Anything else we should know? Will it be in more than one language?

Source: National Cancer Institute. (2001). *Making Health Communication Programs Work* (NIH Pub. No. 02-5145). Bethesda, MD: U.S. Department of Health and Human Services. Retrieved from http://www.cancer.gov/pinkbook

---

Developing a Mental Health Communication and Social Media Plan

The key to effective mental health communication and social media use is consensus on what to say and how to share it. We go back to Sarah Wu's question at the beginning of the chapter: How can you be heard above all of the noise (information) that everyone is constantly receiving? Here are six considerations for creating effective communications (Ammary-Risch, Zambon, & McCormack Brown, 2010):

1. *Understand the concerns and problems.* We know that children and adolescents have mental health concerns and problems. We want to take time to make sure that everyone is current and knowledgeable about the concerns and problems among the members of the teams, partnerships, and collaborations. It is common when communicating about mental programs and services to use statistics generated for a variety of reasons by different groups (e.g., community organizations, government), to quote program and service reports, and to solicit people's personal and professional experiences. Together these create a consensus of what the concerns and problems are that need to be addressed. We want everyone to have a shared understanding of why it is important to address the concerns and problems.

2. *Define communication objectives.* Communication objectives define what we hope to articulate to youth, families, and school community members as well as all of the team, partnership, and collaboration members. Defining the objectives assists with setting priorities. Objectives should be:

    ◆ Aligned with the program and service goals
    ◆ Realistic and reasonable
    ◆ Specific to the change desired, the population affected (i.e., primary, secondary, tertiary program participants and families), and the time period during which change should occur
    ◆ Measurable, in order to track progress
    ◆ Prioritized, to aid in allocation of resources (National Cancer Institute, 2001)

3. *Know your intended audience.* Think about with whom you want to communicate. In a mental health promoting school community we think about communications for groups of individuals (youth, families, school community members, as well as professionals) related to primary, secondary, and tertiary prevention programs and services. Within each of these broad populations, we can define smaller groups of individuals. This process is called **audience segmentation**: division of the target populations into subgroups that share similar qualities or characteristics (Thackeray & McCormack Brown, 2005). Populations can be divided into segments according to multiple factors, including geography, demographics, psychographic traits (e.g., attitudes, beliefs, and self-efficacy), behaviors, and readiness to change (National Cancer Institute, 2001). The goal is to segment the intended population on characteristics that are relevant to the mental health behavior to be changed and to organize and develop our communication efforts around these groups of similar individuals (National Cancer Institute, 2001; Slater, Kelly, & Thackeray, 2006). This information leads to communications that

are developmentally appropriate, gender specific, culturally respectful, and most importantly, useful and user friendly.

4. *Select communication channels and activities.* To reach your intended audience, consider the settings, times, places, and states of mind in which they may be receptive to and able to act on the key message (National Cancer Institute, 2001). Then identify the **channels** (routes of message delivery) through which the message will be delivered and the activities that can be used to deliver it (National Cancer Institute, 2001). Examples of communication channels to consider are:

   ◆ Interpersonal channels are more likely to be trusted and put the message into a personal context. Examples of activities or methods for delivering the message within interpersonal channels are one-on-one counseling, telephone hotlines, informal discussions, and personal coaching and instruction. Interpersonal channels are the most effective for teaching and can be very influential, but they can also be time-consuming and expensive to use and can have a limited reach.

   ◆ Group channels can reach more of the intended audience while still retaining many of the positive aspects of interpersonal channels. Group channels include neighborhood groups, workplaces, churches, or clubs. The activities associated with these channels are classroom instructions, large and small group discussions, recreational and sporting events, and public meetings. As with communicating through interpersonal channels, working with groups requires significant levels of effort and can be time-consuming and expensive.

   ◆ Community channels involve working with community groups to conduct activities such as meetings, conferences, and other events to disseminate the message. Community channels can reach a large intended audience, may be familiar to the audience, may have influence with the audience, and can offer shared experiences. Community channels can also be time-consuming to establish. Another negative aspect is the possibility of losing control of the message if it has to be adapted to fit organizational needs.

5. *Consider your social media options.* Recognize that teams, partnerships and collaborations need to make the most of the social media tools and technology. They have many tools at their disposal. Table 11-1 highlights in the media section the variety of available channels for mental health communications including traditional (i.e., television, radio, newspaper), new (i.e., emails, texts, Facebook, YouTube, apps), and devices (i.e., smartphones, tablets).

6. *Develop and pretest concepts, messages, and materials.* Communicating effectively to an audience (i.e., youth, families, and staff) is a key factor in developing effective mental health communications. It is essential to know how the audience members view their mental health and what they are being asked to do (or not do). One way to understand different audiences and create programs, materials, and messages that resonate with them is to develop and pretest concepts, messages, and materials to see which ones

have the most meaning for them and motivate them to take action. These actions ensure that your brochure, verbal instructions, written communications, announcements, materials, and publications (including e-mailing) are tailored to the group of individuals you want to hear you.

Staff Best Practices as Part of the Health Communication and Social Media Plan

Most youth and family servicing agencies including schools, human service organizations, drug and alcohol programs, after-school programs, and scouts now recognize a need to develop reasonable, user-friendly guidelines to ensure proper use of technology and social media and to prevent its misuse. For example, designate a person on the staff level (not a volunteer) responsible as the equivalent of a Webmaster for social media tools. This person would hold the password to input news items to the Facebook page, for example. Consolidate projects into the same social media site (for each outlet like Facebook) rather than allowing individual programs and services to have their own sites. If youth are posting as part of an organization's health communication and social media plan, proactively work with young people to educate them on how to use social media. You can have the youth update sites under supervision. Use mistakes in posting as teachable moments. (Finkel, 2013).

Most school community agencies will parallel their K–12 school districts in advising staff on the use of social media. For example, most agencies recommend that staff not use their own personal Facebook or other social media accounts to communicate with youth and families in any way, with the goal of maintaining

---

TABLE 11-5   Community Mental Health Agency Staff Social Media Policy: Best Practices

The community mental health agency does not allow social networking between staff members and program participants—children, adolescents, parents, caregivers, family members, or anyone who receives agency services. As a member or prospective member, I agree:

- ❖ Not to "friend" any program participant through any social networking site.
- ❖ To decline any "friend" invitations from any program participants.
- ❖ To make my profile "private" so that program participants cannot view my profile or personal information.
- ❖ Not to post any photographs of (or any information pertaining to) program participants on any social networking site.

It is imperative that staff members understand what is and is not acceptable to post to a social media Web site. We encourage staff to use social media to promote the Community Mental Health Agency. Using social media to fight mental health stigma and support our program participants is an important tool; however, we must be mindful of what we post with regards to program participants.

Source: Adapted from Big Brothers Big Sisters of Greater Memphis. (2011). Social media policy. Retrieved from http://www.msmentor.org/siteC.7gLOK6MGLflWF/b.6571943/k.FFB4/Social _Media_Policy.htm

separation between the staff's professional life and personal life. Social media forces us to address difficult questions about the different ways our personal lives and professional work can intersect. What can you request of staff in terms of their personal accounts? This is a difficult area. Do organizations actually have any rights to define what staff should do with personal accounts? While an organization should never require someone to act a certain way, or to post certain things, it is important to identify some expectations and define boundaries for what the organization can request. Table **11-5** presents a community mental health agency board-approved social media policy.

The evolution of health communication and social media necessitate teams, partnerships, and collaborations to sort out and develop their own best practices. Existing platforms will gain new features and there will always be new platforms. Cell phone are part of the lives of both youth and adults. Smartphones make it possible to have three or four conversations going at one time, texting to different people and posting to blogs and Facebook. Twitter and Instagram have accelerated the speed of communication. Social media will only become more vast and important in all our lives.

Summary

Technology, and especially social media, has made communication increasingly accessible and provides new media for teams, partnerships, collaborations, and mental health programs and services to use. Factors that are key to using social media are mental health literacy and plain language. One negative consequence of social media is cyberbullying, which can involve the use of the Internet or cell phones to harass the recipient. This can take the form of text, video, audio, or any combination of those. Although increased awareness of bullying has led schools to devise policies, plans, and training to cope with it, cyberbullying's reliance on social media presents new issues for mental health programs and services and the larger school community. Social media as part of social marketing can serve as a tool to combat stigma against mental health concerns and problems. Finally, school communities need health communication and social media plans to guide and develop the information exchange between and among the staff, youth, families, and school community members. The plans provide a consistent strategy for what information is communicated and how that communication will occur.

For Practice and Discussion

1. Did you have any preliminary knowledge about the impact of health literacy and how it affects health outcomes prior to reading this chapter? If yes, how does it compare to what you have learned in this chapter? Have you yourself ever experienced low health literacy?
2. **Table 11-6** is a family information sheet on what supportive services are available in a school community. Suggest changes and revisions to make the information sheet accessible for low mental health literacy parents and caregivers.

TABLE 11-6   Family Information on What Supportive Services Are Available

There are a number of mental health support and treatment services available to help you and your child.

Service Coordination. Some children with serious emotional disturbances will require a variety of treatment services. Coordination of these services can quickly become complicated, confusing, and time-consuming for the family. Service coordinators know the mental health system. They can ease the burden and help to coordinate services for you and your child. Children qualify for service coordination support based on their diagnosis and how well they are able to interact at home, in school, and in the community. Any child in Allegheny County with a diagnosed serious emotional disturbance is eligible for service coordination, regardless of their family income or insurance coverage. In fact, many health insurance providers require service coordination. **You will have a choice of who will provide service coordination services.**

There are two levels of service. They are:

1. Administrative Service Coordination: This is usually a starting point for most families. If your child receives treatment from any Service Coordination Unit an administrative service coordinator will help to ensure that an assessment is done, a treatment and service plan is written, referrals are made, and that your child receives the treatment and support services that are needed.
2. Blended Service Coordination: If your child is experiencing more significant serious emotional disturbances that interfere with his or her ability to function at home and he or she needs to receive treatment from two or more mental health providers or publicly-funded systems (such as Education, Child Welfare, or Juvenile Justice), a blended service coordinator would assist you and your child in coordinating these services. A blended service coordinator will also serve as a link and an advocate between multiple systems to ensure that your child gets the services that he or she needs.

Enhanced Service Coordination. There are also three separately funded, unique service coordination programs. They are:

1. The Alliance for Infants and Toddlers: This program coordinates services for children (up to 3 years of age) who have a diagnosis or condition that has a high probability of leading to a developmental delay. "At risk" children include:
   ◆ Children whose birth weight is less than 3 pounds, 5 ounces.
   ◆ Children who were cared for in the hospital's neonatal intensive care unit.
   ◆ Children born to chemically-dependent mothers.
   ◆ Children involved with Children, Youth, and Families (CYF).
   ◆ Children with confirmed lead poisoning.
2. The Life Project: This program is for children between the ages of 2 and 21 years who have serious emotional or behavioral problems and are considered to be at high risk for placement outside of the family home. The Life Project plans, implements, and coordinates:
   ◆ Enhanced service coordination with a focus on multiple system involvement
   ◆ Intensive mental health treatment
   ◆ Advocacy for the needs of the child and family
   ◆ Linking families with community and other natural supports
   ◆ Streamlined funding, offering opportunities for unique and creative treatment and support services

3. Johnson Center Project: This program is for children/adolescents with serious emotional disturbances who are being detained at Johnson Detention Center. The Johnson Center Project provides:

   ◆ A service coordinator who will coordinate mental health services to ensure that services will be in place for the child/adolescent upon release from the detention center
   ◆ Linkages to the probation officer
   ◆ Advocacy for the child/adolescent

Mobile Crisis Services. The goal of this support service is to work with the child with serious emotional disturbances during a crisis (in the home, at school, or in the community) in order to prevent injury or hospitalization. When called, a crisis intervention team will come to the child to assess, coordinate, treat, and refer, if necessary.

Student Support Teams. This is a prevention program provided in every middle and senior high school. Through this program, school personnel are trained to identify potential emotional or behavioral issues that may be causing a child to experience barriers to learning. In collaboration with the family and school personnel, a Student Support Team Liaison will provide treatment suggestions and offer assistance in obtaining mental health services, if needed. The goal of the program is to improve the child's success at school.

Family Support Programs. Family Support Programs are based on the philosophy that the most effective way to ensure the healthy development and growth of small children (up to 5 years of age) is by supporting families in the community where they live. These programs are designed to:

   ◆ Increase the strengths and stability of families
   ◆ Increase parents' confidence and competence in their parenting abilities
   ◆ Afford children a stable and supportive family environment
   ◆ Chart the progress of the child and family

Services offered by the Family Support Programs include:

   ◆ Child development
   ◆ Parenting education
   ◆ Infant and toddler groups
   ◆ Parent support groups
   ◆ Service coordination
   ◆ Resource center
   ◆ Parent leadership and advocacy

Natural Supports. A solid system of natural supports for your child can make a positive difference in his/her life. Natural supports are the relationships that occur in everyday life. These may include family members, friends, and mentors. There are various ways to build up a network of natural supports. Some of these are:

   ◆ Participating in community activities and projects
   ◆ Joining groups and clubs
   ◆ Socializing with immediate and extended family and neighbors

3. Plan your own school community-wide cyberbullying prevention activity and get others to sign on. Set a goal for the minimum number of people you want to participate. When that number of people sign on, take your planned action. Use an online tool, such as the platform provided by www.thepoint.com, to organize and conduct your campaign.
4. Create either a Facebook fan page or a group on Facebook for a campaign to prevent mental health stigma. Compare and contrast how the capabilities of each Facebook tool differ and discuss which might be better, depending on the campaign.
5. Discuss how Twitter, Facebook, YouTube, and LinkedIn might individually and jointly be used to prevent mental health stigma. Which social media channel might work best with what groups of individuals for building the prevention initiative? Why? How could businesses use channels in conjunction with each other?
6. Circle of 6, a mobile phone app, was developed as a tool to promote healthy relationships and prevent violence. The mobile app takes advantage of GPS mapping, group SMS messaging, and preprogrammed resource hotlines to help college students keep themselves and their friends safe. With Circle of 6, you choose six close friends or relatives who you can instantly text when you are feeling unsafe. It also can quickly dial emergency services if there is a need. (http://www.circleof6app.com/wp-content/uploads/2012/09/HealthyRelationshipsToolkit.pdf). Use Circle of 6 as a model to propose a cell phone app to promote child and adolescent mental health.

Key Terms

Audience segmentation 266
Beyondblue 261
Channels 267
Children's Internet Protection
   Act (CIPA) 257
Cyberbullying 256
Mental health communication 247
Mental health communication and social
   media plan 265
Mental health literacy 248
Mental health stigma 259

Like Minds, Like Mine 263
Linguistic competence 249
Plain language 250
Social marketing 259
Social media 246
Stigma 259
StigmaBusters 261
What a Difference a Friend Makes 260
Youth Mental Health First Aid
   (YMHFA) 263

References

Ammary-Risch, N., Zambon, A., & McCormack Brown, K. (2010). Communicating health information effectively. In C. Fertman & D. Allensworth (Eds.), *Health Promotion Programs: From Theory to Practice* (pp.203–232). San Francisco: Jossey-Bass.

Andreason, A. (1995). *Marketing Social Change: Changing Behavior to Promote Health, Social Development, and the Environment.* San Francisco: Jossey-Bass.

Baker, D.W., Williams, M.V., Parker, R.M., Gazmararian, J.A., & Nurss, J. (1999). Development of a brief test to measure functional health literacy. *Patient Education and Counseling,* 38: 33–42.

Bélanger, R., Akre, C., Berchtold, A., Michaud, P. (2011). U-shaped association between intensity of internet use and adolescent health. *Pediatrics*, 127(22), e330–e33.

Berkman, N.D., DeWalt, D.A., Pignone, M.P., Sheridan, S.L., Lohr, K.N., Lux, L., . . ., Bonito, A.J. (2004). *Literacy and Health Outcomes*. Evidence Report/Technology Assessment No. 87 (Prepared by RTI International—University of North Carolina Evidence-Based Practice Center under Contract No. 290-02-0016). AHRQ Pub. No. 04-E007-2. Rockville, MD: Agency for Healthcare Research and Quality.

Beyondblue. (2006). National advertising campaign. Retrieved from http://beyondblue.org.au/index.aspx?link_id=9.750

Centers for Disease Control and Prevention (CDC). (2005). What is health marketing? Retrieved from http://www.cdc.gov/healthmarketing/whatishm.htm

Chisolm, D.J., & Buchanan, L. (2007). Measuring adolescent functional health literacy: A pilot validation of the test of functional health literacy in adults. *Journal of Adolescent Health*, 41(3): 312–314.

Common Sense Media. (2012). Social media, social life: How teens view their digital lives. Retrieved from http://www.commonsensemedia.org/teen-social-media-infographic

Common Sense Media. (2011). Common sense media research documents media use among infants, toddlers, and young children. Retrieved from http://www.commonsensemedia.org/about-us/news/press-releases/common-sense-media-research-documents-media-use-among-infants-toddlers-

Davis, T., Long, S., Jackson, R., Mayeaux, E., George, R., Murphy, P., & Crouch, M. (1993). Rapid estimate of adult literacy in medicine: A shortened screening instrument. *Family Medicine*, 25(6): 391–395.

DeVoe, J.F., & Bauer, L. (2011). *Student Victimization in U.S. Schools: Results from the 2009 School Crime Supplement to the National Crime Victimization Survey* (NCES 2012-314). Washington, DC: U.S. Government Printing Office.

Enough Is Enough. (2010). Pornography statistics. Retrieved from http://www.internetsafety101.org/Pornographystatistics.htm

Finkel, E. (2013) How should kids, youth workers interact virtually. *Youth Today*, 1(22): 6–8.

Glanz, K., Rimer, B.K., & Lewis, F.M. (Eds.). (2002). *Health Behavior and Health Education: Theory, Research and Practice* (3rd ed.). San Francisco: Jossey-Bass.

Goode, T., & Jones, W. (2009). *Linguistic competence*. Washington, DC: National Center for Cultural Competence, Georgetown University Center for Child and Human Development.

Institute of Medicine. (2004). *A Prescription to End Confusion*. Washington, DC: National Academy Press.

Kevorkian, M. (2010). Parents can prevent cyberbullying. *PTA Magazine*. Retrieved from http://www.pta.org/members/content.cfm?ItemNumber=2399

National Cancer Institute. (2001). *Making Health Communication Programs Work*. (NIH Pub. No. 02-5145). Bethesda, MD: U.S. Department of Health and Human Services. Retrieved from http://www.cancer.gov/pinkbook

Ontario Centre of Excellence for Child and Youth Mental Health. (2012). Mental health literacy. Retrieved from http://www.excellenceforchildandyouth.ca/about-mental-health/literacy

Parker, R.M., Baker, D.W., Williams, M.V., & Nurss, J.R. (1995). The test of functional health literacy in adults: A new instrument for measuring patients' literacy skills. *Journal of General Internal Medicine*, 10(10): 537–541.

Perkins, P.H., Craig, D.W. & Perkins, J.M. 2011. Using social norms to reduce bullying: A research intervention in five middle schools. *Group Processes and Intergroup Relations*, 14(5): 703–722.

Pew Research Center (2012). State of the news media in 2012. Retrieved from http://stateofthemedia.org/2012/overview-4/

PlainLanguage.gov. (n.d.). Improving communication from the federal government to the public. Retrieved from http://www.plainlanguage.gov

Pujazon-Zazik, M.A., Manasse, S.M., & Orrell-Valente, J.K. (2012). Adolescents' self-presentation on a teen dating web site: Risk-content analysis. *Journal of Adolescent Health*, 50(5): 517–520.

Romer, D., Bagdasarov, Z., & More, E. (2013). Older versus newer media and the well-being of United States youth: Results from a national longitudinal panel. *Journal of Adolescent Health*, 52(3): 311–332.

Selden, C.R., Zorn, M., Ratzan, S.C., & Parker, R.M. (2000). *National Library of Medicine Current Bibliographies in Medicine: Health Literacy* (NLM Pub. No. CBM 2000-1). Bethesda, MD: National Institutes of Health, U.S. Department of Health and Human Services.

Schiavo, R. (2007). *Health Communication: From Theory to Practice.* San Francisco: Jossey-Bass.

Shanahan, S.J., & Kelly, J.G. (2012). How to protect your students from cyberbullying. *Chronicle of Higher Education.* Retrieved from http://chronicle.com/article/How-to-Protect-Your-Students/131306/

Slater, M.D., Kelly K.J., & Thackeray, R. (2006). Segmentation on a shoestring: Health audience segmentation in limited-budget and local social marketing interventions. *Health Promotion Practice*, 7: 170–173.

Substance Abuse and Mental Health Services Administration. (2007). Mental illness: What a difference a friend makes. Retrieved from http://www.whatadifference.samhsa.gov

Thackeray, R., & McCormack Brown, K. (2005). Social marketing's unique contributions to health promotion practice. *Health Promotion Practice*, 6(4): 365–368.

U.S. Department of Health and Human Services. (2000). *Healthy People 2010: Understanding and Improving Health.* Washington, DC: U.S. Government Printing Office.

U.S. Department of Health and Human Services. (2004). *Prevention: A Blueprint for Action.* Washington, DC: U.S. Government Printing Office.

U.S. Department of Health and Human Services. (n.d.). What is cyberbullying. Retrieved from http://www.stopbullying.gov/cyberbullying/what-is-it/index.html

Willard, N. (2007). *Cyberbullying and Cyberthreats: Responding to the Challenge of Online Social Aggression, Threats, and Distress.* Champaign, IL: Research Press.

Willard, N. (2012). *Cyber Savvy: Embracing Digital Safety and Citizenship.* Thousand Oaks, CA: Corwin Press.

WiredSafety. (2013). Stop cyberbullying. Retrieved from http://www.stopcyberbullying.org/what_is_cyberbullying_exactly.html

EMERGING LEADERSHIP ISSUES

In this chapter, we will:

✦ Define leadership

✦ Describe transactional and transformational leadership

✦ Explain emerging issues for children, adolescents, and families that leaders need to address

✦ Discuss emerging program and service issues that leaders need to address

Scenario

Each member of our partnership is a leader. Even if his or her job title or description never mentions the words leader or leadership, we are leaders. We are a small number of individuals trying to address many concerns and problems. And there are a lot of both [concerns and problems]. Some are pretty hard to deal with. So whether it is leading by speaking up at a meeting, writing a proposal, making decisions, or evaluating a program, leadership is part of what we do. People lead in different ways. And the diversity of styles and strategies adds to our team and to what we can accomplish. It is powerful.

Source: Walter Smith, a member of the West Chester Mental Health Partnership

Leadership Challenge

Most people do not talk much about **leadership**. Many may not perceive themselves as having leadership skills and abilities. However, the need to have professionals who consider themselves leaders has never been greater. The overwhelming nature of the school community and the pace of societal change require that all of us possess a perception of leadership that encompasses our own abilities to influence and to lead people. To be effective, we must answer questions about our own leadership abilities and capacities.

No matter your job title and job responsibilities, as a professional working as a member of a student support team, partnership, or collaboration, some part of your responsibilities will include a leadership element. You will demonstrate leadership in a variety of roles with individuals, organizations, programs, and services. As a leader, you generate new ideas and solutions. You will be innovative and responsive to ever-changing mental health concerns and problems of youth and families. You will be a leader as you listen to individuals, groups, organizations, and communities who bring new ideas, information, resources, and support to bear on youth mental health needs, make decisions, and achieve goals.

Leadership is an elusive concept because people do not often define themselves in leadership terms. For example, we might say that we helped a group or individual take action or that they listened to us. But if asked whether we are leaders, we are apt to answer, "Well, not really." Likewise, it is much easier and acceptable for people to talk about their profession (e.g., teacher, counselor, nurse, director) than to talk about being a leader. Leadership is elusive due to the fact that in the past 50 years, as many as 65 different classification systems have been developed to define the various dimensions of leadership (Fleishman et al., 1991).

Leadership Definition

In summarizing the leadership literature, Northouse (2001) suggests five approaches to defining leadership. First, leadership can be approached from the view of a group process. From this perspective, the leader is at the center of group change and activity and embodies the will of the group. A second group of definitions conceptualizes leadership from a personality perspective that suggests leadership is a combination of special traits or characteristics individuals possess that enable them to induce others to accomplish tasks. A third approach to leadership defines it as an act or behavior—the things leaders do to bring about change in a group. Fourth, leadership is defined in terms of the power relationship that exists between leaders and followers. From this viewpoint, leaders have power and wield it to effect change in others. A fifth view sees leadership as an instrument of goal achievement in helping group members achieve their goals and meet their needs. This view includes leadership that transforms followers through vision setting, role modeling, and individualized attention.

Despite the multitude of ways that leadership has been conceptualized, what is clear from the literature is that leadership is a personal and developmental process.

The development takes place over time, throughout a person's life (Bennis, 1989; van Linden & Fertman, 1998; Wren, 1995). Each person has the potential and capacity to lead (Bennis & Nanus, 1985). As part of the process, people learn and practice a set of skills and attitudes (Bennis & Nanus, 1985; Kouzes & Posner, 1987; Stogdill, 1974). Leadership skills and attitudes are both transactional and transformational (Bass, 1985; Burns, 1978). **Transactional leadership** focuses on the skills and tasks associated with leadership, such as speaking in public, delegating authority, leading meetings, and making decisions. This is what leaders do. **Transformational leadership** focuses on the process of leadership and what it means to be a leader. It is concerned with how individuals use their abilities to influence people. Think of the difference between transactional and transformational leadership as *doing* leadership tasks versus *being* a leader. As leaders, sometimes we focus on "being leaders" and sometimes we focus on "doing leadership tasks." There is no clear separation between doing leadership tasks and being a leader; rather, the two are mixed.

Transformational and Transactional Leadership

Focusing on transactional and transformational leadership can support and guide personal leadership development. It builds awareness of how we influence and lead individuals and organizations that reflect the people, situations, and tasks involved. Transactional and transformational leadership provide a model with which we can examine how we are leaders. Reflecting on these qualities promotes and supports us as leaders. You can use them to reflect on how you can address the emerging issues and make decisions discussed later in the chapter.

Transformational Leadership Qualities

Transformational leadership focuses on the personal qualities of leadership (Bass, 1985; Burns, 1978). It is leadership by example. Often when people are asked if they are leaders, they respond "no." However, if you ask what they did last weekend and how they decided to do it, you can get them to talk about the role they played among their friends in making decisions. As professionals it is critical to think and reflect on how we influence and lead others, to think about how we value people, serve as role models, make good choices, and influence others in positive ways.

The following paragraphs describe eight transformational leadership qualities that can serve as points for reflection and consideration in our professional role. They focus on how we approach requests for information and resources, and the process and care we take in responding to the health needs and questions of individuals and groups (organizations and communities); it is how we share our thinking about our strategies and process. Being a professional involves helping people find and connect with information on the Internet, in the library, and in community health organizations. Furthermore, it is equally important to help people and organizations ask questions and find the answers they want through their own creative actions, reflection, and energies. The transformational qualities are the ways we can support, comfort, and lead people in this process. As you read about each quality, think about how you are able to put into action that quality with the individuals and organizations you serve.

Value the participation and contribution of others. Encourage all members to appreciate their need for others and the value of their efforts. Help individuals and organizations develop a wide network of resources and support that includes colleagues, consumers, friends, and family members. Addressing mental health needs requires looking in as many places as possible. In the search for answers on how to address a concern, often other people have the experience and firsthand knowledge that someone needs. We need to actively empower the people we serve to be thorough in their search for solutions and to appreciate the knowledge and experience of other people and organizations.

Take all viewpoints and advice into account before making decisions. Help people gather the appropriate information, resources, and support so that they can make sound decisions. Strive to view decision making as a data-informed process. Decisions are not made in isolation, but rather are reached after considering the possible consequences and outcomes—both positive and negative. Remind people that their decisions will influence their own and others' future actions and directions.

Consider individuals within their contexts and situations. Help people connect with information, programs, resources, and supports. This means not just tolerating, but understanding and appreciating other people's points of view, culture, and needs. Critical to the process is the ability to listen to another person, and to empathize with and understand another's point of view. Practice key listening behaviors such as being able to paraphrase another's ideas, to empathize, and to accurately express another person's concepts and emotions. As people assess their health needs, plan programs, and search for information, encourage them to listen to other people with care and empathy so as to fully understand the other person's perception of a particular health issue or concern.

Use decisions to test information. Making decisions helps to focus people's energy and effort. The points at which choices are made are opportunities to give and receive useful feedback and new information. Help people feel comfortable defining the decisions they are making and the ways they are working toward their goals in an atmosphere of trust and honesty. Work to be clear about what people can expect to do with the information they receive and how they are going to use it to make a decision. Talk about options and alternatives that might be pursued based on the information, resources, and support that are found in the process of planning, implementing, coordinating, and evaluating programs. Question whether the information is satisfactory and sufficient to help the person or organization address the identified health need.

Focus on personal and organizational development. It is easy to blame others for one's lack of information, coordination, progress, and support. Both individuals and organizations need your help thinking about working as a team, coordinating efforts, communicating their program services, and searching for information and resources. Encourage self-awareness and creativity among team members as they determine how and where to find information, plan programs, coordinate efforts, and evaluate progress toward the goal.

Learn from experiences and generalize to "real life." Seeing the big picture and knowing how to apply what is being learned to "real life" represents a higher level of learning. This perspective adds objectivity and provides motivation to learn even during difficult times. Stepping back from a health need to gain a wider view is difficult. Support people and group efforts to reflect on their experiences and what they are learning.

Recognize the importance of the process. Not everything can, or needs to, be completed today. Individuals and organizations need to take time to interact, learn, and share what they are learning. It is part of the process of learning to be an informed consumer of health information. Likewise, it is part of being a leader and a professional. Focusing on the process will allow everyone to be valued and to have his or her talents highlighted. Ultimately, we want people and organizations to be able to address their health needs independently. Only by focusing on the process can this be accomplished.

Share decision-making responsibilities. Learning when to let go and when to stand firm on decisions is part of working with people to develop, implement, coordinate, and evaluate a health program. Strive to create a trusting and supportive environment to allow others to step forward to share their ideas and suggestions. Such situations allow individuals to feel safe, so that they will be more willing to take risks. When working with individuals, this means encouraging them to pursue ideas and to involve family, friends, and peers in the process. Likewise for organizations, it is a focus on reaching consensus about what ideas and resources to pursue.

Transactional Leadership Qualities

Transactional leadership focuses on the skills and tasks associated with leadership, such as public speaking, delegating authority, providing information, making connections, answering questions, leading meetings, and making decisions (Bass, 1985; Burns, 1978). This is what leaders do. However, transactional leadership emphasizes more than completing tasks. It focuses on how to carry out the tasks of leadership. The following paragraphs describe seven transactional leadership qualities that can serve as points for reflection and consideration in our professional role. As you read each quality, think about how you are able to put into effect that quality with the individuals and organizations you serve. The qualities focus on how professionals help people answer questions and address their needs. They aim at helping professionals to assist the individuals or organizations they serve to clarify what they want to know, even if initially the individuals or organizations are uncertain or anxious about what their needs may be.

Value problem and solution identification. To complete tasks and achieve goals, we must first identify what has to be done. Individuals and organizations can struggle with where to start in addressing issues, designing a program, marketing services, and knowing how to search for information. To support people in the process requires a willingness to be open, to seek help from others, and to share one's own perceptions and feelings. Take time to figure out what individuals or organizations want to know and be willing to deal with the anxiety of looking and finding the answer.

Make decisions—even if everyone has not been heard—in order to move forward. Making decisions and getting a task completed requires action. Priority must be placed on taking steps toward an objective and accomplishing a goal. Information and resource searches may be time limited. Timelines to develop and implement a program may be short. Responsibilities for program coordination may be incomplete. At some point, an organization and individual may need to make a decision based on the available information and resources. Therefore, it is important to learn to be sensitive to the fact that some decisions may not be ideal for each individual, even if they will help to move the project or task at hand to completion.

Use standards and principles as guides. It is critical for individuals to be able to articulate the process they used to make their choices—to be able to identify their information sources, guiding standards, and principles. Likewise, within an organization, everyone does not have to agree with the decisions made, but they should be in agreement regarding how the decisions were made. Provide a clear description of your health education practice to the individuals and groups that seek your help. Be clear about expectations for participation for everyone involved in the process.

Develop yourself to be a better professional. Building trust and support with individuals and organizations is the way to begin addressing their health needs and concerns. This is an ongoing process that involves listening to other people, anticipating results, confronting conflict and anxiety, and soliciting feedback. It is the continual work of managing the stress of making healthy and ethical choices. Individuals and organizations we serve look to us as models in this process. Therefore, our continual efforts to learn more and to search for new ideas and support are indicators of our commitment and dedication to the people and organizations we serve. Personal credibility and integrity are critical to helping people seek and use information, programs, resources, and support.

Get things done. Results count. Consumers of mental health promotion program and services want to work with dependable individuals. They have expectations. As professionals, we need to work hard to ensure that we meet the expectations of those we serve. Likewise, the individuals and organizations we work with need to have clear timelines and tasks to complete if they are to have the information, programs, resources, and support they desire.

Recognize the importance of the product. Outcomes are important. As a professional and leader, it is important to be able to articulate the aims of an activity, program, or task. If people are not clear about where they are headed, they are likely to disengage. Work to have people receive something of value and that they find useful.

Take charge (personal power). Stepping forward requires confidence in one's abilities. Thus it is critical to stress the need for individuals and groups to self-identify that they can do a particular task or participate in an activity, recognizing the challenges and opportunities that exist. Recognition of their self-determination in addressing health issues and concerns is awareness of one's leadership abilities and capacities.

Leadership to Promote Child and Adolescent Mental Health

People do not wake up one day as a leader. Leadership is a personal and developmental process. This development takes place over time, throughout a person's life. However, all people possess leadership potential; they already demonstrate their leadership abilities in small ways in their families, workplaces, and communities. In your teams, partnerships, and collaborations, you will demonstrate leadership promoting child and adolescent mental health. You will be a role model for others helping to develop and shape the leadership abilities and skills of colleagues and peers. Professionals lead in their workplaces, their communities, and their families. Professionals are leaders.

Use the transformational and transactional leadership qualities to reflect on your leadership qualities. We each have a mix of transformational and transactional qualities that we bring to our work. Reflection on these qualities focuses our attention on our abilities to influence and lead others as we work to meet the mental health needs of the youth and families we serve.

Reflecting on these qualities, you are better able to hear and appreciate the thoughts, emotions, and experiences of your peers and colleagues as well as the youth and families with which you work. You get to hear how they feel about the issue and decision. You will be better informed and realistic about the consequences of decisions and changes for youth, families, colleagues, and peers. Reflecting on the leadership qualities helps you add value to the school community.

In the next sections are a few of the emerging issues and decisions that require leadership in promoting child and adolescent mental health in schools and communities. You do not need to have the answers or solutions. What you need to do is be willing to lead the process of consensus building to find a creative solution and make decisions that fit the school, community, youth, and families. The information in the following sections prepares you to lead the process as you talk with others about the issues. It will assist you to assess the options and make a decision.

Emerging Issues for Children, Adolescents, and Families that Leaders Need to Address

Leaders stand up for children, adolescents, and families. Two emerging issues for school community professionals who work directly with youth and families are how best to focus on and build the resilience of young people throughout the school community, and how to respond to **violence** in the school community.

Resilience in Children and Adolescents

For you as a leader promoting child and adolescent mental health, building resilience is part of what you do. It is part of building a school community culture that is caring and nurturing.

Resilience has been defined simply as the ability to bounce back from adversity. It is about our response to stress. When predicting a person's capacity for resiliency, the math is pretty simple. It works out to a highly individualized balance between the risk factors in a child's life and the supports available, both externally and internally (Bluestein, 2001). The supports that you provide through programs, services, parent/family engagement, community engagement, student support teams, school counselors, social workers, mentors, teachers, and other caring adults can make a major difference in a child's life. Those supports are often called assets or **protective factors**.

Researchers have identified traits or characteristics evident in children who have been in high-risk situations and overcome them and succeeded. The profile of the resilient child includes four major characteristics: social competence, problem-solving skills, autonomy, and sense of purpose and future. These are internal (Benard, 1991). Most people have these four attributes to some extent. Whether these attributes are strong enough within the individual to help that person bounce back from adversity depends on having certain protective factors in one's life (Krovetz, 2008). As a mental health promoting leader in a school community, you can provide positive environmental influences and build external and internal protective factors in children to help them overcome stressors in school, home, and life.

One of the simplest ways to build resiliency is by considering what research tells us about routines. Establishing routines is useful for physical school safety as well as for emotional safety, especially during transitions. Establishing anchor points also reduces anxiety and stress. Life's common anchor points are waking up, the main meal of the day, and bedtime. Schools also have anchor points: admission, lunch, and dismissal. Schools that establish consistent rituals for these major transitions seem to have better outcomes (Sanchez, 2008). Classroom teachers know that routines facilitate the instructional day. Schools have established morning and dismissal rituals such as announcements, thought for the day, theme for the week, and other like activities.

Thomsen (2002) provides examples of characteristics found in schools that build resilience (**Table 12-1**). Key actions include support and caring behaviors, high expectations, and opportunities to participate in and contribute to the setting. Use the table as guidance to assess what you want to do or where you want to go in your school community. You can also use the table as a checklist, guiding efforts to create a school environment that fosters resilience. As you use the table, consider that each team's, partnership's, and collaboration's approach to building the resilience of youth and families reflects the leadership of its members. Being aware of your own leadership abilities and capacity helps the school community make decisions that build resiliency in youth and families.

TABLE 12-1 Characteristics of Schools that Build Resilience		
Support and Caring	**High Expectations**	**Opportunities to Participate**
Principals, teachers, and support staff who communicate concern for the whole child	Teachers and staff who believe, and behave as if, all students have potential	Roles and jobs for students that are valued and meaningful
Mechanisms for student support are inclusive and attentive to different groups of students	An academic culture and climate with clear expectations for good performance in all areas of life	Ways for students to shine in addition to academics and athletics
Resources available for youth, both for academics and personal growth	Staff and children who share high expectations for themselves from a positive perspective	Youth voice recognized and encouraged, student leadership opportunities are encouraged
Staff members who feel supported and thereby are supportive of students	Academic support available and accessible	Service learning is part of school culture and climate

Violence in the School Community

Violence in its many manifestations, major or minor, has become such a part of the landscape in the United States that we are often shocked only momentarily by indescribable carnage and are then able to continue leading our daily lives without it having much impact on anything we do. It's minimal effect on us, unfortunately, is reflected in the values of our society in subtle ways, and also permeates our school communities, making us all responsible to a certain degree for the continuing violence. As professionals, we cannot change the world, but we can promote mental health wellness in our schools and communities so that conflicts do not turn into shootouts. We can teach our children social and emotional skills and foster their self-efficacy and resilience. You and your teams can work with students, families, partnerships and collaborations to achieve prevention goals that reflect the consensus of the school community and community at large. All types of violence in the school community, from chronic bullying to relational aggression, threaten the physical, psychological, and emotional well-being of students and school staff (Osher, Dwyer, & Jackson, 2003). These negative effects radiate to all members of the school community. No matter the nature of the violent event, it touches all of our lives.

Violence, the intentional use of force or behavior that causes harm, is a public health problem. As a mental health professional, your leadership is required to address violence in the school community. It is certainly not something you will do alone. It is part of the work that teams, partnerships and collaborations are constantly confronting.

There are many causes for violence: drugs, illiteracy, lack of education, mental illness, bullying, availability of guns, gangs, and countless others. There is no one reason why individuals perform violent acts. Some are mimicking behavior they have seen at home, in their neighborhoods, or in video games, movies, or television. There are some young people that turn to violence because they are victims of bullying who feel they need to do something to make it stop. They feel isolated and rejected by their peers (CDC, 2008).

Mass shootings are another kind of violence that can occur in the school community. While deplorable and pointless, these shootings give Americans the false notion that dramatic increases in school-related violence are happening when in fact national surveys consistently find that school-associated homicides have stayed essentially stable or even decreased slightly over time. According to the CDC's School-Associated Violent Death Study, less than 1% of all homicides among school-age children happen on school grounds or on the way to and from school, meaning that the vast majority of students will never experience lethal violence at school (CDC, 2008).

An essential key to the prevention of violence is planning. School communities need to have policies, procedures, and comprehensive prevention plans in place to address school violence. The implementation of evidenced-based prevention programs that teach social–emotional skills, appropriate behaviors, conflict resolution, the applications of student support teams, and the fair application of discipline when infractions occur all contribute to reduction in violence. A caring and nurturing positive school culture and climate where students and staff feel valued also contributes to less violence. A crisis or emergency response plan that involves in its development the students, staff, local agencies and community-at-large, local law enforcement, local emergency management agencies, and first responders should be in place. There are many templates available on the Web:

Facts About School Violence, Centers for Disease Control and Prevention (CDC) Violence Prevention
http://www.cdc.gov/ViolencePrevention/youthviolence/schoolviolence/index.html
Resources for Crisis Planning, U.S. Department of Education (ED)
http://www2.ed.gov/admins/lead/safety/emergencyplan/crisisplanning.pdf
Resources for Responding to and Preventing School Violence and Suicide, Substance Abuse and Mental Health Services Administration (SAMHSA)
http://www.sshs.samhsa.gov/resources/PreventingViolence.aspx

One of the more comprehensive templates found was developed by the Pennsylvania Emergency Management Agency (2009). The Pennsylvania All Hazards School Safety Planning Toolkit includes responses to individual student emergencies as well as community-wide crises (**Figure 12-1**).

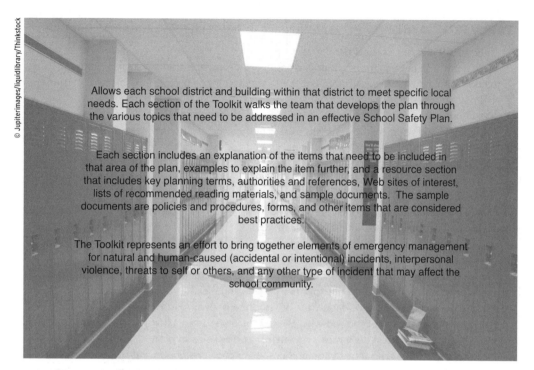

Allows each school district and building within that district to meet specific local needs. Each section of the Toolkit walks the team that develops the plan through the various topics that need to be addressed in an effective School Safety Plan.

Each section includes an explanation of the items that need to be included in that area of the plan, examples to explain the item further, and a resource section that includes key planning terms, authorities and references, Web sites of interest, lists of recommended reading materials, and sample documents. The sample documents are policies and procedures, forms, and other items that are considered best practices.

The Toolkit represents an effort to bring together elements of emergency management for natural and human-caused (accidental or intentional) incidents, interpersonal violence, threats to self or others, and any other type of incident that may affect the school community.

FIGURE 12-1   All Hazards School Safety Planning Toolkit.

As you plan and develop prevention goals, you want to think about and recommend specific actions that everyone can take to prevent violence. The National PTA (**Table 12-2**) has created a checklist of actions for parents. The checklist can guide efforts not merely with parents and caregivers but with students, community members, legislators, and the media.

Finally, as a health professional it is important to learn all that you can about trauma and its effects on learning, and to help the members of your school community create trauma-sensitive schools. The National Child Traumatic Stress Network cites that one in four students attending school has experienced at least one traumatic event (NCTSN, 2008). As a champion, you need to understand that trauma changes the way a child's brain functions, affecting concentration, memory, organizational skills, social relationships, and behavior. **Trauma** occurs when a child is exposed to an event or series of events where physical and/or emotional safety and security are threatened.

Toxic stress damages a child's developing brain (Perry & Pollard, 1998). Children with toxic stress live their lives in fight, flight, or freeze mode. They respond to the world as a place of continuous threat. Their brains are clogged with stress hormones rendering the cognitive and executive function levels of the brain powerless while the alarm center located in the amygdala continuously fires warnings. They cannot focus on schoolwork, remember assignments,

---

TABLE 12-2   Actions to Prevent Violence in Your School Community

1. **Talk with children and adolescents**

   Include children in discussions about current issues, drugs, sex, drinking, their friends, and schoolwork and activities. Let them know you are listening to their opinions, that it matters, and that you care.

2. **Set clear rules and limits for your children and teenagers**

   Let children and youth know what you expect of them; be clear and precise. Explain why you are setting the rule. Follow through and be fair and consistent with the enforcement.

3. **Know the warning signs**

   Know your child. Be aware of changes in moods or activities that seem out of character. Be alert for changes.

4. **Don't be afraid to parent and care give; know when to intervene**

   Be the parent, take care of your child and seek help from school or health professionals when you need it.

5. **Join your school community violence prevention group**

   Join a community-wide violence prevention group. Start a crime watch or other program if there isn't one close by. Reach out to other parents and members of the community.

6. **Help to organize a school community violence prevention forum**

   Rally the troops around school violence prevention; organize an activity.

7. **Help develop a school violence prevention and response plan**

   Make sure that your school has a comprehensive violence prevention and response plan by volunteering to help develop it. Reach out to those community members and agencies who have resources and those that will be responding.

8. **Know how to deal with the media in a crisis**

   Learn what it takes to get media attention and their expectations for press releases and contacts.

9. **Work to influence lawmakers**

   Use the power of your vote and your voice. Work with others to influence those in power to pay attention to violence prevention. Attend meetings, start petitions, write letters or faxes, or use social media to get attention and influence change,

Source: Adapted from National PTA. (2013). Checklist to prevent violence in schools. Retrieved from www.pta.org/content.cfm?ItemNumber=984

---

or organize thoughts. They may perform poorly in school, fail to create healthy relationships with other children, or make trouble with teachers and principals because they do not trust adults. Shaming discipline practices, or exclusion, do not fix the underlying triggers that drive the negative behaviors. For a comprehensive school-wide framework that describes the how-to of creating a trauma sensitive school, download *Helping Traumatized Children Learn* (Massachusetts Advocates for Children, 2005). The book discusses topics such as school community infrastructure and culture, staff training in academic and nonacademic settings for working with traumatized children, and proactive links with mental health treatment. It champions a school-wide effort as critical for addressing the learning, behavioral, and relationship problems that are so necessary for success at school. It also highlights the fact that trauma and violence reach beyond the scope of the school and require engaging communities in holistic prevention efforts. A trauma-sensitive school community can make important contributions to that effort (**Figure 12-2**).

Realistically, as a mental health professional, you cannot address all the aspects of violence in the school community, but you can make a positive contribution to a child's mental health. You can also become a champion for mental health wellness. You can bring leadership and passion and provide insight into how stakeholders work together. You can gather data, identify available

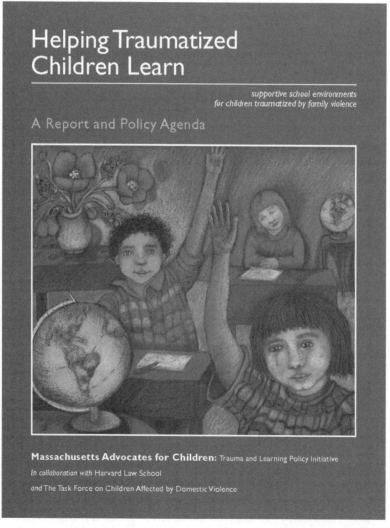

FIGURE 12-2 Helping Traumatized Children Learn.
Source: Courtesy of Massachusetts Advocates for Children.

resources, build a network across agencies, and create opportunities and resources for young people to get support and address their problems and concerns. You can work with local, state, and national legislators to drive the agenda for earlier mental health treatment that emphasizes a system of care approach that is well funded and easily accessible.

One of the things we have learned from recent school shootings is that communities can work to reduce risk factors and they can develop assets that make recovery from violence easier for the school community. There are many dimensions to the issue of violence and most are beyond our individual control or that of the school community. Nonetheless, we must continue to work to improve the mental health of our students, school, and community.

Emerging Program and Service Issues that Leaders Need to Address

Leaders make decisions. One emerging issue for school community professionals that requires making decisions is deciding the mix of programs and services to address addictions within the overall school community mental health programs and services offerings. Another issue is deciding how to evaluate programs and services. In the first example you are deciding how to best meet the needs of youth. In the second example, you are deciding if the school community programs and services are effective. You are deciding if the programs and services work; how well they meet the needs of the youth and families they serve as well as how to make the programs stronger and more responsive.

Balancing Substance Abuse Programs and Services

Your leadership will be required to address the struggles with **substance abuse** (alcohol, tobacco, and other drug abuse) and the tension that exists between mental health and substance abuse **funding**. Furthermore, with the existing school community funding, you will need to prioritize the delicate balance between primary prevention programs and services designed to delay, reduce, or avoid substance abuse during childhood and adolescence with the substance abuse treatment (tertiary prevention) needs of adolescents. As a member of a student support team, partnership, or collaboration, you will encounter a variety of program and service gaps when it comes to substance abuse treatment. Your work is to identify these gaps and advocate with politicians and advisory boards to positively address them.

In this text, we have deliberately chosen the term *mental health* (versus behavioral health) to define the scope of the work of teams, partnerships, and collaborations, and programs and services. Under the umbrella of all of the mental health concerns and problems for youth and families, substance abuse looms large. Substance abuse permeates the school community with consequences for youth and families. Your leadership skills and those of your colleagues and peers will influence the mix of programs and services to address substance abuse within the overall school community mental health programs and services offerings.

Tension exists about the presence and availability of substance abuse programs and services within the mix of school community mental health programs and services. Prior to Jellinek (1960) publishing the first paper on the "disease concept" in 1960, addiction to substances (i.e., tobacco, alcohol, and other drugs) was debated to be a vice, rather than an actual illness with chronic long-term physiological and psychological consequences.

Today, substance abuse or addiction is defined as a chronic, relapsing brain disease that is characterized by compulsive drug seeking and abuse despite harmful consequences. It is considered a brain disease because drugs change the brain structure and how it works. These brain changes can be long lasting and can lead to the harmful behaviors seen in people who abuse drugs (National Institute on Drug Abuse [NIDA], 2010).

The initial decision to take drugs is mostly voluntary. However, when drug abuse takes over, a person's ability to exercise self-control can become impaired. Brain imaging studies from drug-addicted individuals show physical changes in areas of the brain that are critical to judgment, decision making, learning and memory, and behavior control (Fowler, Volkow, Kassed, & Chang, 2007). Scientists believe these changes alter the way the brain works, and may help explain the compulsive and destructive behaviors of addiction.

National drug use surveys indicate some children are already abusing drugs by age 12 or 13. Substance abuse and addiction can refer to any individual who is drinking alcohol or using drugs such as heroin, nicotine, cocaine, marijuana, prescription painkillers, stimulants, or other drugs. In addition, addiction can also refer to compulsive behavior regarding sex, gambling, Internet use, and other activities.

The National Institute on Drug Abuse (NIDA) has concluded that addiction is a developmental disease because it typically begins in childhood or adolescence. One of the brain areas still maturing during adolescence is the prefrontal cortex— the part of the brain that enables us to assess situations, make sound decisions, and keep our emotions and desires under control. The fact that this critical part of an adolescent's brain is still a work in progress puts them at increased risk for poor decisions (such as trying drugs or continued abuse). Also, introducing drugs while the brain is still developing may have profound and long-lasting consequences.

Teens' still-developing judgment and decision-making skills may limit their ability to assess risks accurately and make sound decisions about using drugs. Drug and alcohol abusers can disrupt brain function in areas critical to motivation, memory, learning, judgment, and behavior control. So it is not surprising that teenagers who abuse alcohol and other drugs often have family and school problems, poor academic performance, health-related problems (including mental health), and involvement with the juvenile justice system.

Drug abuse and mental disorders often co-exist. This is called co-morbidity. In some cases, mental diseases may precede substance abuse; in other cases, drug abuse may trigger or exacerbate mental disorders, particularly in individuals with specific vulnerabilities. This is referred to as a bi-directional relationship. For example, an adolescent may begin smoking and find that it relieves feelings of hopelessness and depression. The young person begins to use more nicotine to find that relief, and the nicotine use makes the depression worse.

As a leader in a mental health promoting school community, you have to balance the mix of programs and services to address substance abuse within the overall school community mental health programs and services offerings. The widespread prevalence and consequences of youth substance abuse mean that teams, partnerships, and collaborations need to make priorities and decisions about how best to utilize their staff and funding.

To do this, you will need to use your leadership skills to find out how funding for substance abuse programs and services (primary, secondary, and tertiary prevention) is allocated in your state and local community. You will need to ask questions about state-level funding streams. In some states, a central department of behavioral health has two branches, one for mental health and the other for alcohol/drugs and substance abuse. Other states do not separate the two funding streams. Still other states have separate departments with separate funding streams and authority.

One example of leadership by many members of student support teams, partnerships, and regional collaboration is from a large urban area where there was tension about changing the funding mix for mental health programs and services

Box 12-1
Expanding the Funding for Substance Abuse Programs and Services

The Crisis Center or "CC" provides 24 hour/7 day per week crisis response services to the west side communities via telephone. When necessary, crisis response teams can be sent to the caller's location to assist and stabilize the situation. In addition, they have a 72-hour stabilization unit for adolescents with mental health issues that do not warrant hospitalization. In other sections of the city and county, there was not a comparable unit for substance-abusing adolescents because there was no additional available funding. The local mental health partnerships and regional collaboration decided to advocate with the local elected state representatives, including inviting a few of them to be members of the collaboration. At an emotional meeting, the representatives listened to several parents whose children (ages 15 to 18 years old) had overdosed and died. The parents spoke about how their children had tried to stop abusing prescription medications and heroin but had no resources to help them maintain their beginning recovery. Parents told story after story, explaining that their children might be alive today if there had been a place for them to turn. Currently, parents argued, there is nowhere to go but the streets if an adolescent wants help but has burned bridges with their family because of stealing, lying, and incorrigible behavior. The parents were forceful in championing the need for funding. They repeatedly talked about the difficulty of drug-abusing youth living on the streets with little hope for recovery. After the meetings with the collaboration, the representatives arranged for an inquiry. During the following months, the county commissioners conducted hearings and lobbied for funding to expand programming and services to other communities in the city and county as well as open a 5-day voluntary stabilization unit for substance-abusing teenagers.

to fund more substance abuse programs and services (**Box 12-1**). A change in the mix meant a potential cut in funding for other programs and services. People did not want to cut other funding, but there was a serious gap in programs and services.

As a leader, you listen to the students. You listen to their parents and stay connected. Be certain that students and parents have a space at the table as you advocate for resources and identify the priorities of your teams, partnerships, and collaborations. Reach out to local politicians and managed care organizations, and becertain that those with authority for funding schools and community agencies are represented. Practice the concepts outlined in this chapter and give them energy.

Evaluation

As a member of a team, partnership, or collaboration, you want to have programs and services evaluated. As a leader, you need information about the programs and services to make decisions. We need to know whether the mental health programs and services in the school community have been implemented and are operating as planned. We also need to know how and when they achieve their goals and objectives (or if they did). Lots of time, energy, resources, and effort are spent by many people creating, implementing, and sustaining the school community's primary, secondary, and tertiary prevention programs and services. At a certain point, it is only natural to ask, "Are the programs and services working and addressing the needs of the children, adolescents, and families?"

Evaluation is not the final phase in the process of creating, operating, and sustaining programs and services. It is *one* of the phases, and in the most effective programs and services, it runs parallel to the other phases, starting at the

TABLE 12-3 Types of Program Evaluation
Formative evaluation involves gathering information and materials during program planning and development. It can be used to understand the needs assessment data gathered during the program planning process.
Process evaluation is a snapshot of a program or service. It is about systematically gathering information during implementation. It can be used to describe and assess to what extent the intended program activities and services are being accomplished.
Impact evaluation measures the immediate effects of programs and services. The primary question in an impact evaluation is: What has been the program's immediate effect on the children and adolescents?
Outcome evaluation examines the changes in the children and adolescents during or after their participation in a program and service. We are looking for changes such as knowledge gains, attitude changes, skills acquired, or behavior changes.

very beginning of the process when a program is being planned and continuing in tandem as the program is implemented and sustained, in order to provide continual feedback to program staff, children, adolescents, family, school community members, and funders.

Program evaluation is the systematic collection of information about a program or service in order to answer questions and make decisions about the program. The types of program evaluation are formative evaluation, process evaluation, impact evaluation, and outcome evaluation (**Table 12-3**). Although it is important to know what type of program evaluation needs to be conducted, it is critical to first know what questions are to be answered and what decisions are to be made with the collected information. Once this is known, it is possible to focus on accurately collecting information and on understanding that collected information.

Evaluation often seems like a heavy, complex activity to those who are not familiar with the real nature of evaluation. In essence, however, evaluation means answering some very basic questions and then reporting back to interested individuals and groups (e.g., staff, families, etc.) about what was found. The questions evaluators might ask include:

- ❖ What do children, adolescents, families, and staff funders want to know?
- ❖ What kinds of information are needed? When is the information needed?
- ❖ What decisions will be made based on the evaluation's findings and results?
- ❖ Where can the information be acquired, and how?
- ❖ What resources are available for getting the information, analyzing it, and reporting it?
- ❖ What kind of report would be most useful to youth, families, staff, and funders?

Evaluations are orderly. They follow a set process to make sure that the time and energy spent to ask the questions and collect the information is worthwhile, and that you will be able to use the evaluation results to answer questions and make decisions. A widely used **evaluation framework** is from the Centers for Disease Control and Prevention (1999):

1. Engage stakeholders, especially those involved in program operations (e.g., counselors, teachers, agency staff); those served or affected by the program (e.g., children, adolescents, parents, caregivers); and primary users of the evaluation results. They all have an investment in what will be learned and what will be done with the information.

2. Describe the mental health prevention programs and services, including their mission and objectives; the need or problem addressed; the expected effects of the programs and services; the strategies and activities; the human, material, and time resources available; and the program and services' social, political, and economic context.

3. Focus the evaluation design in order to assess the issues of greatest concern to stakeholders while using time and resources efficiently, accurately, and ethically. Specifically, a focused evaluation design takes into consideration the evaluation's purpose, the users who will receive the results, and how the evaluation will be used. Evaluation design also focuses on developing answerable evaluation questions, developing reasonable evaluation methods, and having agreements on the roles and responsibilities of those conducting the evaluation.

4. Gather credible evidence that will be perceived by stakeholders as believable and relevant for answering questions about the program and service and its implementation or effects. Stakeholders who were involved in planning the evaluation and gathering data are more likely to accept the evaluation's conclusions and to act on its recommendations.

5. Justify conclusions, including recommendations, by ensuring that they are linked to the evidence gathered and to explicit values or standards that were set with the stakeholders. Stakeholders will then use the evaluation results with confidence.

6. Ensure use of the results and share lessons learned by:
   ◆ Having a strong and participatory evaluation design;
   ◆ preparing stakeholders to use the results by exploring the possible positive and negative implications of the findings;
   ◆ promoting stakeholder feedback by holding periodic discussions during the evaluation process and routinely sharing interim findings and possible interpretations and draft reports;
   ◆ engaging with stakeholders and advocating for use of the findings when decisions about the program are being made;
   ◆ and disseminating the findings in a thorough, balanced, and impartial report. This report is tailored to the specific audience and explains the evaluation's focus, its limitations, and its strengths and weaknesses.

A number of terms are used in discussing evaluation, regardless of the evaluation type. They reflect the common purpose of evaluation, in general, to provide the best information to answer people's questions and help them make good decisions.

Quantitative methods involve the gathering and analysis of numerical data. Various techniques are then used to make sense of the numbers or scores in order to interpret the results of a program or service. Numerical data might include a summary of demographic variables, pretest and posttest scores, attitude and self-efficacy ratings, and existing numerical data. Examples include tracking the number of participants in a smoking cessation program, recording participants' scores on a stress survey, and comparing pretest and posttest scores on measures of knowledge before and after a bullying prevention program for children.

Qualitative methods involve the gathering of non-numerical data, including descriptions of the program, often from the perspectives and experiences of the program participants themselves. The data consist primarily of information gathered from interviews with key informants (e.g., parents, teachers, counselors), observations of program activities (e.g., anger management), and focus groups with people who may share common values or experiences (e.g., a gay and lesbian focus group discussing their experience and knowledge of tobacco use in the gay, lesbian, bisexual, and transgender [GLBT] community).

Mixed or integrated methods involve a combination of qualitative and quantitative methods. The mix of methods to use is largely determined by the evaluation's question and purpose.

Reliability refers to the ability of evaluation instruments to provide consistent results each time they are used. Use of reliable instruments is integral to evidence-based practice.

Validity refers to the ability of evaluation instruments to accurately measure what the evaluator wants to measure (e.g., knowledge of how to prevent sexually transmitted diseases). Use of valid instruments is also integral to evidence-based programs.

Cultural relevance means that evaluation instruments have been developed with consideration of how cultural differences (e.g., in language or beliefs) can influence the manner in which qualitative and quantitative questions are perceived and answered.

Finally, most program and service directors do not have the time, personnel resources, or desire to carry out a formal evaluation; therefore it is not uncommon for funding agencies (for example, federal and state agencies and foundations) to require that program directors hire an external evaluator. An external evaluator may be requested if a funding agency feels that an external (and thus objective) evaluator will conduct a stronger evaluation. Selecting a program evaluator is an important task. A good evaluator provides timely information to refine and keep the program and services on track. In addition, a good evaluator accurately documents the program and service experiences and effectiveness. This information is useful for seeking future funding.

Summary

No matter your job title and job responsibilities, as a professional working as a member of a student support team, partnership, or collaboration, some part of your responsibilities will include a leadership element. You will demonstrate leadership in a variety of roles with individuals, organizations, programs, and services. Leadership is an elusive concept because people do not often define themselves in leadership terms. Focusing on transactional and transformational leadership can support and guide personal leadership development. It builds awareness of how we influence and lead individuals and organizations that reflect the people, situations, and tasks involved. Transactional and transformational leadership provide a model with which we can examine our effectiveness as leaders. Transformational leadership focuses on the personal qualities of leadership. It is leadership by example (i.e., being a leader). Transactional leadership focuses on the skills and tasks associated with leadership, such as public speaking, delegating authority, providing information, making connections, answering questions, leading meetings, and making decisions. This is what leaders do (doing leadership tasks).

Two emerging issues for school community professionals that work directly with youth and families are how best to focus on and build the resilience of young people throughout the school community, and how to respond to violence in the school community. Emerging programmatic and service issues for school community professionals are shaping the mix of programs and services to address addictions within the overall school community mental health program and service offerings, and also deciding how to evaluate programs and services.

For Practice and Discussion

1. In your daily life, how are you a transformational and transactional leader? Share examples of your transformational and transactional leadership qualities in your professional and personal lives. Today, where and how were you a leader?
2. How are the programs and services in your school community building resiliency? What more can be done to encourage youth and families support and caring behaviors, high expectations, and opportunities to participate and contribute to the school community?
3. You have decided to plan a community violence prevention forum because your neighborhood has seen a recent rise in bullying incidents when children and youth are on their way to and from school. You have arranged a meeting with the school principal. Make a list of facts and some key questions that you want to share as you discuss your plan with the principal.
4. What are some of the possible manifestations of trauma in the classroom? How would you go about helping the youth in your school who may have experienced trauma?
5. How have the leaders (i.e., team, partnership, and collaboration members) in your school community addressed substance abuse concerns and problems of youth? What is the mix of substance abuse programs and services among the mental health programs and service offerings in your school community? For what programs and services do the local school community leaders need to be advocating for additional funding?
6. Talk with the staff of your school community mental health programs and services to determine how the programs and services are evaluated. Compare and contrast types of evaluations (formative, impact, outcome, and process) and evaluation reports. What questions do the evaluations answer? What questions do you have about the programs and services? What type of evaluation would answer your questions?

Key Terms

Evaluation 291
Evaluation framework 292
Formative evaluation 291
Funding 288
Impact evaluation 291
Leadership 276
Outcome evaluation 291
Process evaluation 291

Protective factors 282
Resilience 282
Substance abuse 288
Transactional leadership 277
Transformational leadership 277
Trauma 285
Violence 281

References

Bass, B.M. (1985). *Leadership and Performance Beyond Expectations*. New York: Free Press.

Benard, B. (1991). *Fostering Resiliency in Kids: Protective Factors in the Family, School, and Community*. Portland, OR: Western Center for Drug-Free Schools and Communities.

Bennis, W.C. (1989). *On Becoming a Leader*. Reading, MA: Addison-Wesley.

Bennis, W.C., & Nanus, B. (1985). *Leaders: The Strategies of Taking Charge*. New York: Harper & Row.

Bluestein, J. (2001). *Creating Emotionally Safe Schools: A Guide for Educators and Parents*. Deerfield Beach, FL: Health Communications, Inc.

Burns, J.M. (1978). *Leadership*. New York: Harper & Row.

Centers for Disease Control and Prevention. (1999). Framework for program evaluation in public health. *Morbidity and Mortality Weekly Report*, 48(RR11): 1–40.

Centers for Disease Control and Prevention. (2008). School-associated student homicides–United States, 1992-2006. *Morbidity and Mortality Weekly Report*, 57(02). Retrieved from http://www.cdc.gov/mmwr/preview/mmwrhtml/mm5702a1.htm

Fleishman, E.A., Mumford, M.D., Zaccaro, S.J., Levin, K.Y., Korotkin, A.L., & Hein, M.B. (1991). Taxonomic efforts in the description of leader behavior: A synthesis and functional interpretation. *Leadership Quarterly*, 2: 245–287.

Fowler, J.S., Volkow, N.D., Kassed, C.A., & Chang, L. (2007). Imaging the addicted human brain. *Science and Practice Perspectives*, 3(2): 4–16.

Jellinek, E.M. (1960). *The Disease Concept of Alcoholism*. New Brunswick, NJ: Hillhouse.

Kouzes, J., & Posner, B. (1987). *The Leadership Challenge*. San Francisco: Jossey-Bass.

Krovetz, M.L. (2008). *Fostering Resilience: Expecting All Students to Use Their Minds and Hearts Well* (2nd ed.). Thousand Oaks, CA: Corwin Press.

Massachusetts Advocates for Children. (2009). *Helping Traumatized Children Learn: Supportive School Environments for Children Traumatized by Family Violence*. Boston, MA: Author. Retrieved from http://www.massadvocates.org/documents/HTCL_9-09.pdf

National Child Traumatic Stress Network Schools Committee (NCTSN). (2008). *Child Trauma Toolkit for Educators*. Los Angeles, CA & Durham, NC: National Center for Child Traumatic Stress. Retrieved from http://www.nctsn.org/sites/default/files/assets/pdfs/Child_Trauma_Toolkit_Final.pdf

National Institute on Drug Abuse (NIDA). (2010). Drugs, brains, and behavior: The science of addiction. Retrieved from http://www.drugabuse.gov/publications/science-addiction/drugs-brain

National PTA. (2013). Checklist to prevent violence in schools. Retrieved from www.pta.org/content.cfm?ItemNumber=984

Northouse, P.G. (2001). *Leadership: Theory and Practice* (2nd ed.). Thousand Oaks, CA: Sage.

Osher, D., Dwyer, K., & Jackson, S. (2003). *Safe, Supportive, and Successful Schools: Step by Step.* Longmont, CO: Sopris West.

Pennsylvania Emergency Management Agency. (2009). Pennsylvania All Hazards School Safety Planning Toolkit. Retrieved from http://www.portal.state.pa.us/portal/server.pt/community /plans,_guides_and_presentations/4625/all-hazards_school_safety_planning_toolkit _(pdf)/541340

Perry, B.D., and Pollard, R.M. (1998). Homeostasis, stress, trauma, and adaptation: A neurodevelopmental view of childhood trauma. *Child and Adolescent Psychiatric Clinics of North America, 7*(1): 33–50.

Sanchez, H. (2008). *A Brain-Based Approach to Closing the Achievement Gap.* Bloomington, IN: Xlibris.

Stogdill, R.M. (1974). *Handbook of Leadership: A Survey of Theory and Research.* New York: Free Press.

Thomsen, K. (2002). *Building Resilient Students: Integrating Resiliency into What You Know and Do.* Thousand Oaks, CA: Corwin Press

van Linden, J., & Fertman, C.I. (1998). *Youth Leadership: A Guide to Understanding Leadership Development in Young People.* San Francisco: Jossey-Bass.

White, W. (2000). Addiction as a disease: Birth of a concept. *Counselor, 1*(1): 46–51, 73.

Wren, J.T. (1995). *The Leader's Companion: Insights on Leadership Through the Ages.* New York: Free Press.

Glossary

Academic concerns teams Teams that operate mainly at the school and are generally comprised of school staff. They address student achievement and develop academic strategies to help students learn successfully.

Adaptation The process by which a program or service undergoes change in its implementation to fit the needs of a particular delivery situation.

Advocacy Action taken in support of a cause or proposal. It is an important part of case and resource management.

Advocate A person who provides leadership and passion in building and sustaining school community mental health programs and services. The advocate fights for resources, knows the systems involved, promotes policies that support programs and services, and engages in shaping public policy.

Alternative education Programs developed and run by school districts to deal with students whose behavioral challenges seriously disrupt the school environment.

Audience segmentation The process of dividing the priority populations into subgroups that share similar qualities or characteristics. The goal is to segment the intended population on characteristics that are relevant to the mental health behavior to be changed and to organize and develop communication efforts around these groups of similar individuals.

Authority The power and right of a collaboration to take action to accomplish agreed-upon goals.

Autonomous organizations Two or more organizations that function independently in parallel fashion, and work toward the identified goals of their respective programs. Autonomous organizations demonstrate a peaceful co-existence, but are neither genuinely interactive nor interdependent.

Barriers Impediments or pitfalls to be eliminated or avoided during case management. Some include biased program and service plans, favoritism, turfism, and neglecting to involve the child or adolescent requesting help.

Behavioral health A concept that integrates practices that deal with the prevention, diagnosis, intervention, and treatment of both mental illness and substance abuse disorders. The term includes addictions (e.g., substance abuse, smoking, and gambling) as well as neurological conditions from attention deficit/hyperactivity disorder to fetal alcohol spectrum disorders, mood disorders and traumatic brain injury.

Beyondblue An organization in Australia that uses social marketing to educate and combat stigmas surrounding depression. Their 2006 national advertising campaign used television commercials and print ads aimed at seven different audiences.

California Strategic Plan on Reducing Mental Health Stigma and Discrimination A plan developed in 2009 by the California Department of Mental Health to prevent and address stigma and discrimination of individuals and their families with a mental illness.

Case and resource management An ongoing process, rather than a single event, through which the youth and family participate in the planned programs and services to achieve the agreed-upon goals. It is confidential and includes the following elements: monitoring, crisis intervention, reassessment, resource management, feedback, and advocacy.

Champion An individual who identifies health issues that need to be addressed, initiates efforts to start programs and services, and provides leadership to ensure programs and services operate effectively.

Channels Routes used to reach the intended audience. They include interpersonal channels, group channels, community channels, mass media channels, and interactive media channels.

Child and Adolescent Needs and Strengths (CANS) CANS is a screening instrument used by community mental health providers to consistently identify mental health problems in children that may not be detected in an interview.

Child and family point of view A focus on the engagement and participation of a child or adolescent in prevention programs at all levels in the school community, not only as consumers, but also as advocates and communicators about service needs, qualities, and improvements.

Child welfare system A group of services designed to promote the well-being of children by ensuring safety, achieving permanency, and strengthening families to care for their children successfully. The primary responsibility for child welfare services rests at the state level.

Children's Internet Protection Act (CIPA) A law enacted in 2000 to protect children using school, college, and library computers from offensive Internet content. It requires that school districts create an Internet safety plan.

Co-occurring disorder A situation where it has been determined that drug abuse and mental health disorders co-exist; also known as co-morbidity.

Code of ethics Standards that are adopted by professional organizations that reflect professional concerns and establish guiding principles. A code of ethics is not law but rather a framework for making decisions in ambiguous circumstances. Codes of ethics vary by profession.

Collaboration A group of independent organizations sharing responsibility for specific changes in practices and policies across a region, state, or group of states. They provide access to a broad scope of knowledge and expertise for program and service planning, implementation, and evaluation. Minimum defining features are shared responsibility and interdependence.

Communities That Care (CTC) An example of a community-based partnership that uses a public health model to prevent youth problem behaviors, including underage drinking, tobacco use, violence, delinquency, school dropout, and substance abuse. CTC is a data-driven process that begins with an assessment risk and protective factors of children grades 6–12.

Community assessment An assessment that collects information about the health risk and protective behaviors of schools and the resources within the community to address these risks. It provides information about what is needed as well as the support, resources, and guidance that are available within any particular organization and system.

Community coalitions Groups consisting of a broad range of community organizations and individuals who share a commitment to a particular concern and identify and agree on needs, and then obtain resources to build effective solutions.

Confidentiality A promise between a counselor and a student, therapist and client, or teacher and student to keep personal information private unless there is a potentially serious and foreseeable threat to the individual's well-being. Confidentiality is very important for establishing and maintaining a strong teacher-student relationship, but has important limits. Threats to harm self or others are nonnegotiable in any setting.

Conflict management The process of taking steps to limit the negative aspects of conflict and to increase the positive aspects of conflict.

Coordinated school health A common approach to addressing students' health needs that includes eight components of wellness. These components are disciplines and services that most schools have, but that have not necessarily been organized to work together.

Crisis determination The first step in any referral to the student support team. It involves the immediate triage of student referrals for crisis indicators so the child can receive immediate intervention and a crisis response plan can be implemented.

Crisis response plans A written plan to address a school community crisis. Plans focus on four key areas: prevention/mitigation, preparedness, response, and recovery, both at the district and school level. These crisis response plans include community and first responders and address responses to the multitude of hazards that can impact a school and its related activities.

Cultural brokers A range of individuals, from immigrant children who negotiate two or more cultures daily to leaders in organizations who serve as catalysts for change. The goal of cultural brokers is to increase the capacity of school communities to design, implement, and evaluate culturally competent mental health promoting programs and services.

Cultural competence   An underlying philosophy that each and every person deserves dignity and respect and has value, and the recognition and acknowledgement that society has not always been fair to everyone and that oppression and discrimination are real.

Cultural competence continuum   A variety of stages or phases toward becoming competent to work with people of other cultures. Not only can individuals travel along this continuum, but also agencies and organizations.

Cyberbullying   When a child, preteen, or teen is tormented, threatened, harassed, humiliated, embarrassed, or otherwise targeted by another child, preteen, or teen using the Internet, interactive and digital technologies, or mobile phones.

Discrimination   Denial of access to services and programs to people from or perceived as from a particular group or class by an individual or institutional practices or policies. It includes stereotypes about people with special needs and prejudices toward them.

Documentation   An accurate written record of the child or adolescent's and family's involvement with the team or case manager.

Duration   A measure of how long certain behaviors have persisted. Duration describes the time frame that the behavior lasts, such as "everyday this week," or "for the last month." Duration is a key term used when discussing student behavior.

Duty to warn   The courts require that anyone in a position to help a student and who becomes aware of a potentially serious and foreseeable threat to the health, welfare, and/or safety of the student or of someone else is bound to report that threat to parents first and then, if necessary, to authorities.

Dynamics   Unarticulated forces that exist "under the surface" and influence the way a team acts, interacts, and performs.

Economics   A social determinant of mental health, because improving the economic health of the family in ways that lead to income stability is an important step in improving developmental outcomes for children in poverty.

Ethics   A system of standards created by a particular profession to give guidance for reasonable decisions and actions in challenging situations.

Evaluation   The systematic collection of information about a program or service to answer questions and make decisions about the program. Four different evaluation types can contribute to the program and its overall success: formative, impact, outcome, and process.

Evaluation framework   The process followed to make sure the time and energy spent to ask the questions and collect the information for an evaluation are worthwhile, and that you will be able to use the evaluation results to answer questions and make decisions.

Evidence-based mental health programs   They identify the priority populations that would benefit from the program and the conditions under which the program works, and may indicate the change mechanisms that account for program effects.

Evidence-based programs   The delivery of optimal care through integration of current best scientific evidence, clinical expertise, experience, and the preferences of individuals, families, organizations, and communities.

Family-centered mental health policy and practice   A model for the delivery of programs and services to youth and their families that links family, community support, and school community organizations to establish a continuum of care.

Family Educational Rights and Privacy Act (FERPA)   Provides parents with privacy rights until a child reaches the age of 18, and allows parents to access all files the school maintains on their children. FERPA promotes sharing of confidential written information when the person has a "legitimate educational interest." This means that only information needed to manage behavior or improve education can be disclosed.

Family engagement   The newer, expanded role of families in the decisions affecting their children, from at-home activities to full partnerships with school community staff and other parents and community members for the overall improvement of the school community.

Family Engagement for High School Success   An initiative with a two-part focus on comprehensive planning and early implementation of a family engagement initiative.

Family network organizations   National, state, and local entities designed to meet the needs of families and consumers to affect national policy and promote mental health issues. They provide a myriad of services to local organizations and individuals, from technical assistance to hotlines.

Family resource centers   Settings that provide caring, affordable, and high-quality health care and supportive services to everyone, with a special commitment to uninsured, low income, and medically underserved persons. These centers promote both the strengthening of families through formal and informal support and the restoration of a strong sense of community.

Fidelity   The extent to which the delivery of a program or service conforms to the curriculum, protocol, or guidelines for implementing that program or service. A program or service delivered exactly as intended by its originator has high fidelity.

Formal connection strategies   Strategies that are offered to students who may benefit from more intensive assistance from a student support team or skill-building group. These approaches may require parental consent.

Formal decisions   Choices made by children, adolescents, and families or caregivers about how to address mental health concerns and problems and their child's participation in secondary and tertiary prevention mental health programs and services.

Formative evaluation   The gathering of information and materials during program planning and development. It can be used to understand the needs assessment data gathered during the program planning process.

Frequency   A measure of how often you see a given action or cluster of behaviors. Frequency is a key term used when discussing student behavior.

Funding   The money to pay for, support, and expand the mental health promoting school community.

Goal setting   The process used to build consensus among family members (children, parents, caregivers) regarding the goals to be addressed in treatment. There are several models commonly used or adapted.

Guide to Community Preventive Services   The U.S. Preventive Services Task Force (USPSTF) recommendations for strategies and policies that healthcare providers can use to improve adolescent health in six areas that contribute to the leading causes of death and disability among youth: alcohol and drug use, injury and violence (including suicide), tobacco use, nutrition, physical activity, and sexual behaviors.

Harvard Family Research Project (HFRP)   An organization that provides leadership to develop school community family engagement.

Health Education Curriculum Analysis Tool (HECAT)   A tool often used to help develop appropriate and effective health education curricula. Educators can customize the HECAT to address the needs of their community and meet curriculum requirements set by their school district and state.

Health Insurance Portability and Accountability Act (HIPAA)   An act that provides for the protection and confidential handling of protected health information.

Helping relationships   The relationships between and among children, youth, parents, schools, and agencies that engender trust and facilitate actions for the completion of goals and the implementation of programs.

Hope   The belief that recovery is real. Hope is internalized. It provides the essential and motivating message of a better future—that people can and do overcome the internal and external challenges, barriers, and obstacles that confront them.

Immigrant and International Advisory Council   A council formed in 2008 as a way to help the Allegheny County (Pa.) Department of Human Services (DHS) staff members increase their understanding of different cultures; it also provides occasional cultural competency trainings. It was designed to make DHS services accessible to all residents of the county, regardless of their country of origin.

Impact evaluation   Measures the immediate effects of programs and services. The primary question in an impact evaluation is: What has been the program's immediate effect on the children and adolescents?

Indicated preventive interventions   A focus on high-risk individuals who are identified as having evident symptoms that have developed, or may develop, into mental illness. Also included are those individuals having genetic markers that put them at risk for a mental illness but who do not meet diagnostic levels at the current time. An IOM classification.

Individual mental health concerns and problems intervention process approach An approach that addresses the mental health and problems of individual children and adolescents within the larger population of youth at a site such as a school. Key elements of the approach include identifying the initial problem, clarifying strengths and needs, consulting and working with the student and family, management of care, and ongoing follow-up and support.

Individualized healthcare plan A form that is completed by the school nurse, which includes concerns, nursing diagnosis, goals, nursing interventions, and expected outcomes, and is used for a student with a physical health problem (and referred to the team by the nurse) identified as needing to address a mental health concern or problem.

Information network A resource that encourages individuals to generate current information on the community mental health programs and services. The content of such a network includes current information, resource updates, and locations of summary information on a wide variety of mental health topics.

Initial information collection The act of collecting all objective and verifiable information that is available in the school about a student's attendance, academic performance, discipline history, and behaviors, as well as health-related concerns.

Institute of Medicine (IOM) intervention classification A classification for mental health promotion and problem prevention interventions based on the populations to be served. There are three levels of interventions: Universal interventions for general population groups; selective interventions for students who are at greater-than-average risk for mental health problems; and indicated interventions for individuals who may already display intense warning signs of mental health problems.

Intensity The amount of disruption a child or adolescent experiences in her or his life stemming from a behavior pattern. Intensity can become so great that it impairs a student's ability to function. Intensity is a key term used when discussing student behavior.

Justice system The U.S. legal system, including the juvenile justice system, which can play an important role in addressing mental health concerns of youth and their families. Two examples of justice system school involvement are school resource officers (SROs) and school-based probation officers (SBPOs).

Key informant A commonly used term for a champion because he or she knows important or key information about an organization.

Laws Systems of rules created by elected representatives and enforced through the courts, either civil or criminal. A government entity usually can enforce compliance.

Leadership The qualities and skills that allow influencing and leading people. It is a personal and developmental process. It is transformational and transactional.

Letter of agreement (LOA)   A statement that clarifies working arrangements between two parties, usually a school district and a community agency. Letters of agreement and releases of information are the policies and procedures that establish the roles and boundaries between the educational and human services domains.

Like Minds, Like Mine   New Zealand's national comprehensive, multilevel, long-term, social marketing-based approach to countering stigma and discrimination. Widely regarded as one of the most successful anti-stigma programs, it is also the longest running national program of its kind.

Linguistic competence   The capacity of an organization and its personnel to communicate effectively and convey information in a manner that is easily understood by diverse audiences, including persons of limited English proficiency/ English language learners, those who have low literacy skills or are not literate, individuals with disabilities, and those who are deaf or hard of hearing.

Mental health   The successful performance of mental functions. The ability to think clearly, feel a variety of feelings, and behave in appropriate ways. This results in productive activities, fulfilling relationships with other people, and the ability to change and to cope with adversity.

Mental Health America   A consumer-based advocacy group committed to helping people affected by mental illness to achieve mental and physical wellness.

Mental health communication   The art and technique of informing, influencing, and motivating individual, institutional, and public audiences about important mental health issues.

Mental health communication and social media plan   A document that guides and develops the information exchange between and among the staff, youth, families, and school community members.

Mental health counselors   Skilled individuals who provide counseling and support in individual or small group counseling sessions, as well as in support groups designed to assist people with specific issues, such as social skills, self-esteem, or depression surrounding divorce, bereavement, or another situation. These individuals can be employed full time by a school district or agency to offer these services.

Mental health diagnostic assessment   A comprehensive, expensive, time-consuming examination of the psychosocial needs and problems identified during the initial mental health screening. The assessment identifies the type and extent of mental health disorders and makes recommendations for treatment interventions.

Mental health literacy   The degree to which individuals have the capacity to obtain, process, and understand basic mental health information and services needed to make appropriate mental health decisions about mentally healthy behaviors, emotional and social functioning, and stress management.

Mental health promoting school community   A school community with mental health programs and services that span schools, families, and the community with primary, secondary, and tertiary prevention. This community is supported and sustained by teams, partnerships, and collaborations.

Mental health screening A relatively brief process designed to identify children and adolescents who are at risk for having disorders that warrant immediate attention, intervention, or more comprehensive review. Identifying the need for further assessment is the primary purpose of screening.

Mental health stigma Synonyms and slang terms used to describe individuals with or without mental health challenges that may or may not be based on clinical terms or diagnoses.

Mosaic of identity Composed of the social determinants of mental health produced by the social differences and social dynamics in children and adolescents' lives. Each child and adolescent is a unique mosaic of identity.

National Alliance for Hispanic Health (NAHH) The leading health agency representing Latino health issues at the national level. It was formed in 1973, and its members are health and human service providers working at the community level, seeking community-based solutions to health and mental health problems.

National Alliance on Mental Illness (NAMI) The largest national grassroots mental health organization. It is dedicated to building better lives for the millions of Americans affected by mental illness. It advocates for access to services, treatment, support, and research.

National Federation of Families for Children's Mental Health (FFCMH) A consumer- (family-) run organization that arose 20 years ago from a grassroots movement. It has more than 120 chapters and state organizations representing the families of children and youth with mental health needs.

National Latino Behavioral Health Association (NLBHA) Formed in 2002, it works to influence policy, improve treatment outcomes and the quality of services, eliminate disparities in access to services and funding, and highlight the underutilization of services and the lack of appropriately trained personnel and practical research.

National Registry of Evidence-Based Programs and Practices (NREPP) A searchable database of interventions for the prevention and treatment of mental and substance use disorders, developed and maintained by the Substance Abuse and Mental Health Services Administration (SAMHSA) in the U.S. Department of Health and Human Services.

Ongoing skill development An approach used to prevent staff burnout and sustain teams, partnerships, and collaborations. It can be system-centered or person-centered.

Organizational capacity The structure and resources, human and otherwise, contained within an organization that enable it to complete a given goal or task.

Outcome evaluation Examines the changes in children and adolescents during or after their participation in a program or service. Changes sought include knowledge gains, attitude changes, skills acquired, or behavior changes.

Out-of-school-time programs   School-related programs that occur after school, on weekends, or during the summer, usually within the community, that provide a wide array of opportunities that support children and youth.

Parent and caregiver conference   A meeting between parents and caregivers and school support team members that is designed to build a working relationship, discuss a student's strengths and challenges, prioritize issues, and develop sound action plans for improvement.

Parent- and caregiver-friendly school communities   Environments that ease tension and create the opportunity for schools and families to partner and collaborate to meet the mental health needs of children and adolescents.

Parent and family education   Programs developed to address families' concerns and to lend support. They are the easiest to implement, low budget, practical, accessible, widely available, and manageable for most schools and community agencies.

Parent checklist   A tool used by many teams when initiating contact with a parent or caregiver and gathering their perspective on the barriers the child is experiencing at school, at home, and/or with friends. The forms are concrete, positive, and strength-based with clear and reader-friendly language.

Parental involvement   A limited view of parents and families' role regarding school issues and their children. Supportive activities that parents and caregivers were previously asked to perform at home in order to support school decisions and programs affecting their child.

Parent or caregiver conference ground rules   In meeting with parents, ground rules help a team use time effectively and remain focused on solution building. These rules structure the meeting and help parents feel more secure and engaged.

Parent engagement   The process whereby school support team members include parents as equal partners, or allies, when interpreting information and creating action plans. Engagement recognizes the parent's right to make decisions that the team may disagree with, yet the team continues to build a trusting relationship and respects the parent's decision.

Parental consent   A document obtained from parents that recognizes their legal right to make decisions about their child's involvement in any process or activity that is beyond the scope of the general curriculum.

Partnership   A group of interdependent local organizations represented by individuals who share responsibility for specific outcomes across organizations. A partnership is typically formed at the school district level or county level, including all district buildings, and joins with a broader range of community-wide agencies, services, and programs.

Partnership models   Approaches to how schools and community organizations work to do something together.

PhotoVoice   A strategy to get youth input by asking young people to represent their point of view by taking photographs, discussing them together, and developing and sharing narratives to go with their photos.

Plain language   Communication the intended audience can understand the first time they read or hear it. Written material is in plain language if the audience can find what they need, understand what they find, and use what they find to meet their needs.

Policy   Written guidelines that meet the legal requirements to operate a school or community organization.

Positive Behavioral Interventions and Supports (PBIS)   A systems approach to establishing the behavioral supports and social culture needed for all students in a school to achieve success. PBIS applies a three-tiered system of support and a problem-solving process to enhance the ability of schools to effectively educate all students.

Poverty   A social determinant of mental health with negative mental health consequences for youth and families and for the school community. Poverty refers to the lack of sufficient economic resources to meet basic food, shelter, medical, and related living expenses.

Primary prevention   The first level of the public health approach addressing the mental health concerns and problems of youth or broader populations. Primary prevention strategies are directed to the entire population and are intended to prevent new incidents of a problem or disorder.

Problem solving   The process used to reach a specific goal or solution to a particular situation. It involves identification of the problem, gathering data, analysis, and formulation of options.

Procedural guidelines   An outline of the steps that staff take when students violate policy. Most procedural guidelines are board approved.

Procedures   See procedural guidelines.

Process evaluation   A snapshot of a program or service. It is about systematically gathering information during implementation. It can be used to describe and assess to what extent the intended program activities and services are being accomplished.

Protective factors   Also called assets, these are the supports provided through programs, services, parent/family engagement, community engagement, student support teams, school counselors, social workers, mentors, and other caring adults that can mitigate or prevent the effects of risk factors that are present in the child or youth's environment, making a major difference in a child's life.

Psychologists   Professionals who offer testing, counseling, and support to students in need of mental health services, particularly those in special education. They are generally employed by school districts and/or private or public agencies.

Public health approach   Primary, secondary, and tertiary prevention strategies that work across systems to forge connections that promote child and adolescent mental health in many types of sites.

Public policy   The result of the interaction of organized political and government structures in the making and administering of public decisions for a society.

Racial and Ethnic Approaches to Community Health (REACH) An initiative started in 1999 as the cornerstone of the Centers for Disease Control and Prevention's efforts to eliminate racial and ethnic disparities in the United States.

Recovery A process of change through which individuals improve their health and wellness with self-defined life goals and paths toward those goals. Self-acceptance, developing a positive and meaningful sense of identity, and regaining belief in one's self are particularly important.

Referral A step that begins the process toward supporting students and their families in taking action to address mental health concerns and problems.

Regional collaborations Organizations that span across a state or region or large number of organizations (i.e., multiple school districts, each with many school buildings) that share a common goal.

Release of information (ROI) Establishes the working roles and boundaries between schools and agencies that work with students and families. Generally, schools must have a parent or caregiver sign a release of information for the school to give information about the student to community providers (i.e., a mental health program).

Research-Tested Intervention Programs (RTIPs) A federal database of evidence-based mental health promotion programs and products that individuals, groups, and organizations can access and use. The database is maintained by the National Cancer Institute.

Resilience The ability to bounce back from adversity; it is about a person's healthy response to stress.

Resources A term referring to human and material support that is available when needed to accomplish goals: funding, infrastructure, skill-base, and services necessary to promote mental health in the school community.

Response to Intervention (RtI) A framework that integrates assessment and intervention within a multilevel prevention system to maximize student achievement and reduce academic problems.

Risk factors Factors associated with an increased potential for mental health concerns or problems. These factors are associated with increases in alcohol and other drug use, delinquency, teen pregnancy, school dropout, and violence.

Roles The part assigned to or assumed by an organization or individual as part of a process that requires responsibility and accountability for actions.

Roles and responsibilities Defined and agreed-upon tasks and activities for partnership members, often with timelines, budgets, and people assigned to complete them.

School climate The quality of everyday life at a school and the way people feel inside the school.

School climate survey An instrument that provides school leaders with data from stakeholders about the school's atmosphere, sense of safety and relationships, teaching and learning, and other major areas.

School community The product of students, school staff, community professionals, parents, caregivers, families, residents, community organizations, public health agencies, government, hospitals, and businesses in a local area working to benefit young people.

School community staff point of view Key information provided by school community professionals to teams, partnerships, and collaborations regarding what is actually occurring among youth in the community and interventions that have proven useful to children and adolescents.

School counselors Individuals who are trained to provide academic as well as personal counseling and support in individual or small group counseling sessions in the school setting, rather than in an agency setting.

School culture A school's persona, which is made up of the attitudes and values of those within the school, and how they treat each other. The culture is reflected in the school's guiding beliefs, norms, and actions and how they promote learning and mental health.

School culture survey An instrument designed to measure the attitudes, relationships, values, and vision of all members of the school community. Results can help administrators and stakeholders understand and shape the values, norms, guiding beliefs, and actions that occur in the school as well as provide information on how best to promote and improve student learning and mental health.

School Health Index (SHI) A self-assessment and planning guide that helps schools identify the strengths and weaknesses of their health and safety policies and programs, and develop an action plan for improving student health.

School nurse An individual who performs a critical role by addressing the major health problems experienced by children. This role includes providing preventive and screening services, health education, assistance with decision making about health, and immunization against preventable diseases.

School resource officer (SRO) A law enforcement officer who conducts programs in schools to help bridge the gap between police officers and young people through law-related education, student counseling, and law enforcement.

School-based probation officer (SBPO) A court-approved probation officer who is placed in a school to work with students who are under court supervision.

Secondary prevention The second level of the public health approach addressing the mental health concerns and problems of youth or broader population. Secondary prevention strategies focus on a subpopulation with elevated risk and/ or with a disorder. The goal is to identify the disorder early, reduce symptoms, cure the disorder and/or limit disability, and reduce the frequency of disruptive behaviors.

Selective preventive interventions A focus on individuals or a population subgroup whose risk of developing mental disorders is significantly higher than average or who already demonstrate some warning signs. An IOM classification.

Self-efficacy   A person's confidence in his or her ability to pursue a behavior, take a specific action, and/or perform a specific task.

Shared responsibility   Families, school community staff, and community members share the responsibility for child and adolescent mental health outcomes.

SMART goals   A widely used model whose acronym means specific, measurable, attainable, realistic, and time delineated.

Social and emotional learning (SEL)   The process of developing fundamental social and emotional competencies in children. SEL programs develop five core social and emotional competencies in students: self-awareness, social awareness, self-management, relationship skills, and responsible decision making.

Social conditions   Multifaceted, complex, and dynamic system that includes social differences and social dynamics affecting youth and families; it is part of the mosaic of identity.

Social determinants of health   Factors, such as economics, social conditions, and culture, in which we are born, live, learn, work, and play that have significant impact on our mental and physical health. They include gender, economics, education, disability, geographic location, culture, identity, social conditions, and sexual orientation.

Social marketing   The application of commercial marketing technologies to the analysis, planning, execution, and evaluation of programs designed to influence the voluntary behavior of individuals in order to improve their personal welfare and that of society.

Social media   Online media for social interaction, using highly accessible and scalable publishing techniques and web-based platforms.

Social support   An important protective factor and buffer to stress.

Social workers   One of the three professional pupil services groups that provide counseling services to children and adolescents in schools. Social workers have different training from school counselors and school psychologists, and often work more closely with families.

Socio-ecological approach   An approach that looks beyond the school. Teams, partnerships, and collaborations take a socio-ecological approach to promoting child and adolescent mental health by building a mental health promoting culture and climate within the school community.

Special education   Specially designed instruction and the related services needed by a student to benefit from that instruction. As part of special education, teachers adapt the content (what is taught), methodology (the process used to teach), or delivery of the curriculum to take into account a student's learning needs and to ensure that the student has access to the general curriculum provided to children without disabilities.

Staff burnout   When staff experience physical and emotional exhaustion involving the development of negative job attitudes, a poor professional self-concept, and a loss of empathic concern for the youth and families they are trying to help.

State School Health Policy Database   A resource that contains brief descriptions of laws, legal codes, rules, regulations, administrative orders, mandates, standards, resolutions, and other written means of exercising authority from 50 states on more than 40 health topics.

Statewide Family Network Program   A program, supported by the Substance Abuse and Mental Health Services Administration, to enhance states' capacity and infrastructure to address the needs of children and adolescents with serious emotional disturbances and their families and to create a mechanism for families to participate in state and local mental health services planning and policy development.

Stigma   Attitudes and beliefs that lead people to reject, avoid, or fear those they perceive as being different.

StigmaBusters   A social media campaign to fight stigma developed by the National Alliance on Mental Illness.

Structural connection strategies   Strategies that are available to all students, and do not require parental consent.

Structural decisions   Decisions that affect primary prevention programs and services that all students are being offered in school and do not require parent/caregiver permission for access or participation.

Student self-referral   A situation in which a student voluntarily requests help for a mental health problem and is ensured access to programs and services without penalty.

Student support team flyer   A tool that schools use to explain the purpose and boundaries of the student support team to parents, caregivers, and families.

Student support teams   Teams that are concerned with student behavioral health and school climate reflective of the system of care available within the school community.

Substance abuse   A chronic, relapsing brain disease that is characterized by compulsive drug seeking and abuse, despite harmful consequences.

Sustainability   Having the capacity to support and continue to improve the existing program, team, partnership, or collaboration.

System of care   An adaptive network of different systems, collaborations, organizations, and groups that interface to provide children and youth with serious emotional disturbance and their families access to optimal services and supports. Schools are one part of a system of care, but it involves multiple organizations with many different types of services, such as intensive case management, family-based treatment, and partial hospitalization programs.

Team   A group that is present mostly at the school building level with participation of families and youth, building educators, and local community human service agencies and programs. There are many different types of teams in a school.

Tertiary prevention   The third level of the public health approach to addressing the mental health concerns and problems of youth. Tertiary prevention strategies focus on a subpopulation showing symptoms of a diagnosable disorder. The goal is to promote wellness, slow the progression of a disorder while minimizing complications, and reduce the intensity of problem behaviors.

Transactional leadership   Focuses on the skills and tasks associated with leadership, such as public speaking, delegating authority, providing information, making connections, answering questions, leading meetings, and making decisions.

Transformational leadership   Focuses on the personal qualities of leadership, such as valuing the participation and contributions of others, taking all viewpoints and advice into account before making decisions, and considering individuals within their contexts and situations.

Trauma   Exposure to an event or series of events where physical and/or emotional safety and security are threatened.

Universal preventive interventions   A focus on the general public or a whole population that has not been identified on the basis of individual risk. The intervention is desirable for everyone in that group, such as all students in a school.

Violence   The intentional use of force that causes physical or emotional damage to another person, group, or community.

What a Difference a Friend Makes   An example of how social marketing principles are used for a successful health education program to reduce stigma. One of the primary goals of this SAMHSA program is to provide information and resources for friends of those with mental health issues so that they can learn to be supportive and accepting. Materials are available in Spanish and English.

Youth Mental Health First Aid (YMHFA)   An example of a social marketing course designed to teach adults how to support adolescents who might be developing a mental health problem or in a mental health crisis, and to help them receive professional help. It is an interactive public education program designed to increase mental health literacy.

Youth Risk Behavior Surveillance System (YRBSS)   A national survey that monitors priority health risk behaviors that contribute to the leading causes of death, disability, and social problems among youth and adults in the United States. The survey, conducted by the Centers for Disease Control and Prevention, provides data representative of 9th- through 12th-grade students in public and private schools in the United States.

Youth voice   The distinct ideas, opinions, attitudes, knowledge, and actions of young people as a collective body. The term often groups together a diversity of perspectives and experiences, regardless of backgrounds, identities, and cultural differences.

Index